Nanotechnology in Drug Discovery

Authored by

Laksiri Weerasinghe

Imalka Munaweera

&

Senuri Kumarage

Department of Chemistry University of Sri Jayewardenepura, Gangodawila, Nugegoda 10250, Sri Lanka

Nanotechnology in Drug Discovery

Authors: Laksiri Weerasinghe, Imalka Munaweera & Senuri Kumarage

ISBN (Online): 978-981-5238-81-5

ISBN (Print): 978-981-5238-82-2

ISBN (Paperback): 978-981-5238-83-9

Published by Bentham Science Publishers Pte. Ltd. Singapore. All Rights Reserved.

First published in 2024.

need for a court order if at any point you breach any terms of this License Agreement. In no event will any delay or failure by Bentham Science Publishers in enforcing your compliance with this License Agreement constitute a waiver of any of its rights.

3. You acknowledge that you have read this License Agreement, and agree to be bound by its terms and conditions. To the extent that any other terms and conditions presented on any website of Bentham Science Publishers conflict with, or are inconsistent with, the terms and conditions set out in this License Agreement, you acknowledge that the terms and conditions set out in this License Agreement shall prevail.

Bentham Science Publishers Pte. Ltd.
80 Robinson Road #02-00
Singapore 068898
Singapore
Email: subscriptions@benthamscience.net

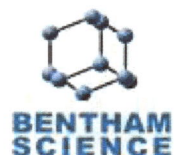

**BENTHAM
SCIENCE**

CONTENTS

PREFACE

Drug discovery is a critical step in the treatment and cure of diseases, involving identifying drug targets, lead identification, modification, synthesis, characterisation, validation, optimization, screening, and tests for therapeutic efficacy. Drug research and development have been greatly impacted by nanotechnology, resulting in the development of novel medicines for diseases that were previously incurable. At present, the pharmaceutical industry is attempting to minimize the time needed for medication development in response to the growing demand for fast drug development. Nanotechnology has allowed for the evolution of critical processes in traditional drug discovery, with an emphasis on enhancing lead identification, modifications, synthesis, stability, and target selectivity. There has been a surge in nanomedicine research over the last few decades, which is now being translated into commercialization endeavours throughout the world, leading to the marketing of various nano-drugs.

This book is intended for students and researchers who are just starting out in the modern drug development sector, where nanotechnology has taken up a significant space. The book will progressively expose readers to the topic of nanotechnology-based drug research by first examining the fundamentals of nanoparticles. Then this book will cover the utilization of nanotechnology throughout the drug development process from lab to market, focusing on lead identification and synthesis, drug delivery, nano-drug toxicity, in-vivo fate of NPs, and finally regulations on NPs-based drugs in various countries. The work then finally focuses on the future perspective of nanotechnology in drug discovery. Eventually, the readers will have an overall idea of how nanotechnology has improved the conventional drug development process. The abstract and conclusion given at the beginning and end of each chapter will provide the readers with concise information that is elaborated throughout the chapters.

We anticipate that this book will serve as a reference book, offering an in-depth account of how nanotechnology has revolutionized the drug development process while highlighting the intriguing recent findings in the field.

Laksiri Weerasinghe

Imalka Munaweera

&

Senuri Kumarage
Department of Chemistry University of Sri Jayewardenepura
Gangodawila, Nugegoda 10250
Sri Lanka

CHAPTER 1

Fundamentals of Nanotechnology

Abstract: Nanomaterials, a category of materials with a dimension in the nanometric range (1 nm-100 nm), were first recognized in 1959. They have unique physical, chemical, and mechanical properties, with nanoparticle size affecting properties like melting temperature, ionization potential, colour, electron affinity, electrical conductivity, and magnetism which is different from their bulk material. Nanotechnology improves biomarker development and aids in developing more sensitive treatments in medicine using nanodevices which enhances drug discovery by improving the understanding of biological processes, disease mechanisms, and signalling pathways.

This chapter provides an overview of nanomaterials and examines their distinct properties. The key top-down and bottom-up methods for synthesizing nanomaterials are also explained along with specific examples. The chapter will also include a summary of several nanoparticle characterization methods and the attributes associated with each method. In addition, comprehensive information about advanced devices that have been inspired by nanotechnology to increase the efficiency of the drug development process through a better understanding of the biological mechanisms underlying diseases, signalling pathways, and the precise effects of medications have also been discussed. The chapter will conclude by outlining the advantages and challenges of using nanotechnology in drug development and treatment.

Keywords: Challenges, Characterisation, Drug discovery, Nanomedicine, Nanomaterials, Nanodevices, Opportunities, Synthesis.

1. INTRODUCTION TO NANOMATERIALS

Although nanomaterials are not a new phenomenon in nature, interest in engineering at a very tiny scale arose following Richard P Feynman's legendary talk titled "There's plenty of space at the bottom" on 29th December 1959, at the annual meeting of the American Physical Society, when he spoke of manipulating and controlling things on a microscopic scale. Feynman is often considered as the first visionary of nanotechnology due to his clairvoyance. Unfortunately, it took the scientific community more than three decades to turn his vision into reality due to a lack of suitable tools and processes.

The prefix "nano" is derived from the Greek word for "dwarf." Nanomaterials represent a category of special materials that have at least one dimension in the nanometric range (1 nm-100 nm). The size comparison of nanomaterials is given in Fig. (**1**). Nanomaterials are classified into four types as zero-dimensional (0D), one-dimensional (1D), two-dimensional (2D), and three-dimensional (3D) nanostructures. All three dimensions are present at the nanoscale in zero-dimensional nanostructures. These nanoparticles resemble point particles and display quantum confinement. 1D nanoparticles have at least one dimension bigger than nanoscales (*i.e.* 100 nm), with the remaining dimensions occurring within the nano range. Nanofibers, nanotubes, and nanorods are the most frequent types of one-dimensional nanoparticles. The most popular examples of 2D nanomaterials are nanofilms, nanolayers, and nanocoatings, which are plate-like structures having two dimensions larger than the nanoscale. Although the constituents of 3D nanomaterials are smaller than 100 nm, none of their dimensions are less than the nanoscale. Nanomaterials with three dimensions are formed when the nanoscale particles are combined. These substances are typically nonporous and have a wide range of uses. The most common types of three-dimensional nanomaterials include nanocomposites, bundles of nanofibers, and multi-nanolayer structures [1, 2].

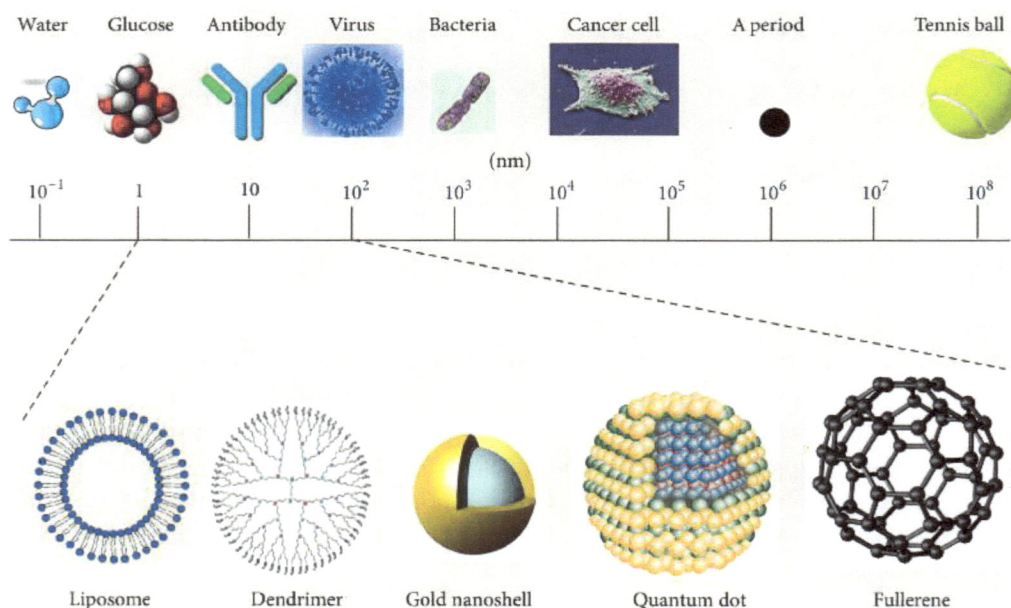

Fig. (1). Length scale showing size of nanomaterials. Reproduced with permission from [6] © 2015, Neha Pradhan *et al.* published by Hindawi Publishing Corporation, distributed under the terms of the Creative Commons Attribution 3.0 International. https://creativecommons.org/licenses/by/3.0/.

Beyond mere miniaturisation, nanotechnology has other applications. Materials at the nanoscale have distinctly different physical, chemical, and mechanical properties from bulk materials. When grain size is reduced to nanoscale dimensions, considerable changes are made to the properties, and the resulting qualities typically outperform those of conventional materials. The fact that nanoparticles are used in so many different applications is not surprising. The potential applications of nanomaterials are being discovered in ever-greater quantities.

Nature is undoubtedly the most important source of inspiration for nanoscientists and nanotechnologists. Many nanoparticles and nano-based systems have been refined by nature over millions of years through the process of evolution. Practically all fields of science and technology, including nanoscience and nanotechnology, can benefit from simple observation of the natural occurrences occurring around us. The cell membranes, as well as various other functioning organelles and enzymes, which are responsible for all metabolic activity in the body, are all nanometric in size. It is unsurprising that nanoparticles are employed in so many different applications [3 - 5].

Quantum phenomena, increased surface area, and self-assembly are mostly credited for the special features of nanomaterials. At the nanoscale, quantum effects may appear to govern how matter behaves, influencing how materials behave electrically, optically, and magnetically. This is because, at the nanoscale, matter no longer complies with Newtonian physics but rather with quantum mechanics, which is explicated by quantum confinement, size effect, and density of states. The bulk properties of a material are set by the average of all the quantum forces acting on all the atoms simultaneously. Yet, as structures get progressively smaller, eventually there comes a moment where averaging is no longer effective. Moreover, compared to bulk materials generated from the same mass, nanoparticles have a considerably greater surface area. When the fraction of surface atoms becomes greater, reactivity of the material is enhanced due to an increased number of active sites. In certain circumstances, inert materials in their bulk form turn out to be reactive when manufactured at the nanoscale level. All nanomaterials, regardless of their shape, including nanoparticles, nanowires, nanotubes, and nanocoatings, are affected by the increasing surface area. Finally, self-assembly is a process that relies on the arrangement of individual components to create structured or ordered patterns.

It reflects the information contained in each individual molecule, including shape, charge, polarizability, and other characteristics that affect their attracting or repelling interactions, particularly at the nanoscale. Whilst it can also exploit kinetically labile covalent connections, molecular self-assembly often benefits from supramolecular interactions such as ionic, van der Waals, hydrogen, hydrophobic, and coordination bonds. Ordered nanostructures develop as a result of ordered nanoparticles' inherent mobility as they equilibrate between aggregated and non-aggregated states, giving rise to a number of intriguing properties like error correction, self-healing, and great sensitivity to environmental cues [7].

When a particle size falls below the nanoscale in at least one dimension, properties that are not generally size dependent, such as melting temperature, ionisation potential, colour, and electron affinity, electrical conductivity, or magnetism, start to change with size. In this case, the properties of matter may be tailored to their desired values by varying the size of nanoparticles and the thickness of thin layers or wires. The ability to alter and change dimensions at the nanoscale has significantly improved by making it feasible to achieve the interesting features of nanostructures.

1.1. Changes in Thermal Properties

In bulk metals, electrons are the principal thermal energy carriers, and their distribution could be manipulated by nano structuring. The narrower energy bands generated by quantum confinement as a result of changed electron distribution can alter the temperature-related properties including melting point, phase transitions, thermal conductivity, and heat capacity [8].

1.2. Changes in Optical Properties

Nanomaterials have unique optical characteristics like colour, luminescence, and non-linear optical properties that are governed by "plasmons" and quantum size confinement. Certain inorganic NPs have intriguing optical characteristics based on their surface functionalization and particle size [9]. Their emission wavelengths may be controlled from the UV through the visible to the near-infrared parts of the spectrum by altering the size and composition of the nanomaterials. The emission wavelength of colloidal CdSe-CdS core-shell nanoparticles, for instance, may be changed to emit light at different wavelengths in the visible spectrum by varying their size from 2 to 6 nm in diameter, with the smaller particles generating blue light and the larger particles red light [10].

1.3. Changes in Electronic Properties

The shifts in electronic characteristics that take place as the system length scale shrinks are mostly attributable to the rising influence of the electrons' wave-like quality owing to quantum mechanical effects and the dearth of scattering centres [11]. The discrete aspect of the energy levels re-emerges when the system size approaches the de Broglie wavelength of the electrons, yet a completely discrete energy spectrum is only seen in systems that are restricted in all three dimensions. Because of their wave-like nature, electrons may tunnel quantum mechanically between two closely neighbouring nanostructures, and if a voltage is supplied between two nanostructures that have coinciding discrete energy levels, resonant tunnelling occurs, boosting the tunnelling current. Quantum dots display conductivity that is reliant on the presence of other charge carriers and, subsequently, the charge state of the dot due to their extreme confinement. Single-electron conduction processes produced by these Coulomb blockade effects only need a small amount of energy to turn on a switch, transistor, or memory device [12].

1.4. Changes in Electrical Properties

Materials are classified into three categories based on their electrical properties: conductors, semiconductors, and insulators. The ability to fill the energy separation between the valence band and the conduction band determines whether a material is a conductor, semiconductor, or an insulator. A metal becomes a semiconductor as its size is reduced because the quantum confinement effect causes the band gap to widen when a particle's size decreases in the nanoscale domain. Some nanoparticles exhibit electrical properties that are absolutely extraordinary and are related to their unique architectures. Carbon nanotubes, for instance, can be either conductors or semiconductors depending on their nanostructure [13, 14].

1.5. Changes in Magnetic Properties

The magnetic behaviour is determined by the structure and temperature of a material, and the regular size of traditionally anticipated domains is about 1 μm. Surface effects, the ratio of surface atoms to total atoms, and quantum effects start to take precedence as the dimension of a magnetic material is reduced. Due to the high surface-to-volume ratio, a large number of atoms have different magnetic couplings with their surroundings, giving rise to diverse magnetic properties [15].

1.6. Changes in Chemical Properties

With the predominance of surface effects at nanoscale the chemical properties also change in nano-materials compared to their bulk counterparts. Significantly the reactivity of the materials are enhanced substantially at nanoscale [16]. Nanomaterials are more energetic and catalytically active than bulk materials, due to the presence of more atoms on their surface than larger structures. The enhanced chemical activity is brought on by the large number of atoms that are exposed on the surface. Because of the high surface reactivity, contaminants may potentially interact more with nanomaterials; the nature of this interaction depends on the surface structure and the type of chemical bonding [17].

2. SYNTHESIS AND CHARACTERIZATION METHODS OF NANOMATERIALS

The "bottom-up" and "top-down" techniques are the most common ways to categorize the synthesis of nanostructures. Individual atoms and molecules are brought together or self-assembled to create nanostructured materials in the bottom-up method. Liquids and gases are used as the starting material in this process. With the top-down method, a microcrystalline substance is broken up into a nanocrystalline substance. This category includes all solid state routes. If the process parameters are well controlled, bottom-up approaches may often produce very small nanostructures of individual nanoparticles, nanoshells, *etc.*, with narrow size distributions. The top-down approaches can result in bulk nanostructured materials. While top-down techniques can be scaled up easily, many bottom-up systems are finding it difficult to scale up. Consequently, depending on the needs of a specific application, it is clear that both of these techniques complement one another [18].

2.1. Bottom-up Synthesis Methods

The two main types of bottom-up techniques for the synthesis of nanomaterials are known as solid-phase and liquid-phase techniques. Chemical vapour deposition (CVD), thermal decomposition and physical vapour deposition (PVD) approaches are available for solid phase methods. Nevertheless, most bottom-up techniques for nanomaterial production, such as liquid/liquid procedures (chemical reduction, biological reduction, solvothermal, spray drying, and spray pyrolysis) and sedimentation methods (sol-gel, alkaline precipitation, co-precipitation, and hydrolysis), are performed in the liquid phase [19].

2.1.1. Chemical Vapour Deposition

In CVD processes, a precursor gas is heated to form thin coatings on heated surfaces inside a reaction chamber, where at the end volatile by-products and unreacted precursor gases are subsequently removed by gas flow. Plasmas, ions, hot filaments, lasers, photons, and combustion reactions are used in modern CVD procedures to speed up deposition and reduce reaction temperature [19]. CVD is one of the standard methods for producing CNTs by chemical breakdown of a gaseous hydrocarbon on a substrate using a metal catalyst. This breakdown of the gaseous hydrocarbon at the surface of catalyst particles will cause the availability of carbon at the edges of the nanoparticles where nanotubes can develop [20]. CNT has demonstrated effectiveness and safety in the treatment of a number of illnesses, including cancer and brain tumours, using phototherapy, gene therapy, antiviral, antifungal, and antibacterial therapies, as well as other biomedical applications based on nanotechnology. Furthermore Titanium Nitride NPs which shows potential photothermal therapeutic ability for cancer treatment has also been synthesized frequently using CVD method [21].

2.1.2. Physical Vapour Deposition

A thin layer is deposited using the PVD technology, which builds the coating on the substrate atom by atom. PVD involves the vaporisation or atomization of substance from a solid source, also known as the target. Deposited thin films usually range in thickness from a few atomic layers to many microns. This procedure changes the surface's properties as well as the region between the substrate and the deposited substance. On the other hand, the properties of the films can also be influenced by the qualities of the substrate. Atomic deposits can be produced in a variety of conditions, including vacuum, gaseous, plasma, and electrolytic. A further benefit of the vacuum in the deposition chamber is that it will reduce gaseous contamination when the material is being deposited [22]. Graphitic NPs which are extensively used in medical applications have been synthesized using PVD methods like arc discharge, irradiation, vaporisation, and sputtering techniques [23].

2.1.3. Thermal Decomposition

This is a type of chemical decomposition process that is mediated by heat and results in the generation of nanoparticles with high crystallinity and limited size distribution. Organometallic compounds are decomposed in this process at high refluxing temperatures in solvents with high boiling points and with the assistance of stabilizing surfactants. Thermal decomposition is commonly utilized in the creation of metal oxide nanoparticles such as ZnO [24], Fe_3O_4 [25], CuO [26], Co_3O_4 [27], metal nanoparticles such as Fe [28], Ni [29] and Co [30], and alloys such as $CoPt_3$ [31] and $FePt$ [32]. The size, shape, and polydispersity of the resulting nanoparticles may be controlled by adjusting the ratios of the precursors, solvents, and surfactants [33, 34].

2.1.4. Chemical Reduction

This is one of the most adaptable procedures. In the majority of situations, with the Brust-Schiffrin two-phase process, in which chemical reduction occurs at the oil-water interface. As the precursor in the chemical reduction technique, an aqueous solution containing metal ions is employed. The ions are reduced to their metallic form by adding sodium borohydrate [35], sodium citrate [36, 37], sodium ascorbate [38] or hydrazine hydrate [39] in a volatile organic solvent such as toluene [40] or chloroform [41] to the reaction mixture. Nanoparticles aggregate and form clusters as a result of this process. Therefore, it is necessary to utilise capping agents to stop colloidal nanoparticle aggregation. Otherwise, it can be impossible to control the sizes of the final nanoparticle [42]. The most commonly used stabilizing agents include amines and thiols such as dodecylamine [43], dodecanethiol [44], alkanethiolates [45], surfactants [46], polymers [47], carboxylic acids [48] and organic compounds [49]. For instance gold nanoparticles (AuNPs) which is widely applied as biosensors, anticancer agents and in drug delivery are synthesized frequently by chemical reduction in major two steps. A reduction agent will provide electrons to reduce the gold ions, Au^{3+} and Au^+ to Au^0 which is the electric state for nanoparticles. Then a stabilizing agent will stabilize nanoparticles against aggregation [50].

2.1.5. Photo-reduction

One of the downsides of the chemical reduction process is the use of large amounts of reducing and stabilising chemicals, which must be eliminated from the finished product in the last step. A feasible solution to this issue is photo-reduction, which includes exposing the reaction mixture to a light source and photoreducing agents without the use of stabilising or capping compounds [51]. The photoreduction process has the advantage of largely eliminating undesirable by-products, and it may be used in both the solid and liquid phases [19]. AgNPs synthesized by the photoreduction of Leaves and Fruit Extracts of *Plinia cauliflora* and *Punica granatum* has shown high antimicrobial activity against Gram-negative and Gram-positive bacteria and yeast as well.

2.1.6. Biological Synthesis

The concepts of green chemistry are the foundation of the biological synthesis method, which is also known as "green synthesis." The primary solvent in the reaction mixture is water, however methanol and ethanol may also be employed. This approach has the benefit of using the reducing agent as a capping agent. The two main categories of reducing and capping agents employed in the green synthesis process are microorganisms and plant extracts [19]. For instance palladium NPs synthesized using the extract from brown alga, *Padina boryana* as a bio-capping and bio-reduction agent, has exhibited strong antibacterial/antibiofilm activities against *Staphylococcus aureus*, *Escherichia fergusonii*, *Acinetobacter pittii*, *Pseudomonas aeruginosa*, *Aeromonas enteropelogenes*, and *Proteus mirabilis* [52].

2.1.7. Solvothermal

The solvothermal approach has the potential to produce novel materials by using a variety of organic solvents as a reaction medium. The molecular weight, dipole moment, polarity, density, boiling point, melting point, heat of evaporation, and dielectric constant are just a few of the qualities that are impacted by the solvent of choice. Benzyl alcohol, propanol, butanol, heptanol, ethyl alcohol, and others are examples of the solvents used in the solvothermal process [53]. Leucine coated cobalt ferrite ($CoFe_2O_4$) nanoparticles loaded with DOX has been synthesized using solvothermal method with ethylene glycol and it has shown high cell viability towards the HeLa cells [54].

2.1.8. Sol-gel

This is a method for producing metal oxide nanoparticles and oxide composites. When the reaction media involves water, the term aqueous sol-gel is used and the procedure is known as the non-aqueous sol-gel method when organic solvents are involved. The non-aqueous sol-gel approach produces superior metal-oxides in terms of surface characteristics, nanoparticle size, morphological features, and chemical composition. The qualities of the final product are significantly influenced by the solvent and precursor metal salt used in the sol-gel process. The procedure is frequently carried out in three steps: hydrolysis (which creates the hydroxides of the precursors), condensation (which condenses the hydroxides into a 3D gel), and drying (leading to a xerogel or aerogel depending on the drying method) [55]. Teicoplanin drug loaded chitosan nanoparticles crosslinked with tripolyphosphate ion have been syntheized by *Kahdestani et al.*, and accessed for its ability of sustained drug delivery [56]. It is observed that 28.2% of teicoplanin was released in the frst 10 h and the release is continued gradually to receive 37.4% in 100 h.

2.1.9. Co-precipitation

One of the earliest wet chemical processes to produce nanomaterials is co-precipitation. In this approach, more than one compound is precipitated simultaneously from a salt precursor. Hydroxides, carbonates, chlorides, sulphates, and oxalates are the most regularly employed precipitants [19]. Co-precipitation is an efficient, rapid, and simple technique that may be readily scaled up for commercial use. It is an effective way to make nanomaterials without using hazardous organic solvents or high temperatures and pressures. Other benefits of this approach is its simplicity in controlling particle size and composition. However, this approach has certain drawbacks, including issues with batch-t--batch repeatability, time consumption, and contamination of the samples with trace contaminants that will precipitate simultaneously [57]. Magnetite nanoparticles used in therapeutic applications can be synthesized using this method. For instance, magnetite (Fe_3O_4) has been synthesized by co-precipitating $FeCl_2.4H_2O$ and $FeCl_3.6H_2O$ in distilled water that was previously purged by nitrogen. The synthesized Fe_3O_4 were directly coated with organic (Oleic Acid), inorganic (SiO_2) and polymeric (PEG) coatings and cell viability has been assessed with MTT assay for Hepatoma G2 cells [58].

2.2. Top-down Synthesis Methods

2.2.1. Mechanical Ball Milling

In comparison to alternative top-down approaches, mechanical ball milling is typically advantageous to produce various types of nanoparticles. This synthesis method is particularly useful when the synthesis procedure begins on a micrometre scale. A suitable milling medium and powder made up of a mixture of materials are often added to the mill with the goal of blending and particle-size reduction of the constituents. Charge ratio, milling time, drum rotation speed, brittleness of basic materials, size and size distribution, and ball building material are the key elements influencing the size of nanoparticles created from the milling process [59]. Additionally, milling temperature has a substantial impact on diffusivity. Higher temperatures are predicted to produce atomically mobile phases such as intermetallics, whereas lower temperatures mostly produce amorphous structures [60]. Peptides are prospective medicine candidates due to their efficiency, selectivity, and biodegradability. Mechanochemical peptide synthesis necessitates a modest amount of low-impact solvent (such as EtOAc or tBuOAc) and is a generally eco-friendly workup with better safety. Pure N-(--methoxyphenyl)-benzamide which can be used for the synthesis of the drug candidates of Benzimidazole derivatives has been synthesized by ball milling a crude mixture of benzoic acid, p-anisidine, anhydrous nitromethane, 4-dimethylaminopyridine (DMAP) and N-ethyl-N'-(3-dimethylaminopropyl)carbodiimide·HCl for 10-30 minutes [61]. Furthermore, within 180 minutes of milling with a single 12 mm diameter stainless steel ball at 30 Hz frequency, five homo- and hetero-dipeptides were produced starting with N-Boc-protected glycine or alanine and benzyl esters of glycine or alanine in the form of tosylate salts. Procainamide which is an antiarrhythmic drug has been synthesized successfully using K_2CO_3-assisted ball milling of p-nitrobenzoyl chloride with N,N-diethylenediamine for amide coupling followed by catalytic transfer hydrogenation under liquid assisted grinding [62].

2.2.2. Nanolithography

The study of producing nanometric-scale particles from bulk materials is referred to as nanolithography. The size of the synthesized nanoparticles obtained by this process ranges from 1 to 100 nm. To produce nanomaterials, a variety of nanolithography techniques have been utilized, including electron beam, optical process, nanoimprint, and high energy proton beams. In general, lithography is the process of producing nanoparticles of a certain form and size from light-sensitive bulk materials by selectively removing a portion of the bulk materials. The capacity to create single-size nanoparticle clusters in any desired form and size is the main advantage of this technique [63 - 65]. Rod-shaped docetaxel-loaded Poly(D,L-lactide-co-glycolide) nanoparticles has been synthesized using imprint lithography based technique referred to as Particle Replication in Nonwetting Templates which was then tested in the C3(1)-T-antigen (C3Tag) genetically engineered mouse model (GEMM) of breast cancer that represented the taxane resistant, basal-like subtype of triple-negative breast cancer [66]. The nanosystem of the drug has shown improved tumour growth inhibition and significantly increased median survival time.

2.2.3. Laser Ablation

One of the primary techniques for creating nanoparticles from different precursor liquids is laser ablation. When the metallic solution is combined with the liquid medium and subjected to a laser beam, the metallic solution condenses to form nanoparticles with sizes ranging from 1-100 nm. This procedure does not produce any toxic by-products, is cost-effective, and does not involve any hazardous chemicals or stabilizing agents. This is considered as a green synthesis method since both water and organic liquids can be used to form stable nanoparticles [67 - 71]. Al-Kinani *et al.*, synthesized a new formula of curcumin loaded, chitosan, gold and folic acid -coated Fe magnetic nanoparticles Fe@Au-CS-CU-FA nanoparticle by pulsed laser ablation in liquid by forming a water-in-oil microemulsion [72]. The NPs has shown sustained releasing behaviour, good stability and resulted in decrease of T-47D cell viability and induced 85% apoptosis.

2.2.4. Electrospinning

This is a common top-down technique that uses electrostatic forces to propel a conductive fluid to produce fibrous structures ranging from few nanometres to tens of micrometres. In this process a high voltage is supplied to the spinneret to charge the polymer solution, forming a potential gradient between the polymer droplet and the ground collector. When the voltage is high enough, the polymer jet will reach the ground collector, forming ultrafine fibers. These fibers will be deposited on a grounded collector plate to produce a nanofibrous membrane. The capability to control the surface morphology and chemical functionality of the produced fiber membranes have allowed the use of electrospun nanofibers in variety of disciplines [73, 74] Depending on the field of application electrospun fibers can be engineered to be core-shell [75], hollow [76], anisotropic [77], or biphasic structures [78].

Farkas et al., have developed a doxycycline (DOX) loaded polylactic acid-hydroxyapatite electrospun membrane as a drug delivery vehicle [79]. The Doxy-loaded PLA-HAP nanofiber system prepared by physical adsorption was found to be the most acceptable membrane to provide a prolonged release of DOX, in simulated body fluid and phosphate buffer solution rather than an immediate release of DOX. A Resveratrol-loaded polylactic acid (PLA) electrospun membrane has been employed as a pH-responsive drug delivery vessel which exhibited antibacterial and antibiofilm properties against *Pseudomonas aeruginosa* PAO1, and *Streptococcus mutans* [80]. The data acquired indicated that in acidic conditions, the RSV release rate from the PLA-membrane was significantly higher than in neutral pH. Furthermore, there has been a notable increase in RSV release during a pH shift from neutral to slightly acidic. Thus when the pH of the surrounding environment is neutral, PLA-RSV membranes can function as drug reservoirs. When the pH drops, as happens when an oral bacterial infection is present, the membranes begin to release bioactive compounds.

2.3. Characterisation of Nanomaterials

Throughout the last three decades, a variety of analytical tools for the characterization of nanomaterials have been developed. They have assisted in structural characterisation and understand the behaviour of nanomaterials and nanostructures. Different methods have been used to describe various physical and chemical aspects of nanomaterials, including size, shape, crystal structure, elemental content, and other nano-structural features. Therefore, it is possible to evaluate a single physical attribute of nanoparticles using more than one approach. In other words, the outcomes of various characterization approaches may be related to or complementary. Therefore, choosing the optimum method for nanomaterial characterization is undoubtedly crucial. Herein, we have summarized the different methods for nanomaterial characterization and the characteristic property analysed. (Table 1)

Table 1. The most important characterization techniques to characterize nanomaterials.

Characterization Technique	Characteristic Analysed	Refs.
FT-IR	Molecular structure (functional groups)	[81]
Raman scattering spectroscopy	Molecular structure (functional groups)	[81]
Ultraviolet-visible (UV-Vis) spectroscopy	Optical properties of nanoparticles	[81]

(Table 1) cont.....

Characterization Technique	Characteristic Analysed	Refs.
X-ray diffraction (XRD)	Crystalline structure, preferred crystalline orientations, average crystallite/grain size, chemical composition, and physical properties of nanomaterials	[81]
X-ray fluorescence (XRF)	Elemental composition of solid nanomaterials	[82]
X-ray photoelectron spectroscopy (XPS)	Surface chemical composition, binding states of the elements (under ultra-high vacuum conditions), ligand exchange interactions in the nanomaterials	[81]
Energy dispersive X-ray spectroscopy (EDX)	Elemental composition, atomic and weight percentage of the containing elements in the nanomaterials	[81]
Nuclear magnetic resonance (NMR) spectroscopy	Surface molecular structure, composition, molecular weight, dynamics, stoichiometry, *etc.* in the nanomaterials	[83]
Scanning Electron Microscopy / Field Emission Scanning Electron Microscopy (SEM)	Surface topology of nanomaterials	[81]
Transmission electron microscopy / High-resolution transmission electron microscopy (TEM)	Internal structure of the nanomaterials	[81]
Atomic Force Microscopy (AFM)	Three-dimensional characterization of nanomaterials such as geometries of nanoparticles, probing into hydrated nanoparticles, physical properties, studying the properties of soft and hard nanomaterials, and the surface roughness	[81]
The Brunauer–Emmett–Teller (BET)	Pore size distribution, pore volume, and the surface area measurement of nanomaterials	[84]
Zeta potential analyser	Stability of nanocolloids and nanomaterials suspensions	[81]
Vibrating Sample Magnetometer	Magnetic properties of the nanomaterials	[85]
Superconducting Quantum Interference Device (SQUID)	Magnetic properties of the nanomaterials	[84]

3. NANODEVICES

Drug discovery requires a thorough grasp of biological processes, from the molecular to the physiological, as well as a comprehension of disease in terms of protein synthesis, gene expression, and specific cellular and tissue responses. Technological advancements have been sparked by nanotechnology to increase the efficiency of the drug development process. Additionally, nanotechnology has given scientists a number of techniques to better understand the biological mechanisms underlying disease, signaling pathways, and the precise effects of medications [86].

Analysis of signalling pathways by using nanobiotechnology techniques might provide new insights into disease management processes. Identification of more efficient biomarkers and understanding the mechanism of action in drugs tremendously help in drug discovery. Harnessing the strategies of nanotechnology for diagnostic purposes is successfully obtained in medicine. New dimensions of diagnostic tools have been explored with the aid of this cutting-edge technique. More sensitive diagnostic kits, with the capability of probing the bodily problems at cellular pores and receptor level than existing ones were developed. Additionally, the degree of hazardous and harmful effects has been significantly decreased as a result of the use of miniature diagnostic materials. Below, we've covered a number of nano-enabled diagnostic tools used in the medical field.

3.1. Atomic Force Microscopy

Atomic force microscopy (AFM) is a versatile nanoscale technology that enables high-resolution imaging of biological macromolecules in their natural environment with a high signal-to-noise ratio. Additionally, AFM offers a delicate method for working with biomolecular machinery and aids in comprehending the molecular interactions and functionality of cell structures. The advancement of the AFM is the application of nanomechanical cantilevers, where a cantilever with a sharp tip at one end is used to image surfaces on molecular and atomic size [87]. As a result of the research and development done thus far, it has been discovered that high-rate AFM has entered the realm of time at the nanoscale and millisecond resolution in chemical processes, such as the visualization of the real-time motion of myosin on an actin filament [88]. AFM allows for the application and measurement of stresses in the piconewton to micronewton on spatially defined areas with dimensions ranging from a few nanometers to several tens of micrometers. AFM can measure mechanical properties such as force, pressure, adhesion, elasticity, tension, viscosity, and energy dissipation [89].

The significance of AFM lies in several key factors. First off, because of its extraordinarily high resolution, molecular- and even atomic-scale structures may be directly imaged in three dimensions. Second, sample preparation for AFM is simple, there is minimal harm to the original structure, and the sample's original structure may be precisely and objectively assessed. Thirdly, because samples can be examined in close to physiological settings, real-time AFM recordings of the dynamic activities of molecules, organelles, and other structures in living cells are possible [90]. Furthermore, intermolecular forces, charge, pH, and other physicochemical properties of sample materials may all be measured using AFM. Additionally, specific molecules or forces of interaction, such as ligand-receptor interactions, can be located using the functionalized probe. AFM thus has a significant chance of being used in biomedicine and clinical medicine, especially in the diagnosis and treatment of cancer [91]. AFM also makes it possible to investigate the mechanisms of anticancer medications at the cellular and molecular levels, enabling the assessment of their effectiveness and providing new opportunities for the prevention of tumour cell proliferation [92 - 94]. For instance, alterations in cell and tissue mechanics are among the traits of cancer, however, it is unclear how the stiffening of the tissue affects the growth of tumours. Mammary tumour cells and surrounding tissues have been measured for stiffness *in situ* using AFM to better understand this process, and it was discovered that tumour tissues are stiffer than isolated tumour cells [95 - 97].These studies show how AFM may be used to study mechanical characteristics associated with illness in settings that retain the physiological milieu. Alzheimer's disease is identified by intracellular neurofibrillary lesions and β-Amyloid (Aβ) plaques in the brain. Song *et al.* [98] investigated the interactions between vanillin and Aβ polypeptide using AFM in conjunction with fluorescence spectroscopy. Their findings showed that vanillin depolymerized Aβ1-42 aggregates in a dose-dependent manner, and the authors hypothesized that vanillin would be a promising pharmacological therapy for Alzheimer's disease.

3.2. Nanoarrays/nanochips

Micro- and nanoarrays are increasingly used as analytical instruments and platforms for evaluating chemical libraries, analyzing reactions at nanoliter scales, and attaining densities of thousands of spots/cm^2, surpassing the scale and density restrictions of well plates. These nanoarrays are miniature versions of microarrays, dispersed in micron or sub-micron spatial ranges [99].

Nanoarrays are static, regulated systems that have a high level of sensitivity and selectivity by nature [100]. Given these properties, nanoarrays have been employed for biomolecular analysis which are difficult to study *in vitro* due to their dynamic structure and have been used for the detection of pathogens in trace amounts [101, 102]. Nanoarrays are employed in bio-affinity testing for proteins, nucleic acids, and receptor-ligand pairs because they can quantify interactions between individual molecules with resolutions as low as one nanometre [86]. Nanoarray technology is expanding rapidly and has the potential for advancing pharmaceutical research and development.

Nanoarrays can store 10^4–10^5 more characteristics than traditional microarrays. Consequently, several targets may be promptly and simultaneously screened in a single experiment. Additionally, just a few target molecules may be identified for a given analyte concentration, and only extremely small amounts of sample and reagent are needed resulting in much lower detection limits than microarrays. Furthermore, just 1/10000 of the surface area needed by traditional microarray devices is needed for nanoarrays, and around 1500 nanoarray devices may be fitted into the same space as one microarray device. Last but not least, since biorecognition is intrinsically a nanoscopic phenomenon rather than a microscopic or macroscopic event, nanoarrays can be utilized to shed light on crucial problems surrounding biomolecular recognition [103].

The Nano Chip System has achieved 100% accuracy in the detection of nanoparticles by electrically enhancing the hybridization of complementary DNA strands. The Nano Chip System combines contemporary microelectronics and molecular biology into a platform technology with widespread commercial applications in the domains of genomic diagnostics. This method facilitates the investigation of DNA sequences or the pairing of separated DNA strands by using complementary DNA strands from the known collection that act as probes. DNA microarray experiments, which use the power of a digital device to separate DNA probes to particular websites at the array depending on charge and size, are currently conducted using DNA chips. Using these probes to analyze test sample (blood) data, DNA sequences may then be found [104].

3.3. Nanofluidics

Research tools for the explication of essential phenomena in nanoscale confined fluids have been made available by nanofluidics [105]. It is a particularly ideal platform for high-throughput biological Screening of single cell sample analysis because the volume of the nanospace is between aL $(= (100 \text{ nm})^3)$ and fL $(= (1000 \text{ nm})^3)$, which is 10^4 to 10^3 times smaller than the volume of a single cell [106].

Small molecules and particles including NPs, DNA fragments, and proteins have been effectively separated using nanofluidic devices [107, 108]. For cell biology, disease pathology, drug development, and medical therapies, living single-cell analysis is essential for identifying genes in cells, proteomics, and the temporal and spatial variety of physiology and pathology. Understanding the causes of life-threatening serious diseases is extremely important. For obtaining the average information about cells, the traditional single cell analysis concentrates on a large number of cells or cell lysis. As a result, it is unable to assess the actual, real-time data on variations between individual cells, which restricts the growth of several industries, including the biomedical sector. Small sample volumes, fast response times, easy operation, and effective processing, which have been widely employed in complicated procedures such single cell capture, separation, and detection, distinguish nanofluidics-based biochemical analysis from conventional approaches [106].

In a recent study, a nanofluidic device that has great sensitivity, resolution, and speed was established to continually assess the purity and bioactivity of biologics.

A continuous size-based examination of biologics was carried out using periodic and angled nanofilter arrays as molecular sieve structures. The supernatant of the cell culture can be directly used to continually assess several important safety and effectiveness measures, including binding, folding, and aggregation [109]. Additionally, they are enhancing the created nanofluidic device's capacity to track additional crucial quality characteristics during bio-manufacturing, such as binding affinity and glycosylation of monoclonal antibodies. To accomplish "real-time" and "multi-modal" quality analytics, the monitoring system will be further optimized [110]. Future bio-manufacturing processes are expected to be safer and more effective and broad applications in systems biology, personalized medicine, pathogen detection, drug development, and clinical research are expected with nanofluidic technology [111].

Additionally, drug delivery systems that are remotely controlled have included nanofluidics as actuators. For example, using electrostatic gating, Di Trani *et al.* have created a SiC-coated nanofluidic membrane that can reliably regulate the distribution of quantum dots and methotrexate, a first-line treatment for rheumatoid arthritis [112]. Hence, it has been proposed as a remedy for the inadequacy of sophisticated systems for the controlled and customized delivery of therapeutic interventions, which hinders the best possible management of conditions like diabetes, hypertension, and rheumatoid arthritis.

3.4. Nano Biosensors

Diagnostics are now provided in a personalized manner by considering the needs of disease management and the patient's disease profile. On this note, the advancements in point-of-care (POC) sensing unit fabrication, device integration, interfacing, packaging, and sensing performance have been enabled by nanotechnology. Modern biosensing technology is being actively marketed as the next generation of non-invasive illness detection techniques [113]. A biosensor is a biological component that detects and signals the activity, presence, or concentration of a specific biological molecule in solution through biochemical changes. The biological signal is changed into a measurable signal using a transducer. The selectivity and sensitivity of biosensors are essential traits. Nanoparticles are crucial in medical diagnostics because they are physiologically and chemically sensitive and may identify certain cells or body regions. Utilizing markers and distinctive biomolecules, nanobiosensors may distinguish between various cell types and recognize cancer cells. This makes it possible to monitor how different body parts are growing, and developing on delivering drugs. Even from outside the body, nanobiosensors are capable of detecting large-scale variations and signals linked to identical molecules within the body. By locating the fluoresced nanodot that was previously injected, a doctor might detect malignancies within the body by using the fluorescence characteristics of quantum dots of specific metals. Due to its capacity to detect specific DNA, genetic abnormalities might be identified specifically and sooner [114, 115]. Using metastasis-initiating cells (MIC), Ganesh *et al.* created a self-functionalized nanosensor for the early detection and forecasting of cancer metastasis. The nanosensor was generated by interacting a laser pulse with a carbon substrate in an oxygen-rich environment. By examining intracellular biological functions and tumour microenvironment features, it can identify MIC.

3.5. Nanobiopsy

Nano biopsy is a less invasive technique used in nanosurgery to examine live cells. It can serve as a platform for evaluating the prevalence of mitochondrial mutations in cancer research and clinical cancer care. Therefore, a nano biopsy might serve as the basis for a dynamic subcellular genetic study [116]. And it will help the researchers to track disease progression.

The system is based on scanning ion conductance microscopy, which has lately received attention for its capacity to capture high-resolution images of live cells in both space and time [117, 118]. The specimen is extracted using a glass nanopipette that is between 50 and 100 nm in size. The nanopipette is permitted to descend to a depth of around 1 nm to penetrate the cell membrane to enter the cell. The fluid can then enter the pipette once a voltage is introduced across the tip. The cell and cell membrane are both intact after the pipette has been removed from the cell. The electrolyte solution is then poured into the nanopipette, and the size of the ion current is evaluated at its tip. The size of the ion current diminishes when the nanopipette gets closer to a cell membrane [117, 119, 120].

Recently, nanopipettes have been used to localize delivery molecules to various subcellular locations, monitor the electrophysiology at tiny synaptic buttons, and trap molecules in lipid bilayers. Briefly, a liquid-liquid interface forms at the nanopipette aperture when an organic solution is placed within and submerged in an aqueous solution. The force created by applying a voltage across this contact can cause the aqueous solution to flow into and out of the nanopipette. [117, 121 - 123] The few copies of mitochondrial DNA that may be aspirated from a live cell using nanopipettes may serve as the foundation for less invasive and more precise disease progression monitoring. Nanobiopsy could pave the way for the creation of new therapeutic classes that will lessen a variety of illnesses, including Parkinson's and Alzheimer's disease. The nanopipette may be utilized as a platform for cancer research and therapeutic care, clarifying the function of heterogeneity in primary tumour tissues and systematically identifying important factors in disease development and possible metastatic states [124, 125]. The most difficult malignancies to identify in a person are frequently brain tumours. Biopsies allow for to diagnose if a tumour is benign or malignant in other tissues. However because the brain is such a unique organ, it is best to avoid removing brain tissue. However, the less intrusive nature of nanobiopsy provides an option [126]. By integrating the nanopipette platform with downstream sequencing technology, gene expression in individual cells can be fully examined and the influence of pharmacological processes on mutation-selection can be more thoroughly addressed [127].

4. ADVANTAGES OF EMPLOYING NANOMATERIALS AND NANODEVICES IN DRUG DISCOVERY

This rapidly developing field enables multidisciplinary researchers to create multifunctional nanoparticles that can target, identify, and treat a range of diseases. The development of improved diagnostic methods, therapeutic formulations, and drug delivery systems is one of the main objectives of nanotechnology in the field of drug research and development. The scientific community is increasingly focusing on the unique chemical and physical properties of nanoscale materials in search of potential applications to improve human health.

In general, nanoparticles can differ physicochemically from their bulk counterparts, leading to the creation of materials with unique properties that are distinct from those of products created conventionally. The development of innovative materials seeks to overcome challenges from conventional medicine, such as the use of weakly water-soluble chemicals encapsulated in water-soluble matrices, the targeted delivery of medications to tissues reducing the dose necessary, and the influence in other body parts, the delivery of numerous pharmaceuticals for combined therapy or the potential for theranostics, integrated diagnostic and treatment. The similar size of these structures to biological structures essential to the organism, such as proteins, is one of the intriguing benefits of employing nanomaterials in medicine [128].

Nanoparticles have more adaptable optical and magnetic properties than bulk materials because of the sophisticated quantum mechanics at the nanoscale. As a result, characteristics like colour can be adjusted by only changing the nanoparticle size. One of the most important aspects of medical diagnostics is the detection and identification of the material used for diagnostic outcomes. Since multiple colours may be produced by varying the nanoparticle's size, this is especially advantageous for the colour coding and labelling of materials used during diagnostic testing.

Another significant advantage of the tailorable properties of nanoparticles is the capacity to target nanoparticles or devices to deliver drugs selectively to illness sites. This allows for increased pharmacological effectiveness and a reduction in unwanted side effects. The attachment of biological moieties facilitates the distribution of functionalized nanomaterials to diseased tissues expressing biomarkers that differentiate it from surrounding healthy tissue. Several biomarkers, such as membrane receptors and mutated cellular proteins, are examples. As a result, less healthy tissues and organ systems are exposed to the systemic effects of drugs, which might diminish side effects. For instance, tumour necrosis factor alpha (TNF-α) was administered in its free form earlier and was discontinued during clinical trials due to severe immunotoxicity. Now it is in the market as Aurimune® which contains TNF-α bound to polyethylene glycol (PEG)-coated nanosized colloidal gold and is associated with minimal ill effects [129, 130].

Additionally, the nano drug delivery systems have significant benefits like the ability to achieve longer circulation times by modifying the surface charges, rapid response to environmental condition variations bringing out the stimulus-responsive behaviour, inherent antimicrobial properties, regulated drug distribution, enhanced pharmacokinetic characteristics, immune system resistance, high degree of encapsulation efficiency, strong stability of the drug and formulation, and improved drug delivery. A variety of drug delivery nano platforms with these properties are further explained in chapter 4.

The use of nanodevices in drug development helps create diagnostic instruments that are more sensitive than those that are now available. Furthermore, the degree of hazardous and negative effects has been greatly reduced due to the small size of the diagnostic materials. This state-of-the-art technology has enabled the investigation of novel diagnostic tool aspects. As mentioned in section 1.3, the pharmaceutical industry has made extensive use of nanodevices at various stages of drug development, including AFM, Nanoarrays, Nanochips, and Nanosensors.

Nano biosensors are being employed in target identification, validation, assay development, lead optimization, and ADMET (Absorption, Distribution, Metabolism, Excretion, and Toxicity) evaluation, however they are ideally suited for applications involving soluble molecules. Nano biosensors can solve many issues with the cell-based assays currently in use. Since biosensors do not require the removal of the receptor from the cell's lipid membranes, as other test techniques do, they are very useful in the research of receptors. Nanoarrays can be used to examine the bioaffinity of proteins, nucleic acids, and receptor-ligand combinations by measuring interactions between individual molecules with a one nanometer accuracy. For the last few decades, optical biosensors with the ability to employ resonant mirrors, wave guides, and surface plasmon resonance (SPR) have been extensively used to study biomolecular interactions. Without the requirement for a molecular tag or label, these sensors enable the real-time assessment of the affinity and kinetics of a wide range of chemical interactions. For biosensing devices, conventional SPR is used. For the immobilisation of ligands or proteins, these devices need complex chemistry, as well as pricey sensor chips with limited reusability. Cost savings are achieved by the use of nanoliter amounts in nanoscale experiments [86, 131].

5. CHALLENGES AND OPPORTUNITIES IN NANOSCALE

Nanoscale material has been embraced by interdisciplinary scientists because of its enormous potential, but it is not without difficulties. The manufacture, use, disposal, and waste treatment of products containing nanoparticles are the main causes of nanoparticulate environmental discharge in their original or modified forms.

5.1. Challenges

- The tiny size of NPs allows active chemical species to cross biological barriers such as the skin, lungs, body tissues, and organs. NPs can induce permanent oxidative stress, asthma, organelle damage, and cancer depending on their composition. The common acute toxic effects of NPs and nanostructured materials include protein denaturation, reactive oxygen species production, mitochondrial disruption, and phagocytic function interruption. The uptake of NPs by the reticuloendothelial system, nucleus, and neuronal tissue, and the formation of neoantigens, which can cause organ swelling and dysfunction, are common chronic adverse effects of NPs [1].
- With their cellular penetration and translocation capacity, foreign NPs cause permanent cell harm through oxidative stress or/and organelle injury. Along with entering cells, NPs also interact with their constituent parts through steric contact, interfacial tension effects, van der Waals forces, electrostatic charges, and van der Waals interactions that result in cell death. Numerous NPs have the potential to create reactive oxygen species, which can damage cells by changing lipids, proteins, DNA, signalling mechanisms, and gene transcription. How the oxidative products are disposed of depends on the NPs' chemistry, shape, size, and location. The cytoplasm, cytoplasmic components, and nucleus are just a few of the many biological places where nanoparticles might shift or spread. Due to their cellular localization impact, NPs can damage cell organelles or DNA and result in cell death [1, 132].
- Because of their high intrinsic reactivity, nanomaterials interact with harmful substances. When biological systems are exposed to chemically active

nanomaterials, some extraneous compounds and dangerous materials that are attached to those nanoparticles will also enter the biological systems and exacerbate the harmful effects.

- It is still largely unknown how nanomaterials may affect the ecosystem, both positively and negatively. Negatively, removing nanoparticles from the environment will be extremely difficult or impossible. One illustration of the ambiguous nature of nanomaterials is nano-silver. Although nano-silver is employed in many items because of its anti-microbial capabilities, those same qualities might be dangerous to the environment and waste-treatment facilities that use microorganisms to clean sewage [133].

- In addition to the issues with toxicology, scaling up the synthesis is a key drawback of nanoscale materials. With very few exceptions, nanoparticles used in preclinical research are nearly always synthesised in very small batches, and it is not always feasible to scale them up for synthesis in large volumes. Due to the complexity of human diseases, it is essential to produce a consistent and highly repeatable formulation before reaching the stage of clinical trials. Synthesis problems have occasionally occurred in clinical settings, as in the case of LipoDox, which was swiftly approved and used in place of Doxil due to a scarcity of the latter drug. Nonetheless, despite assurances that the drugs were equal, effectiveness variations between these two formulations were documented [134, 135]. It is likely that reliable synthesis and scale-up processes were involved, even though the exact origin of these variances is unknown.

5.2. Opportunities

- The primary possibility at the nanoscale for advancing drug discovery is the development of detecting devices that will lead to more accurate, efficient in terms of both time and money, safe, and portable ways of illness diagnosis, management, and treatment.

- Exceptional capabilities of nano instruments such as electron microscopes and AFM allow not only in-depth analysis of virus structure and function but also investigation of virus impact on host cells and extracellular environment, useful in drug discovery applications [136]. These methods do not require organism-specific reagents for detecting the pathogenic agent, in contrast to the molecular and serological methodologies used for viral diagnosis, which requires a particular probe to recognize the virus.

- The opportunity for the introduction of improved sensing mechanisms with a multidisciplinary approach has arisen as a result of the rapid development of nanotechnology. These mechanisms will enable the quick and on-site detection of viruses for point-of-care diagnostics, the early prevention of epidemics, and the early detection of ailments such as cancers, which will save more lives.

- Furthermore, the synergistic fusion of several other technologies and medical treatment modalities with nanotechnology can open up new possibilities. For instance, Liu *et al.* have discussed the opportunities for nanotechnology in a digital age by combining plasma medicine, nano- and digital technology, in the health care sector [137]. Investigations, such as the utilization of plasma to efficiently transport nanocapsules past the epidermal barrier [138], in polymer nanocomposites coated with antibacterial coatings *via* plasma [139] and in the combined use of plasma-nanomaterials for oncotherapies [140] have already revealed the potential synergistic effects of plasma-nano.

- Atmospheric pressure plasma alterations of printed nanomaterials present intriguing potential for the fusion of plasma, nano, and digital technologies for use in healthcare-related applications. Integrating plasma, nano, and digital technologies into a single multimodal healthcare package could significantly enhance patient comfort and outcomes, as well as provide a chance to lessen the financial burden on community healthcare and deal with a variety of problems related to overburdened healthcare systems [137].

CONCLUSION

Nanomaterials, a category of special materials with at least one dimension in the nanometric range (1 nm-100 nm), were first recognized by Richard P Feynman in 1959. Nanotechnology has various applications, with nanoparticles having distinctly different physical, chemical, and mechanical properties from bulk materials. Quantum phenomena, increased surface area, and self-assembly are key features of nanomaterials. Nanoparticle size affects properties like melting temperature, ionization potential, colour, electron affinity, electrical conductivity, and magnetism, allowing for the customization of matter properties through size. Bottom-up and top-down techniques are commonly used for synthesizing nanostructures. Bottom-up methods involve self-assembling atoms and molecules into nano size, while top-down methods break down microcrystalline substances, producing bulk nanostructures. Over the past three decades, various analytical tools have been developed for the characterization of nanomaterials, aiding in structural and behavioural understanding. These methods describe the physical and chemical aspects of nanomaterials, including size, shape, crystal structure, and elemental content.

Nanotechnology enhances drug discovery by improving the understanding of biological processes, disease mechanisms, and signalling pathways. It also aids in the development of efficient biomarkers and diagnostic tools, enabling more sensitive and less harmful treatments in medicine. In this chapter, various nanodevices such as AFM, nanoarrays/nanochips, nanofluidics, nanobiopsys, and nanobiosensors have been discussed. Nanomaterials in medicine offer advantages like the similar size to biological structures, colour coding, selective drug delivery, and enhanced pharmacokinetic characteristics. They also provide longer circulation times, rapid response to environmental conditions, and improved diagnostic instruments. However, there are still many challenges that need to be addressed when using nanoparticles and nanotechnology in medicinal applications.

PRACTICE QUESTIONS

1. Discuss how nanomaterials are involved in natural phenomena in biological systems.
2. Discuss the reason for the significant changes of properties during size reduction of a material to nanoscale, compared to its bulk component.
3. Define 'top-down' and 'bottom-up' approaches for the synthesis of nanomaterials.
4. List out the nanomaterial synthesis methods that are most prominently utilized in the drug development sector.
5. List different nanodevices used through the process of drug development and how they are utilized in the process.
6. Discuss the benefits and challenges of using nanoscale in drug development.

REFERENCES

[1]   Jeevanandam, J.; Barhoum, A.; Chan, Y.S.; Dufresne, A.; Danquah, M.K. Review on nanoparticles and nanostructured materials: history, sources, toxicity and regulations. *Beilstein J. Nanotechnol.,* **2018**, *9*(1), 1050-1074.
        [http://dx.doi.org/10.3762/bjnano.9.98] [PMID: 29719757]

[2]   Byakodi, M.; Shrikrishna, N. S.; Sharma, R.; Bhansali, S.; Mishra, Y.; Kaushik, A.; Gandhi, S. Emerging 0D, 1D, 2D, and 3D nanostructures for efficient point-of-care biosensing. *Biosensors and Bioelectronics: X,* **2022**, *12*, 100284.

[3]   Prammitha, R.; Jeice, A.R.; Jayakumar, K. Review of multifaceted application based green synthesized TiO_2 nanoparticles. *Surfaces and Interfaces,* **2023**, 102912.

[4]   Aziz, T.; Farid, A.; Haq, F.; Kiran, M.; Ullah, A.; Zhang, K.; Li, C.; Ghazanfar, S.; Sun, H.; Ullah, R.; Ali, A.; Muzammal, M.; Shah, M.; Akhtar, N.; Selim, S.; Hagagy, N.; Samy, M.; Al Jaouni, S.K. A review on the modification of cellulose and its applications. *Polymers,* **2022**, *14*(15), 3206.
        [http://dx.doi.org/10.3390/polym14153206] [PMID: 35956720]

[5]   Aziz, T.; Fan, H.; Zhang, X.; Haq, F.; Ullah, A.; Ullah, R.; Khan, F.U.; Iqbal, M. Advance study of cellulose nanocrystals properties and applications. *J. Polym. Environ.,* **2020**, *28*(4), 1117-1128.
        [http://dx.doi.org/10.1007/s10924-020-01674-2]

[6]   Pradhan, N.; Singh, S.; Ojha, N.; Shrivastava, A.; Barla, A.; Rai, V.; Bose, S. Facets of Nanotechnology as Seen in Food Processing, Packaging, and Preservation Industry. *BioMed Res. Int.,* **2015**, *2015*, 1-17.
        [http://dx.doi.org/10.1155/2015/365672] [PMID: 26613082]

[7]   Kumar, N.; Kumbhat, S. Unique properties. *Essentials in nanoscience and nanotechnology*; John Wiley & Sons: New Jersey, **2016**, pp. 326-360.
        [http://dx.doi.org/10.1002/9781119096122.ch8]

[8]   Roduner, E. Nucleation, Phase Transitions and Dynamics of Clusters. *Nanoscopic materials size-dependent phenomena*; RCS publishing: Cambridge, **2006**, pp. 209-232.

[http://dx.doi.org/10.1039/9781847557636-00209]

[9]   Quinten, M. *Optical properties of nanoparticle systems: Mie and beyond*; John Wiley & Sons, **2010**.

[10]   Roduner, E. Size matters: why nanomaterials are different. *Chem. Soc. Rev.,* **2006**, *35*(7), 583-592.
        [http://dx.doi.org/10.1039/b502142c] [PMID: 16791330]

[11]   Bhushan, B.; Luo, D.; Schricker, S.R.; Sigmund, W.; Zauscher, S. *Handbook of Nanomaterials Properties*; Springer: Heidelberg, **2014**, p. 1463.
        [http://dx.doi.org/10.1007/978-3-642-31107-9]

[12]   Kumar, N.; Kumbhat, S. Unique Properties. In Essentials in Nanoscience and Nanotechnology, First Edition ed.; Wiley: 2016; pp 326-356.
        [http://dx.doi.org/10.1002/9781119096122.ch8]

[13]   Barhoum, A.; García-Betancourt, M.L. Physicochemical characterization of nanomaterials: Size, morphology, optical, magnetic, and electrical properties. *Emerging applications of nanoparticles and architecture nanostructures*; Elsevier, **2018**, pp. 279-304.
        [http://dx.doi.org/10.1016/B978-0-323-51254-1.00010-5]

[14]   Yurkov, G.Y.; Fionov, A.S.; Koksharov, Y.A.; Koleso, V.V.; Gubin, S.P. Electrical and magnetic properties of nanomaterials containing iron or cobalt nanoparticles. *Inorg. Mater.,* **2007**, *43*(8), 834-844.
        [http://dx.doi.org/10.1134/S0020168507080055]

[15]   Lu, A.H.; Salabas, E.L.; Schüth, F. Magnetic nanoparticles: synthesis, protection, functionalization, and application. *Angew. Chem. Int. Ed.,* **2007**, *46*(8), 1222-1244.
        [http://dx.doi.org/10.1002/anie.200602866] [PMID: 17278160]

[16]   Neus, G.B.; Eudald, C.; Isaac, O.; Miriam, V.; Victor, P. *The Delivery of Nanoparticles*; Abbass, A.H., Ed.; IntechOpen: Rijeka, **2012**.

[17]   Singh, V.; Yadav, P.; Mishra, V. Recent advances on classification, properties, synthesis, and characterization of nanomaterials. *Green synthesis of nanomaterials for bioenergy applications,* **2020**, 83-97.

[18]   Murty, B.S.; Shankar, P.; Raj, B.; Rath, B.B.; Murday, J. Synthesis Routes. *Textbook of nanoscience and nanotechnology*; Raj, B., Ed.; Springer Science & Business Media, **2013**, pp. 66-100.
        [http://dx.doi.org/10.1007/978-3-642-28030-6_3]

[19]   Vaseghi, Z.; Nematollahzadeh, A. Nanomaterials: types, synthesis, and characterization. In Green Synthesis of Nanomaterials for Bioenergy Applications, Neha Srivastava; Manish Srivastava; P. K. Mishra; Gupta, V. K., Eds. John Wiley & Sons: 2020; pp 23-82.
        [http://dx.doi.org/10.1002/9781119576785.ch2]

[20]   Rahamathulla, M.; Bhosale, R.R.; Osmani, R.A.M.; Mahima, K.C.; Johnson, A.P.; Hani, U.; Ghazwani, M.; Begum, M.Y.; Alshehri, S.; Ghoneim, M.M.; Shakeel, F.; Gangadharappa, H.V. Carbon Nanotubes: Current perspectives on diverse applications in targeted drug delivery and therapies. *Materials,* **2021**, *14*(21), 6707.
        [http://dx.doi.org/10.3390/ma14216707] [PMID: 34772234]

[21]   Ifijen, I.H.; Maliki, M. A comprehensive review on the synthesis and photothermal cancer therapy of titanium nitride nanostructures. *Inorganic and Nano-Metal Chemistry,* **2023**, *53*(4), 366-387.
        [http://dx.doi.org/10.1080/24701556.2022.2068596]

[22]   Baptista, A.; Silva, F.J.G.; Porteiro, J.; Míguez, J.L.; Pinto, G.; Fernandes, L. On the physical vapour deposition (PVD): evolution of magnetron sputtering processes for industrial applications. *Procedia Manuf.,* **2018**, *17*, 746-757.
        [http://dx.doi.org/10.1016/j.promfg.2018.10.125]

[23]   Zia, A.W.; Birkett, M.; Badshah, M.A.; Iqbal, M. Progress in-situ synthesis of graphitic carbon nanoparticles with physical vapour deposition. *Prog. Cryst. Growth Charact. Mater.,* **2021**, *67*(3), 100534.

[http://dx.doi.org/10.1016/j.pcrysgrow.2021.100534]

[24]   Saravanan, R.; Gupta, V.K.; Prakash, T.; Narayanan, V.; Stephen, A. Synthesis, characterization and photocatalytic activity of novel Hg doped ZnO nanorods prepared by thermal decomposition method. *J. Mol. Liq.,* **2013**, *178*, 88-93.
[http://dx.doi.org/10.1016/j.molliq.2012.11.012]

[25]   Amara, D.; Felner, I.; Nowik, I.; Margel, S. Synthesis and characterization of Fe and Fe_3O_4 nanoparticles by thermal decomposition of triiron dodecacarbonyl. *Colloids Surf. A Physicochem. Eng. Asp.,* **2009**, *339*(1-3), 106-110.
[http://dx.doi.org/10.1016/j.colsurfa.2009.02.003]

[26]   Ibrahim, E.M.M.; Abdel-Rahman, L.H.; Abu-Dief, A.M.; Elshafaie, A.; Hamdan, S.K.; Ahmed, A.M. The synthesis of CuO and NiO nanoparticles by facile thermal decomposition of metal-Schiff base complexes and an examination of their electric, thermoelectric and magnetic Properties. *Mater. Res. Bull.,* **2018**, *107*, 492-497.
[http://dx.doi.org/10.1016/j.materresbull.2018.08.020]

[27]   Momeni, B.Z.; Rahimi, F.; Rominger, F. Preparation of Co_3O_4 Nanoparticles *via* Thermal Decomposition of Three New Supramolecular Structures of Co(II) and (III) Containing 4'-Hydrox--2,2':6',2''-Terpyridine: Crystal Structures and Thermal Analysis Studies. *J. Inorg. Organomet. Polym. Mater.,* **2018**, *28*(1), 235-250.
[http://dx.doi.org/10.1007/s10904-017-0706-6]

[28]   Simeonidis, K.; Mourdikoudis, S.; Moulla, M.; Tsiaoussis, I.; Martinez-Boubeta, C.; Angelakeris, M.; Dendrinou-Samara, C.; Kalogirou, O. Controlled synthesis and phase characterization of Fe-based nanoparticles obtained by thermal decomposition. *J. Magn. Magn. Mater.,* **2007**, *316*(2), e1-e4.
[http://dx.doi.org/10.1016/j.jmmm.2007.02.009]

[29]   He, X.; Zhong, W.; Au, C.T.; Du, Y. Size dependence of the magnetic properties of Ni nanoparticles prepared by thermal decomposition method. *Nanoscale Res. Lett.,* **2013**, *8*(1), 446.
[http://dx.doi.org/10.1186/1556-276X-8-446] [PMID: 24164907]

[30]   Shao, H.; Huang, Y.; Lee, H.; Suh, Y.J.; Kim, C.O. Cobalt nanoparticles synthesis from $Co(CH_3COO)_2$ by thermal decomposition. *J. Magn. Magn. Mater.,* **2006**, *304*(1), e28-e30.
[http://dx.doi.org/10.1016/j.jmmm.2006.02.032]

[31]   Tzitzios, V.; Niarchos, D.; Gjoka, M.; Boukos, N.; Petridis, D. Synthesis and characterization of 3D CoPt nanostructures. *J. Am. Chem. Soc.,* **2005**, *127*(40), 13756-13757.
[http://dx.doi.org/10.1021/ja053044m] [PMID: 16201773]

[32]   Nandwana, V.; Elkins, K.E.; Poudyal, N.; Chaubey, G.S.; Yano, K.; Liu, J.P. Size and shape control of monodisperse FePt nanoparticles. *J. Phys. Chem. C,* **2007**, *111*(11), 4185-4189.
[http://dx.doi.org/10.1021/jp068330e]

[33]   Khan, L.U.; Khan, Z.U. *Bifunctional nanomaterials: Magnetism, luminescence and multimodal biomedical applications. Complex Magnetic Nanostructures: Synthesis*; Assembly and Applications, **2017**, pp. 121-171.

[34]   Unni, M.; Uhl, A.M.; Savliwala, S.; Savitzky, B.H.; Dhavalikar, R.; Garraud, N.; Arnold, D.P.; Kourkoutis, L.F.; Andrew, J.S.; Rinaldi, C. Thermal decomposition synthesis of iron oxide nanoparticles with diminished magnetic dead layer by controlled addition of oxygen. *ACS Nano,* **2017**, *11*(2), 2284-2303.
[http://dx.doi.org/10.1021/acsnano.7b00609] [PMID: 28178419]

[35]   Mehr, F.; Khanjani, M.; Vatani, P. Synthesis of nano-Ag particles using sodium borohydride. *Orient. J. Chem.,* **2015**, *31*(3), 1831-1833.
[http://dx.doi.org/10.13005/ojc/310367]

[36]   Piella, J.; Bastús, N.G.; Puntes, V. Size-Controlled Synthesis of Sub-10-nanometer Citrate-Stabilized Gold Nanoparticles and Related Optical Properties. *Chem. Mater.,* **2016**, *28*(4), 1066-1075.
[http://dx.doi.org/10.1021/acs.chemmater.5b04406]

[37]   Biz, H. M.; da Silva Moraes, D.; de Campos Rocha, T. L. A. Gold Nanoparticles Synthesis with Different Reducing Agents Characterized by UV-Visible Spectroscopy and FTIR. *Journal of bioengineering of and tecchnology applied to health,* **2022**, *5*(1), 44-51.

[38]   Kumar, M.; Pakshirajan, K. Immobilized biogenic copper nanoparticles from metallic wastewater as a catalyst for triazole synthesis by a click reaction using water as a solvent. *New J. Chem.,* **2022**, *46*(29), 13953-13962.
[http://dx.doi.org/10.1039/D2NJ02882D]

[39]   Azharul Islam, D.; Acharya, H. Pd-Nanoparticles@layered double hydroxide/reduced graphene oxide (Pd NPs@LDH/rGO) nanocomposite catalysts for highly efficient green reduction of aromatic nitro compounds. *New J. Chem.,* **2022**, *46*(11), 5346-5354.
[http://dx.doi.org/10.1039/D1NJ05377A]

[40]   Zhai, Y.; Whitten, J.J.; Zetterlund, P.B.; Granville, A.M. Synthesis of hollow polydopamine nanoparticles using miniemulsion templating. *Polymer,* **2016**, *105*, 276-283.
[http://dx.doi.org/10.1016/j.polymer.2016.10.038]

[41]   Shankar, S.; Rhim, J.W. Tocopherol-mediated synthesis of silver nanoparticles and preparation of antimicrobial PBAT/silver nanoparticles composite films. *Lebensm. Wiss. Technol.,* **2016**, *72*, 149-156.
[http://dx.doi.org/10.1016/j.lwt.2016.04.054]

[42]   Pandey, A.; Manivannan, R. A study on synthesis of nickel nanoparticles using chemical reduction technique. *Recent Pat. Nanomed.,* **2015**, *5*(1), 33-37.
[http://dx.doi.org/10.2174/1877912305666150417232717]

[43]   Morán-Lázaro, J.; López-Urías, F.; Muñoz-Sandoval, E.; Blanco-Alonso, O.; Sanchez-Tizapa, M.; Carreon-Alvarez, A.; Guillén-Bonilla, H.; Olvera-Amador, M.; Guillén-Bonilla, A.; Rodríguez-Betancourtt, V. Synthesis, characterization, and sensor applications of spinel ZnCo2O4 nanoparticles. *Sensors,* **2016**, *16*(12), 2162.
[http://dx.doi.org/10.3390/s16122162] [PMID: 27999315]

[44]   Mancini, G.F.; Latychevskaia, T.; Pennacchio, F.; Reguera, J.; Stellacci, F.; Carbone, F. Order/disorder dynamics in a dodecanethiol-capped gold nanoparticles supracrystal by small-angle ultrafast electron diffraction. *Nano Lett.,* **2016**, *16*(4), 2705-2713.
[http://dx.doi.org/10.1021/acs.nanolett.6b00355] [PMID: 26918756]

[45]   San, K.A.; Chen, V.; Shon, Y.S. Preparation of partially poisoned alkanethiolate-capped platinum nanoparticles for hydrogenation of activated terminal alkynes. *ACS Appl. Mater. Interfaces,* **2017**, *9*(11), 9823-9832.
[http://dx.doi.org/10.1021/acsami.7b02765] [PMID: 28252941]

[46]   Sun, Z.; Zhang, L.; Dang, F.; Liu, Y.; Fei, Z.; Shao, Q.; Lin, H.; Guo, J.; Xiang, L.; Yerra, N.; Guo, Z. Experimental and simulation-based understanding of morphology controlled barium titanate nanoparticles under co-adsorption of surfactants. *CrystEngComm,* **2017**, *19*(24), 3288-3298.
[http://dx.doi.org/10.1039/C7CE00279C]

[47]   Pourmasoud, S.; Sobhani-Nasab, A.; Behpour, M.; Rahimi-Nasrabadi, M.; Ahmadi, F. Investigation of optical properties and the photocatalytic activity of synthesized YbYO$_4$ nanoparticles and YbVO$_4$/NiWO$_4$ nanocomposites by polymeric capping agents. *J. Mol. Struct.,* **2018**, *1157*, 607-615.
[http://dx.doi.org/10.1016/j.molstruc.2017.12.077]

[48]   Shombe, G.B.; Mubofu, E.B.; Mlowe, S.; Revaprasadu, N. Synthesis and characterization of castor oil and ricinoleic acid capped CdS nanoparticles using single source precursors. *Mater. Sci. Semicond. Process.,* **2016**, *43*, 230-237.
[http://dx.doi.org/10.1016/j.mssp.2015.11.011]

[49]   Sun, J.K.; Zhan, W.W.; Akita, T.; Xu, Q. Toward homogenization of heterogeneous metal nanoparticle catalysts with enhanced catalytic performance: soluble porous organic cage as a stabilizer and homogenizer. *J. Am. Chem. Soc.,* **2015**, *137*(22), 7063-7066.

[http://dx.doi.org/10.1021/jacs.5b04029] [PMID: 26020572]

[50]   Daruich De Souza, C.; Ribeiro Nogueira, B.; Rostelato, M.E.C.M. Review of the methodologies used in the synthesis gold nanoparticles by chemical reduction. *J. Alloys Compd.,* **2019**, *798*, 714-740.
[http://dx.doi.org/10.1016/j.jallcom.2019.05.153]

[51]   Zaarour, M.; El Roz, M.; Dong, B.; Retoux, R.; Aad, R.; Cardin, J.; Dufour, C.; Gourbilleau, F.; Gilson, J.P.; Mintova, S. Photochemical preparation of silver nanoparticles supported on zeolite crystals. *Langmuir,* **2014**, *30*(21), 6250-6256.
[http://dx.doi.org/10.1021/la5006743] [PMID: 24810992]

[52]   Sonbol, H.; Ameen, F.; AlYahya, S.; Almansob, A.; Alwakeel, S. Padina boryana mediated green synthesis of crystalline palladium nanoparticles as potential nanodrug against multidrug resistant bacteria and cancer cells. *Sci. Rep.,* **2021**, *11*(1), 5444.
[http://dx.doi.org/10.1038/s41598-021-84794-6] [PMID: 33686169]

[53]   Feng, S-H.; Li, G-H. Hydrothermal and solvothermal syntheses. *Modern inorganic synthetic chemistry*; Elsevier, **2017**, pp. 73-104.
[http://dx.doi.org/10.1016/B978-0-444-63591-4.00004-5]

[54]   Zhang, H.; Wang, J.; Zeng, Y.; Wang, G.; Han, S.; Yang, Z.; Li, B.; Wang, X.; Gao, J.; Zheng, L.; Liu, X.; Huo, Z.; Yu, R. Leucine-coated cobalt ferrite nanoparticles: Synthesis, characterization and potential biomedical applications for drug delivery. *Phys. Lett. A,* **2020**, *384*(24), 126600.
[http://dx.doi.org/10.1016/j.physleta.2020.126600]

[55]   Bokov, D.; Turki Jalil, A.; Chupradit, S.; Suksatan, W.; Javed Ansari, M.; Shewael, I.H.; Valiev, G.H.; Kianfar, E. Nanomaterial by sol-gel method: synthesis and application. *Adv. Mater. Sci. Eng.,* **2021**, *2021*, 1-21.
[http://dx.doi.org/10.1155/2021/5102014]

[56]   Kahdestani, S.A.; Shahriari, M.H.; Abdouss, M. Synthesis and characterization of chitosan nanoparticles containing teicoplanin using sol–gel. *Polym. Bull.,* **2021**, *78*(2), 1133-1148.
[http://dx.doi.org/10.1007/s00289-020-03134-2]

[57]   Rane, A.V.; Kanny, K.; Abitha, V.K.; Thomas, S. Methods for Synthesis of Nanoparticles and Fabrication of Nanocomposites. *Synthesis of Inorganic Nanomaterials*; Mohan Bhagyaraj, S.; Oluwafemi, O.S.; Kalarikkal, N.; Thomas, S., Eds.; Woodhead Publishing, **2018**, pp. 121-139.
[http://dx.doi.org/10.1016/B978-0-08-101975-7.00005-1]

[58]   Mohammadi, H.; Nekobahr, E.; Akhtari, J.; Saeedi, M.; Akbari, J.; Fathi, F. Synthesis and characterization of magnetite nanoparticles by co-precipitation method coated with biocompatible compounds and evaluation of in-vitro cytotoxicity. *Toxicol. Rep.,* **2021**, *8*, 331-336.
[http://dx.doi.org/10.1016/j.toxrep.2021.01.012] [PMID: 33659189]

[59]   Bello, S.A.; Agunsoye, J.O.; Hassan, S.B. Synthesis of coconut shell nanoparticles *via* a top down approach: Assessment of milling duration on the particle sizes and morphologies of coconut shell nanoparticles. *Mater. Lett.,* **2015**, *159*, 514-519.
[http://dx.doi.org/10.1016/j.matlet.2015.07.063]

[60]   Prasad Yadav, T.; Manohar Yadav, R.; Pratap Singh, D. Mechanical milling: A top down approach for the synthesis of nanomaterials and nanocomposites. *Nanoscience and Nanotechnology,* **2012**, *2*(3), 22-48.
[http://dx.doi.org/10.5923/j.nn.20120203.01]

[61]   Štrukil, V.; Bartolec, B.; Portada, T.; Đilović, I.; Halasz, I.; Margetić, D. One-pot mechanosynthesis of aromatic amides and dipeptides from carboxylic acids and amines. *Chem. Commun.,* **2012**, *48*(99), 12100-12102.
[http://dx.doi.org/10.1039/c2cc36613d] [PMID: 23135220]

[62]   Portada, T.; Margetić, D.; Štrukil, V. Mechanochemical Catalytic Transfer Hydrogenation of Aromatic Nitro Derivatives. *Molecules,* **2018**, *23*(12), 3163.
[http://dx.doi.org/10.3390/molecules23123163] [PMID: 30513686]

[63]   Ding, L.; Li, Y.; Chu, H.; Li, X.; Liu, J. Creation of cadmium sulfide nanostructures using AFM dip-pen nanolithography. *J. Phys. Chem. B,* **2005**, *109*(47), 22337-22340.
[http://dx.doi.org/10.1021/jp053389r] [PMID: 16853909]

[64]   Duan, X. *Nanowire nanoelectronics assembled from the bottom-up*; Harvard University, **2002**.

[65]   Pimpin, A.; Srituravanich, W. Review on micro-and nanolithography techniques and their applications. *Eng. J.,* **2012**, *16*(1), 37-56.
[http://dx.doi.org/10.4186/ej.2012.16.1.37]

[66]   Bowerman, C.J.; Byrne, J.D.; Chu, K.S.; Schorzman, A.N.; Keeler, A.W.; Sherwood, C.A.; Perry, J.L.; Luft, J.C.; Darr, D.B.; Deal, A.M.; Napier, M.E.; Zamboni, W.C.; Sharpless, N.E.; Perou, C.M.; DeSimone, J.M. Docetaxel-Loaded PLGA Nanoparticles Improve Efficacy in Taxane-Resistant Triple-Negative Breast Cancer. *Nano Lett.,* **2017**, *17*(1), 242-248.
[http://dx.doi.org/10.1021/acs.nanolett.6b03971] [PMID: 27966988]

[67]   Amendola, V.; Meneghetti, M. Laser ablation synthesis in solution and size manipulation of noble metal nanoparticles. *Phys. Chem. Chem. Phys.,* **2009**, *11*(20), 3805-3821.
[http://dx.doi.org/10.1039/b900654k] [PMID: 19440607]

[68]   Delmée, M.; Mertz, G.; Bardon, J.; Marguier, A.; Ploux, L.; Roucoules, V.; Ruch, D. Laser ablation of silver in liquid organic monomer: influence of experimental parameters on the synthesized silver nanoparticles/graphite colloids. *J. Phys. Chem. B,* **2017**, *121*(27), 6646-6654.
[http://dx.doi.org/10.1021/acs.jpcb.7b05409] [PMID: 28628747]

[69]   Fong, Y.Y.; Gascooke, J.R.; Visser, B.R.; Harris, H.H.; Cowie, B.C.C.; Thomsen, L.; Metha, G.F.; Buntine, M.A. Influence of cationic surfactants on the formation and surface oxidation states of gold nanoparticles produced *via* laser ablation. *Langmuir,* **2013**, *29*(40), 12452-12462.
[http://dx.doi.org/10.1021/la402234k] [PMID: 24015926]

[70]   Saitow, K.; Okamoto, Y.; Yano, Y.F. Fractal of gold nanoparticles controlled by ambient dielectricity: synthesis by laser ablation as a function of permittivity. *J. Phys. Chem. C,* **2012**, *116*(32), 17252-17258.
[http://dx.doi.org/10.1021/jp304109h]

[71]   Zhang, D.; Gökce, B.; Barcikowski, S. Laser synthesis and processing of colloids: fundamentals and applications. *Chem. Rev.,* **2017**, *117*(5), 3990-4103.
[http://dx.doi.org/10.1021/acs.chemrev.6b00468] [PMID: 28191931]

[72]   Al-Kinani, M.A.; Haider, A.J.; Al-Musawi, S. Design and Synthesis of Nanoencapsulation with a New Formulation of Fe@Au-CS-CU-FA NPs by Pulsed Laser Ablation in Liquid (PLAL) Method in Breast Cancer Therapy: *In Vitro* and *In Vivo. Plasmonics,* **2021**, *16*(4), 1107-1117.
[http://dx.doi.org/10.1007/s11468-021-01371-3]

[73]   Kumarage, S.; Madhusha, C.; Munaweera, I.; Kottegoda, N. Application of Metal/Metal Oxide Doped Electrospun Nanofiber Membranes in Sustainable Catalysis. *Vidyodaya Journal of Science,* **2022**, *25*(01)

[74]   Kumarage, S.; Munaweera, I.; Kottegoda, N. A comprehensive review on electrospun nanohybrid membranes for wastewater treatment. *Beilstein J. Nanotechnol.,* **2022**, *13*(1), 137-159.
[http://dx.doi.org/10.3762/bjnano.13.10] [PMID: 35186649]

[75]   Xiao, Y.; Xie, F.; Luo, H.; Tang, R.; Hou, J.; Electrospinning, S.A. Electrospinning SA@PVDF-HFP Core–Shell Nanofibers Based on a Visual Light Transmission Response to Alcohol for Intelligent Packaging. *ACS Appl. Mater. Interfaces,* **2022**, *14*(6), 8437-8447.
[http://dx.doi.org/10.1021/acsami.1c23055] [PMID: 35129949]

[76]   Ghaedi Dehaghi, N.; Kokabi, M. Polyvinylidene fluoride/ barium titanate nanocomposite aligned hollow electrospun fibers as an actuator. *Mater. Res. Bull.,* **2023**, *158*, 112052.
[http://dx.doi.org/10.1016/j.materresbull.2022.112052]

[77]   Mondésert, H.; Bossard, F.; Favier, D. Anisotropic electrospun honeycomb polycaprolactone

scaffolds: Elaboration, morphological and mechanical properties. *J. Mech. Behav. Biomed. Mater.,* **2021**, *113*, 104124.
[http://dx.doi.org/10.1016/j.jmbbm.2020.104124] [PMID: 33091720]

[78]   Tang, Y.; Tian, J.; Li, L.; Huang, L.; Shen, Q.; Guo, S.; Jiang, Y. Biomimetic biphasic electrospun scaffold for anterior cruciate ligament tissue engineering. *Tissue Eng. Regen. Med.,* **2021**, *18*(5), 819-830.
[http://dx.doi.org/10.1007/s13770-021-00376-7] [PMID: 34355341]

[79]   Farkas, N.I.; Marincaş, L.; Barabás, R.; Bizo, L.; Ilea, A.; Turdean, G.L.; Toşa, M.; Cadar, O.; Barbu-Tudoran, L. Preparation and Characterization of Doxycycline-Loaded Electrospun PLA/HAP Nanofibers as a Drug Delivery System. *Materials,* **2022**, *15*(6), 2105.
[http://dx.doi.org/10.3390/ma15062105] [PMID: 35329557]

[80]   Bonadies, I.; Di Cristo, F.; Valentino, A.; Peluso, G.; Calarco, A.; Di Salle, A. pH-Responsive Resveratrol-Loaded Electrospun Membranes for the Prevention of Implant-Associated Infections. *Nanomaterials,* **2020**, *10*(6), 1175.
[http://dx.doi.org/10.3390/nano10061175] [PMID: 32560209]

[81]   Titus, D.; James Jebaseelan Samuel, E.; Roopan, S.M. Nanoparticle characterization techniques.*Green Synthesis, Characterization and Applications of Nanoparticles*; Shukla, A.K.; Iravani, S., Eds.; Elsevier, **2019**, pp. 303-319.
[http://dx.doi.org/10.1016/B978-0-08-102579-6.00012-5]

[82]   McCarron, E.; Chambers, G. A review of suitable analytical technology for physio-chemical characterisation of nanomaterials in the customs laboratory. *Talanta Open,* **2021**, *4*, 100069.
[http://dx.doi.org/10.1016/j.talo.2021.100069]

[83]   Kaliva, M.; Vamvakaki, M. Nanomaterials characterization. *Polymer Science and Nanotechnology*; Narain, R., Ed.; Elsevier, **2020**, pp. 401-433.
[http://dx.doi.org/10.1016/B978-0-12-816806-6.00017-0]

[84]   Singh, V.; Yadav, P.; Mishra, V. Recent advances on classification, properties, synthesis, and characterization of nanomaterials. *Green synthesis of nanomaterials for bioenergy applications*; Srivastava, N.; Srivastava, M.; Mishra, P.K.; Gupta, V.K., Eds.; Wiley Online Library, **2020**, pp. 83-97.
[http://dx.doi.org/10.1002/9781119576785.ch3]

[85]   Alfredo Reyes Villegas, V.; Isaías De León Ramírez, J.; Hernandez Guevara, E.; Perez Sicairos, S.; Angelica Hurtado Ayala, L.; Landeros Sanchez, B. Synthesis and characterization of magnetite nanoparticles for photocatalysis of nitrobenzene. *J. Saudi Chem. Soc.,* **2020**, *24*(2), 223-235.
[http://dx.doi.org/10.1016/j.jscs.2019.12.004]

[86]   Jain, K.K. The role of nanobiotechnology in drug discovery. *Drug Discov. Today,* **2005**, *10*(21), 1435-1442.
[http://dx.doi.org/10.1016/S1359-6446(05)03573-7] [PMID: 16243263]

[87]   Binnig, G.; Quate, C.F.; Gerber, C. Atomic force microscope. *Phys. Rev. Lett.,* **1986**, *56*(9), 930-933.
[http://dx.doi.org/10.1103/PhysRevLett.56.930] [PMID: 10033323]

[88]   Kodera, N.; Yamamoto, D.; Ishikawa, R.; Ando, T. Video imaging of walking myosin V by high-speed atomic force microscopy. *Nature,* **2010**, *468*(7320), 72-76.
[http://dx.doi.org/10.1038/nature09450] [PMID: 20935627]

[89]   Krieg, M.; Fläschner, G.; Alsteens, D.; Gaub, B.M.; Roos, W.H.; Wuite, G.J.L.; Gaub, H.E.; Gerber, C.; Dufrêne, Y.F.; Müller, D.J. Atomic force microscopy-based mechanobiology. *Nature Reviews Physics,* **2018**, *1*(1), 41-57.
[http://dx.doi.org/10.1038/s42254-018-0001-7]

[90]   Yang, F.; Riedel, R.; del Pino, P.; Pelaz, B.; Said, A.H.; Soliman, M.; Pinnapireddy, S.R.; Feliu, N.; Parak, W.J.; Bakowsky, U.; Hampp, N. Real-time, label-free monitoring of cell viability based on cell adhesion measurements with an atomic force microscope. *J. Nanobiotechnology,* **2017**, *15*(1), 23.

[http://dx.doi.org/10.1186/s12951-017-0256-7] [PMID: 28330480]

[91]   Deng, X.; Xiong, F.; Li, X.; Xiang, B.; Li, Z.; Wu, X.; Guo, C.; Li, X.; Li, Y.; Li, G.; Xiong, W.;
        Zeng, Z. Application of atomic force microscopy in cancer research. *J. Nanobiotechnology,* **2018**,
        16(1), 102.
        [http://dx.doi.org/10.1186/s12951-018-0428-0] [PMID: 30538002]

[92]   He, Y.; Jing, Y.; Wei, F.; Tang, Y.; Yang, L.; Luo, J.; Yang, P.; Ni, Q.; Pang, J.; Liao, Q.; Xiong, F.;
        Guo, C.; Xiang, B.; Li, X.; Zhou, M.; Li, Y.; Xiong, W.; Zeng, Z.; Li, G. Long non-coding RNA
        PVT1 predicts poor prognosis and induces radioresistance by regulating DNA repair and cell apoptosis
        in nasopharyngeal carcinoma. *Cell Death Dis.,* **2018**, *9*(2), 235.
        [http://dx.doi.org/10.1038/s41419-018-0265-y] [PMID: 29445147]

[93]   Tang, L.; Wei, F.; Wu, Y.; He, Y.; Shi, L.; Xiong, F.; Gong, Z.; Guo, C.; Li, X.; Deng, H.; Cao, K.;
        Zhou, M.; Xiang, B.; Li, X.; Li, Y.; Li, G.; Xiong, W.; Zeng, Z. Role of metabolism in cancer cell
        radioresistance and radiosensitization methods. *J. Exp. Clin. Cancer Res.,* **2018**, *37*(1), 87.
        [http://dx.doi.org/10.1186/s13046-018-0758-7] [PMID: 29688867]

[94]   Tang, Y.; He, Y.; Zhang, P.; Wang, J.; Fan, C.; Yang, L.; Xiong, F.; Zhang, S.; Gong, Z.; Nie, S.;
        Liao, Q.; Li, X.; Li, X.; Li, Y.; Li, G.; Zeng, Z.; Xiong, W.; Guo, C. LncRNAs regulate the
        cytoskeleton and related Rho/ROCK signaling in cancer metastasis. *Mol. Cancer,* **2018**, *17*(1), 77.
        [http://dx.doi.org/10.1186/s12943-018-0825-x] [PMID: 29618386]

[95]   Lopez, J.I.; Kang, I.; You, W.K.; McDonald, D.M.; Weaver, V.M. *In situ* force mapping of mammary
        gland transformation. *Integr. Biol.,* **2011**, *3*(9), 910-921.
        [http://dx.doi.org/10.1039/c1ib00043h] [PMID: 21842067]

[96]   Staunton, J.R.; Doss, B.L.; Lindsay, S.; Ros, R. Correlating confocal microscopy and atomic force
        indentation reveals metastatic cancer cells stiffen during invasion into collagen I matrices. *Sci. Rep.,*
        2016, *6*(1), 19686.
        [http://dx.doi.org/10.1038/srep19686] [PMID: 26813872]

[97]   Plodinec, M.; Loparic, M.; Monnier, C.A.; Obermann, E.C.; Zanetti-Dallenbach, R.; Oertle, P.;
        Hyotyla, J.T.; Aebi, U.; Bentires-Alj, M.; Lim, R.Y.H.; Schoenenberger, C.A. The nanomechanical
        signature of breast cancer. *Nat. Nanotechnol.,* **2012**, *7*(11), 757-765.
        [http://dx.doi.org/10.1038/nnano.2012.167] [PMID: 23085644]

[98]   Song, S.; Ma, X.; Zhou, Y.; Xu, M.; Shuang, S.; Dong, C. Studies on the interaction between vanillin
        and β-Amyloid protein *via* fluorescence spectroscopy and atomic force microscopy. *Chem. Res. Chin.
        Univ.,* **2016**, *32*(2), 172-177.
        [http://dx.doi.org/10.1007/s40242-016-5347-8]

[99]   Pereira, S.A.P.; Dyson, P.J.; Saraiva, M.L.M.F.S. Miniaturized technologies for high-throughput drug
        screening enzymatic assays and diagnostics – A review. *Trends Analyt. Chem.,* **2020**, *126*, 115862.
        [http://dx.doi.org/10.1016/j.trac.2020.115862]

[100]   Sitharaman, B. *Nanobiomaterials handbook*; CRC Press, **2016**.
        [http://dx.doi.org/10.1201/b10970]

[101]   Chen, H.; Li, J. *Nanobiomaterials handbook*; n Microarrays: Volume 1: Synthesis Methods, Rampal,
        J. B., Ed. Humana Press: Totowa, NJ, 2007; pp 411-436.

[102]   Pereira, S.A.P.; Dyson, P.J.; Saraiva, M.L.M.F.S. Miniaturized technologies for high-throughput drug
        screening enzymatic assays and diagnostics – A review. *Trends Analyt. Chem.,* **2020**, *126*, 115862.
        [http://dx.doi.org/10.1016/j.trac.2020.115862]

[103]   Kumar, C.S.S.R. *Semiconductor nanomaterials*; John Wiley & Sons, **2010**, 6, .

[104]   Estes, R. Semiconductor packaging technologies advance DNA analysis systems. *IVD Technology,*
        2005, *4*, 1-5.

[105]   Kazoe, Y.; Xu, Y. Advances in Nanofluidics. *Micromachines,* **2021**, *12*(4), 427.
        [http://dx.doi.org/10.3390/mi12040427] [PMID: 33919709]

[106] Wu, Z.; Lin, L. Nanofluidics for single-cell analysis. *Chin. Chem. Lett.,* **2022**, *33*(4), 1752-1756.
[http://dx.doi.org/10.1016/j.cclet.2021.08.100]

[107] Wang, Y.C.; Stevens, A.L.; Han, J. Million-fold preconcentration of proteins and peptides by nanofluidic filter. *Anal. Chem.,* **2005**, *77*(14), 4293-4299.
[http://dx.doi.org/10.1021/ac050321z] [PMID: 16013838]

[108] Fu, J.; Schoch, R.B.; Stevens, A.L.; Tannenbaum, S.R.; Han, J. A patterned anisotropic nanofluidic sieving structure for continuous-flow separation of DNA and proteins. *Nat. Nanotechnol.,* **2007**, *2*(2), 121-128.
[http://dx.doi.org/10.1038/nnano.2006.206] [PMID: 18654231]

[109] Ko, S.H.; Chandra, D.; Ouyang, W.; Kwon, T.; Karande, P.; Han, J. Nanofluidic device for continuous multiparameter quality assurance of biologics. *Nat. Nanotechnol.,* **2017**, *12*(8), 804-812.
[http://dx.doi.org/10.1038/nnano.2017.74] [PMID: 28530715]

[110] Kwon, T.; Ko, S.H.; Hamel, J.F.P.; Han, J. Continuous Online Protein Quality Monitoring during Perfusion Culture Production Using an Integrated Micro/Nanofluidic System. *Anal. Chem.,* **2020**, *92*(7), 5267-5275.
[http://dx.doi.org/10.1021/acs.analchem.9b05835] [PMID: 32167286]

[111] Rajasundari, K.; Ilamurugu, K. Nanotechnology and its applications in medical diagnosis. *J Basic Appl Chem,* **2011**, *1*(2), 26-32.

[112] Di Trani, N.; Silvestri, A.; Wang, Y.; Demarchi, D.; Liu, X.; Grattoni, A. Silicon Nanofluidic Membrane for Electrostatic Control of Drugs and Analytes Elution. *Pharmaceutics,* **2020**, *12*(7), 679.
[http://dx.doi.org/10.3390/pharmaceutics12070679] [PMID: 32707665]

[113] Mujawar, M.A.; Gohel, H.; Bhardwaj, S.K.; Srinivasan, S.; Hickman, N.; Kaushik, A. Nano-enabled biosensing systems for intelligent healthcare: towards COVID-19 management. *Mater. Today Chem.,* **2020**, *17*, 100306.
[http://dx.doi.org/10.1016/j.mtchem.2020.100306] [PMID: 32835155]

[114] Beishon, M. Exploiting a nano-sized breach in cancer's defences. *Cancer World,* **2013**, *55*, 14-21.

[115] Jackson, T.C.; Patani, B.O.; Ekpa, D.E. Nanotechnology in diagnosis: a review. *Adv. Nanopart.,* **2017**, *6*(3), 93-102.
[http://dx.doi.org/10.4236/anp.2017.63008]

[116] Joshi, P.S.; Chougule, M.; Hongal, B.; Agnihotri, N. Nanobiopsy: An emerging innovative tool for interrogating living cells. *European Journal of Molecular Biology and Biochemistry and Biophysics Reports,* **2015**, *2*(4), 160-162.

[117] Actis, P.; Maalouf, M.M.; Kim, H.J.; Lohith, A.; Vilozny, B.; Seger, R.A.; Pourmand, N. Compartmental genomics in living cells revealed by single-cell nanobiopsy. *ACS Nano,* **2014**, *8*(1), 546-553.
[http://dx.doi.org/10.1021/nn405097u] [PMID: 24279711]

[118] Tian, B.; Cohen-Karni, T.; Qing, Q.; Duan, X.; Xie, P.; Lieber, C.M. Three-dimensional, flexible nanoscale field-effect transistors as localized bioprobes. *Science,* **2010**, *329*(5993), 830-834.
[http://dx.doi.org/10.1126/science.1192033] [PMID: 20705858]

[119] Chen, C.C.; Zhou, Y.; Baker, L.A. Scanning ion conductance microscopy. *Annu. Rev. Anal. Chem. (Palo Alto, Calif.),* **2012**, *5*(1), 207-228.
[http://dx.doi.org/10.1146/annurev-anchem-062011-143203] [PMID: 22524219]

[120] Rheinlaender, J.; Geisse, N.A.; Proksch, R.; Schäffer, T.E. Comparison of scanning ion conductance microscopy with atomic force microscopy for cell imaging. *Langmuir,* **2011**, *27*(2), 697-704.
[http://dx.doi.org/10.1021/la103275y] [PMID: 21158392]

[121] Novak, P.; Gorelik, J.; Vivekananda, U.; Shevchuk, A.I.; Ermolyuk, Y.S.; Bailey, R.J.; Bushby, A.J.; Moss, G.W.J.; Rusakov, D.A.; Klenerman, D.; Kullmann, D.M.; Volynski, K.E.; Korchev, Y.E.

Nanoscale-targeted patch-clamp recordings of functional presynaptic ion channels. *Neuron,* **2013**, *79*(6), 1067-1077.
[http://dx.doi.org/10.1016/j.neuron.2013.07.012] [PMID: 24050398]

[122] Jönsson, P.; McColl, J.; Clarke, R.W.; Ostanin, V.P.; Jönsson, B.; Klenerman, D. Hydrodynamic trapping of molecules in lipid bilayers. *Proc. Natl. Acad. Sci. USA,* **2012**, *109*(26), 10328-10333.
[http://dx.doi.org/10.1073/pnas.1202858109] [PMID: 22699491]

[123] Dale, S.E.C.; Unwin, P.R. Polarised liquid/liquid micro-interfaces move during charge transfer. *Electrochem. Commun.,* **2008**, *10*(5), 723-726.
[http://dx.doi.org/10.1016/j.elecom.2008.02.023]

[124] Clark, I.E.; Dodson, M.W.; Jiang, C.; Cao, J.H.; Huh, J.R.; Seol, J.H.; Yoo, S.J.; Hay, B.A.; Guo, M. Drosophila pink1 is required for mitochondrial function and interacts genetically with parkin. *Nature,* **2006**, *441*(7097), 1162-1166.
[http://dx.doi.org/10.1038/nature04779] [PMID: 16672981]

[125] Ståhlberg, A.; Thomsen, C.; Ruff, D.; Aman, P. Quantitative PCR analysis of DNA, RNAs, and proteins in the same single cell. *Clin. Chem.,* **2012**, *58*(12), 1682-1691.
[http://dx.doi.org/10.1373/clinchem.2012.191445] [PMID: 23014600]

[126] Boisseau, P.; Loubaton, B. Nanomedicine, nanotechnology in medicine. *C. R. Phys.,* **2011**, *12*(7), 620-636.
[http://dx.doi.org/10.1016/j.crhy.2011.06.001]

[127] Bulbul, G.; Chaves, G.; Olivier, J.; Ozel, R.; Pourmand, N. Nanopipettes as Monitoring Probes for the Single Living Cell: State of the Art and Future Directions in Molecular Biology. *Cells,* **2018**, *7*(6), 55.
[http://dx.doi.org/10.3390/cells7060055] [PMID: 29882813]

[128] Whitesides, G.M. The 'right' size in nanobiotechnology. *Nat. Biotechnol.,* **2003**, *21*(10), 1161-1165.
[http://dx.doi.org/10.1038/nbt872] [PMID: 14520400]

[129] Min, Y.; Caster, J.M.; Eblan, M.J.; Wang, A.Z. Clinical translation of nanomedicine. *Chem. Rev.,* **2015**, *115*(19), 11147-11190.
[http://dx.doi.org/10.1021/acs.chemrev.5b00116] [PMID: 26088284]

[130] Paciotti, G.F.; Myer, L.; Weinreich, D.; Goia, D.; Pavel, N.; McLaughlin, R.E.; Tamarkin, L. Colloidal gold: a novel nanoparticle vector for tumor directed drug delivery. *Drug Deliv.,* **2004**, *11*(3), 169-183.
[http://dx.doi.org/10.1080/10717540490433895] [PMID: 15204636]

[131] Hsu, H.Y.; Huang, Y.Y. RCA combined nanoparticle-based optical detection technique for protein microarray: a novel approach. *Biosens. Bioelectron.,* **2004**, *20*(1), 123-126.
[http://dx.doi.org/10.1016/j.bios.2003.10.015] [PMID: 15142584]

[132] Buzea, C.; Pacheco, I.I.; Robbie, K. Nanomaterials and nanoparticles: Sources and toxicity. *Biointerphases,* **2007**, *2*(4), MR17-MR71.
[http://dx.doi.org/10.1116/1.2815690] [PMID: 20419892]

[133] Murty, B.S.; Shankar, P.; Raj, B.; Rath, B.B.; Murday, J. Concerns and Challenges of Nanotechnology. *Textbook of nanoscience and nanotechnology*; Raj, B., Ed.; Springer Science & Business Media, **2013**, pp. 214-223.
[http://dx.doi.org/10.1007/978-3-642-28030-6_7]

[134] Barlas, S. FDA strategies to prevent and respond to drug shortages: finding a better way to predict and prevent company closures. *P&T,* **2013**, *38*(5), 261-263.
[PMID: 23946619]

[135] Smith, J.A.; Costales, A.B.; Jaffari, M.; Urbauer, D.L.; Frumovitz, M.; Kutac, C.K.; Tran, H.; Coleman, R.L. *Is it equivalent?* Evaluation of the clinical activity of single agent Lipodox® compared to single agent Doxil® in ovarian cancer treatment. *J. Oncol. Pharm. Pract.,* **2016**, *22*(4), 599-604.
[http://dx.doi.org/10.1177/1078155215594415] [PMID: 26183293]

[136] Bhalla, N.; Pan, Y.; Yang, Z.; Payam, A.F. Opportunities and Challenges for Biosensors and

Nanoscale Analytical Tools for Pandemics: COVID-19. *ACS Nano,* **2020**, *14*(7), 7783-7807.
[http://dx.doi.org/10.1021/acsnano.0c04421] [PMID: 32551559]

[137] Liu, D.; Szili, E.J.; Ostrikov, K.K. Plasma medicine: Opportunities for nanotechnology in a digital age. *Plasma Process. Polym.,* **2020**, *17*(10), 2000097.
[http://dx.doi.org/10.1002/ppap.202000097] [PMID: 32837492]

[138] Lademann, J.; Patzelt, A.; Richter, H.; Lademann, O.; Baier, G.; Breucker, L.; Landfester, K. Nanocapsules for drug delivery through the skin barrier by tissue-tolerable plasma. *Laser Phys. Lett.,* **2013**, *10*(8), 083001.
[http://dx.doi.org/10.1088/1612-2011/10/8/083001]

[139] Sardella, E.; Palumbo, F.; Camporeale, G.; Favia, P. Non-equilibrium plasma processing for the preparation of antibacterial surfaces. *Materials,* **2016**, *9*(7), 515.
[http://dx.doi.org/10.3390/ma9070515] [PMID: 28773637]

[140] Rasouli, M.; Fallah, N.; Ostrikov, K.K. Lung cancer oncotherapy through novel modalities: gas plasma and nanoparticle technologies. *Lung Cancer-Modern Multidisciplinary Management*; Park, H.S., Ed.; IntechOpen: London, UK, **2020**, pp. 185-212.

CHAPTER 2

Nanotechnology in Drug Development

Abstract: Nanotechnology plays a key role in the development of new drugs, from start to end through target identification, lead identification, lead optimization, and synthesis of active pharmaceutical ingredients (API) as well. Nanodevices and nanoparticles have been extensively utilized in discovering new drug targets in illness sites or blood and for swift screening of interactions of molecular compounds with therapeutic targets for lead identification/optimization. In addition, API development employing nanoparticle catalysts to expedite the drug development process and investigating pure nanomaterials as drugs are two further areas on which the pharmaceutical industry is concentrating. This chapter will go into great detail on how nanotechnology is used in the drug development process, starting with the identification of drug targets, moving on to the identification and optimization of leads, and concluding with the synthesis of API.

Keywords: Active pharmaceutical ingredients, Drug target, Lead optimization, Nanotechnology, Nanoparticles, Nanosensors, Nanocatalysts, Nano-drugs.

1. INTRODUCTION

Due to the availability of several competing alternative medical markets, pharmaceutical companies are always challenged to create improved drug discovery technologies. For the efficient treatment of a wide range of disorders, the pharmaceutical industry needs to find and develop novel medications. Nanotechnology has become an area of enormous relevance to pharmaceutical corporations and their drug development programs.

Nanotechnology plays a key role in the development of new drugs, from start to end through target identification, lead identification, lead optimization, and synthesis of active pharmaceutical ingredients (API) as well. Nanotechnology is focused on developing better medication formulations and diagnostic techniques for more efficient and effective therapy in the realm of drug research and development. The utilization of nanodevices and nanoparticles has been widespread in the search for new drug targets because of their unique advantages. These advantages include enhanced biomarker detection sensitivity for early identification of diseases and diagnosis, the production of safer drug formulations, and the development of intriguing medical devices.

Laksiri Weerasinghe, Imalka Munaweera and Senuri Kumarage

Nanotechnology has been utilized for the swift screening of interactions of molecular compounds with therapeutic targets for lead identification/optimization as well. For instance, nanosensors to detect protein activity in drug-treated cells have been created. By effectively suppressing background noise from irrelevant sources and drastically enhancing signals for specific biomolecular binding, these nanosensors have higher sensitivity and consume less sample. Investigating real-time dynamic processes in living cells, such as protein interactions inside cells, intracellular signal transmission systems, and cell proliferation, is made possible by fluorescent nanoparticles' special optical feature. This expedites the process of optimizing lead compounds chemically by the use of in vivo biological consequences. Such nanosystems are appropriate for probing biological disorders at the cellular pore and receptor levels. Furthermore, there has been a noticeable decrease in the degree of harmful and negative consequences because of the small size of diagnostic materials. New dimensions of diagnostic tools that have been explored with the aid of these cutting-edge nanotechniques will be discussed in this chapter. In addition, API development employing nanoparticle catalysts to expedite the drug development process and investigating pure nanomaterials as drugs are two further areas on which the pharmaceutical industry is concentrating. To meet the increased demand of drug production, it is extremely promising to restructure and optimize the development process of APIs as early as feasible. In comparison to small-molecule medicines, which frequently have poor pharmacokinetic profiles and extensive secondary effects, nanotherapeutics have been proven to improve therapeutic effectiveness and decrease off-target toxicity by modifying drug biodistribution.

2. NANOTECHNOLOGY IN DRUG TARGET IDENTIFICATION

The first crucial steps in the process of discovering new drugs are the identification and validation of targets. Therefore, this first stage of the drug development process is of utmost importance to researchers. The goal of target identification is to find new targets, which are typically hormones, proteins, enzymes, genes, and DNA/RNA, whose modulation might slow or reverse disease development. In the past, scientists tended to focus on a small number of preferred genes that could be studied using low-throughput methods and were often discovered in the literature by academia. Due to the relatively modest number of protein classes that have proven susceptible to pharmaceutical development, most of the effective drug discovery initiatives have focused on these selected classes. With the use of modern technology, researchers can look for novel targets by attempting to link variations in gene (genomics) and protein (proteomics) expressions with human ailments [1]. To find new targets in illness sites or blood, nanotechnology is a potential technique in the biomedical industry.

Single-molecule fluorescence (SMF) nanosensors have been widely used to identify a variety of drug targets, including proteins, nucleic acids (including DNAs and microRNAs), enzymes, viruses, and living cells [2]. A tricyclic ligase chain reaction (LCR)-mediated QD-based Förster resonance energy transfer (FRET) nanosensor, for example, was created by Wang *et al.* to detect DNA methylation, an epigenetic mutation linked to a number of hereditary illnesses in humans [3]. Changes in microRNA expression are strongly associated with a number of human disorders, including cancer [4]. Zhang *et al.* developed an enzyme-free toehold-mediated strand displacement cascade-based QD-SMF nanosensor to detect microRNA [5]. Without any protein enzyme requirement, for target signal amplification, in this nanosensor, microRNA itself operates as the signal catalyzer. A SMF nanosensor based on AuNP and the same above mechanism was created by Liu *et al.* to detect microRNA [6]. Additionally, as one disease is typically associated with the deregulation of numerous microRNAs, simultaneous detection of multiple microRNAs is crucial for clinical diagnosis [7]. In this regard, Zhang *et al.* created a siRNA-directed self-assembled QDs nanosensor for the simultaneous single-molecule detection of many microRNAs [8]. TdT is a DNA-modifying enzyme that has the potential to serve as a biomarker for the leukaemia illness disease [9], since it can catalyze the random integration of nucleotides into the 30 -OH termini of DNA strands without the need of any DNA templates [10]. To measure TdT activity, Wang *et al.* created a QD-based SMF nanosensor [11].

SMF nanosensors have also been used in the detection of deregulated proteins and protein-modifying enzyme biomarkers associated with various diseases as drug targets. A single-molecule immunosorbent nanosensor based on upconversion nanoparticles (UCNPs) was created by Farka *et al.* to detect prostate-specific antigen (PSA), a crucial oncological biomarker for the detection of prostate cancer [12]. In addition, Wang *et al.* developed an SMF nanosensor based on a magnetic nanobead-assisted dual bar-code method to concurrently detect the tumour necrosis factor-α (TNF-α) and cytokines interferon-γ (IFN-γ) [13]. As the deregulation of OGT activity is intimately associated with several human disorders including malignancies and Alzheimer's disease, Zhang *et al.* developed a single QD-based fluorescent nanosensor to detect OGT activity [14]. For label-free quantitative detection of Acetylcholinesterase activity, which is directly related to Alzheimer's disease, a fluorescent conjugated polymer nanoparticle and manganese dioxide (MnO_2)-based SMF nanosensor have been created [15]. It has been discovered that inhibiting acetylcholinesterase activity is a successful method for treating the symptoms of Alzheimer's disease [16].

For the clinical diagnosis and treatment of illnesses caused by viruses, reliable viral detection is crucial [17]. Using fluorescent magnetic multifunctional nanospheres, Zhang *et al.* created an SMF nanosensor that can concurrently detect various viruses, including the avian influenza viruses; H9N2, H7N9, and H1N1 [18]. The simultaneous detection of all three viruses at the single-particle level was made possible by this nanosensor, which has the benefits of high specificity and robust anti-interference capacity.

To identify seven distinct proteins, including acid phosphatase, bovine serum albumin, lipase, cytochrome C, subtilisin A, alkaline phosphatase and β –galactosidase, You and colleagues devised an array technique employing highly fluorescent AuNPs. Each of the six distinct cationic AuNPs was coupled to the fluorescent polymer PPE-CO$_2$, a derivative of the poly p-phenylene. When a protein interacted with the AuNP-conjugate, reversal quenching brought back the fluorescence that had been lost when the polymer was conjugated to the AuNP. Even at nanomolar concentrations, fluorescence patterns were extremely distinctive for each unique protein, enabling a very flexible way to identify these specific proteins in biomedical applications [19].

Another technique that examines the protein corona (PC), a biological covering created when proteins interact with nanoparticles exposed to biological fluids, is available. Finding the proteins that make up the PC may reveal vital details about the medical conditions present in the particular individuals to whom NPs are administered. For instance, identifying biomarkers in patient samples at the beginning of a disease might help choose appropriate therapies. Hepatoma derived growth factor (HDGF) was discovered as a biomarker for ovarian cancer in one such study by Arvizo *et al.*, who investigated the PC around positively charged gold NPs [20]. The proteins PPA1 and SMNDC1 have also been found by Giri *et al.* as possible therapeutic targets for ovarian cancer after they examined the PC of 20 nm self-therapeutic gold NPs [21]. Furthermore, Schrittwieser *et al.* reported a biosensing device based on cobalt nanorods to identify sHER2, the breast cancer biomarker, in human serum and saliva [22].

A gold nanotechnology sensing technique was disclosed by Hajipour *et al.* to identify Alzheimer's disease and multiple sclerosis in patient plasma. Following the incubation of A uNPs coated with spherical citrate, p olyethylene glycol, cysteine, and cysteamine, with 10% and 100% patient serum, the protein corona responses were assessed. The assessing was carried out using hierarchical cluster analysis (HCA), UV-visible spectra, colorimetric differential profile (CDP) and principal component analysis (PCA).

Thus, nanotechnology and nanoparticles constitute a significant resource for interrogating biological systems in order to identify novel molecular actors that might serve as diagnostic biomarkers and/or therapeutic intervention targets.

3. NANOTECHNOLOGY IN LEAD IDENTIFICATION AND LEAD OPTIMIZATION

A lead compound is a synthetic or natural substance with biological activity against a pharmacological target. The identification and optimization of leads is a critical phase in the drug development process. Lead optimization involves chemical refinement of a viable drug target to enhance biological activity, drug-like qualities and reduce toxicity. To improve activity, selectivity, and minimize negative effects, this method improves interactions with active sites.

Current applications of biosensors include target validation, assay development, lead optimization, and absorption, distribution, metabolism, excretion, and toxicity (ADMET). The optimization of limited-scope drug libraries against specific targets is one of the main applications of the current biosensor technology. They circumvent many of the issues that emerge with cell-based assays. They are especially helpful in studying receptors since they avoid the need to take the receptor out of the cell's lipid membrane, which is often essential with other test techniques.

To swiftly screen anticancer drugs, Zheng *et al.*developed an ultrasensitive dynamic light scattering (DLS) based biosensor that employs gold nanoparticles as plasmon-enhanced sensing probes. The nanobiosensor detects protein activity in drug-treated cells by using DNA-conjugated dumbbell-shaped gold nanoprobes. By measuring the hydrodynamic size of the nanoprobes using DLS, they have confirmed the effectiveness of their nanosensor for screening for substances known to activate mutant p53, a tumour suppressor protein, for DNA binding in complicated biological contexts. The binding of p53 had resulted in an increase in the hydrodynamic size of the nano probes. This special nanoplasmonic biosensor improves sensitivity and uses less sample and reduced the consumption of the probe because it efficiently suppresses background noise from unrelated entities while simultaneously dramatically boosting the DLS signal for particular biomolecular binding. Additionally, a test was designed to analyze the relative DNA binding strengths of p53 using the same sensing probes that enable a concurrent evaluation of responsive p53 pathways downstream or cell destiny. Most importantly, their nanosensor offered on-target confirmation during phenotypic screenings by enabling direct probing of endogenous protein activity after drug treatment in live cells [24]. You *et al.* have created a DNA probe that may be utilized to research the dynamics of interactions between diverse membrane components [25]. Using flow cytometry and fluorescence microscopy, they have effectively observed the swift encounter events of membrane lipid domains.

Because of developments in microscopic imaging platform technology, optical biosensor design, and image interpretation tools, live cell imaging applications in drug discovery have expanded. These methods can shorten preclinical lead optimization cycles and enhance treatment and candidate translation from *in vitro* to *in vivo*. *In vitro* and *In vivo* research on real-time image-based drug response can shorten drug development timeframes, save costs, reveal new insights on adaptive response, and improve clinical predictability. Rapid image-based medication response evaluations in real animals enable for more exact scheduling, dosing, and acceleration of preclinical response evaluations. This speeds up the chemical optimization of lead compounds based on *in vivo* biological outcomes [26].

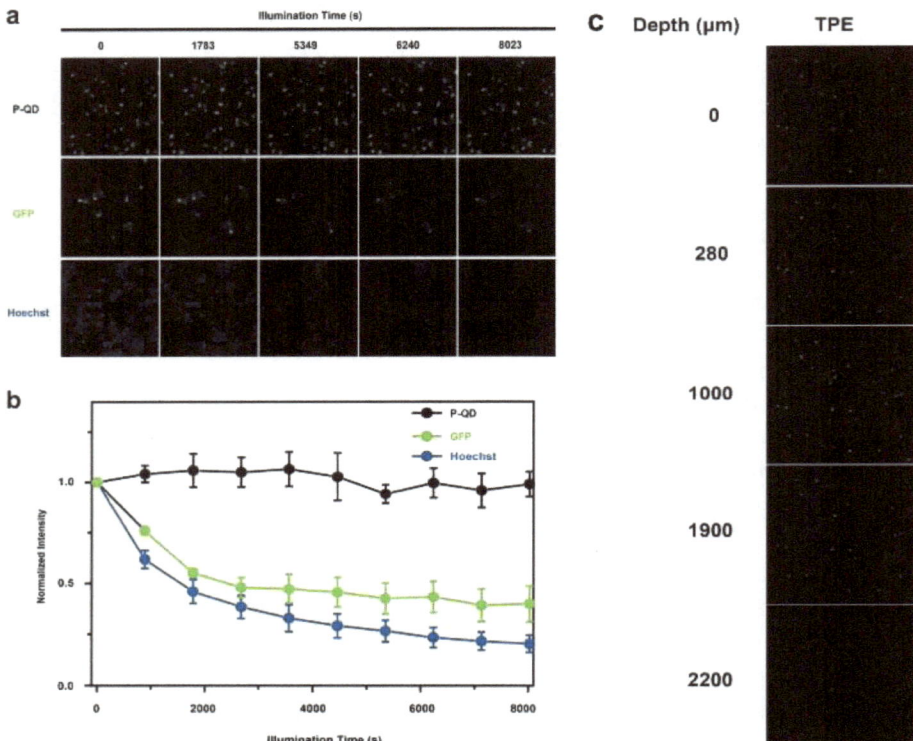

Fig. (1). (a) Typical Two Photon (TP) images of Polymer encapsulated -QD (P-QD)-treated HepG2 after different time intervals 800 nm femtosecond laser illumination. For comparison, the TP images of conventional dyes Hoechst 33342 and Green Fluorescent Protein (GFP) under the same conditions are shown. (b) The intensity of P-QD as a function of illumination time. For comparison, the fluorescence decay curves of Hoechst 33342 and Green Fluorescent Protein (GFP) under the same conditions are shown. (c) Imaging depth of P-QD in tissue phantom under 800 nm femtosecond laser excitation. Adapted from [40] Copyright (2015) Yanyan Fan *et al.* published by Springer Nature distributed under the terms of the Creative Commons Attribution 4.0 International http://creativecommons.org/licenses/by/4.0/.

Nanotechnology advancements have produced light-emitting nanoparticles like quantum dots, which have higher spectrum qualities and more versatility as functional reporters [27]. Tiny nanocrystals termed as quantum dots (QDs) possess greater brightness and photostability than fluorescent proteins or dyes, due to their high extinction coefficients and quantum yields. The near infrared fluorescence (NIRF) window, which allows for the best tissue penetration, may be designed using quantum dots to create nanoparticles with broad excitation but limited emission features. When compared to traditional fluorescent proteins and organic dyes, the ability of deep tissue imaging and long-term successive imaging in living samples may be attributed to the enhanced brightness and high sensitivity due to the customizable NIRF emission wavelengths (Fig. **1**) [28]. Novel fluorescent nanomaterials, such as bioinspired metal nanoclusters [29 - 31], carbon dots [32 - 36], aggregation-induced emission dyes [37, 38], and fluorescent conjugated polymers, can also be employed in place of semiconductor quantum dots to observe the interactions between biomolecules [39].

Through fluorescence anisotropy or fluorescence resonance energy transfer (FRET), it is simple to examine how fluorescent chemical molecules are oriented in relation to DNA base pairs. For instance, quantum dot (QD)-based FRET sensor developed by Zhao *et al.* demonstrated promising potential for detecting interactions between molecules and DNA as well as in biochemical detections and was capable of determining the interaction of common platinum drugs (cisplatin, oxaliplatin, and carboplatin) with DNAs [41].

4. NANOMATERIALS IN ACTIVE PHARMACEUTICAL INGREDIENT (API) DEVELOPMENT

4.1. Nanomaterials in the Synthesis of API

The need for the expeditious creation of pharmaceuticals has substantially risen as a result of the advent of new diseases, the formation of drug resistance, and our improved understanding of health conditions, enabling the treatment of previously incurable diseases. As the need for more drugs grows, the pharmaceutical industry is striving to reduce drug development time and the time to market. The initial step of drug designing is the identification and synthesis of the desirable active pharmaceutical ingredients (APIs), which are the biologically active component of the drug product (tablets, cream, capsule *etc.*) To meet the increased demand of drug production. It is extremely promising to restructure, and optimize the development process of APIs as early as feasible.

Heterocyclic compounds have long been a key component in the synthesis of APIs [42] as antitumour, antidiabetic, antimicrobial, antibacterial, antibiotic, antiviral, antifungal, anti-inflammatory, anti-HIV, antimalarial and antidepressant agents in drug molecules [43 - 46].The conventional synthesis method of the APIs includes complex synthetic pathways which is time consuming, expensive, has low reaction efficiency, with non-recyclable catalysts, and require toxic organic solvents. Hence there is an urgent need to create low-cost and simple alternative synthetic routes for the efficient large-scale synthesis of these potential heterocyclic compounds. In current synthetic organic chemistry, multicomponent reactions (MCRs) have evolved as an efficient and potent technique. By lowering the number of synthetic stages, energy consumption, and waste creation, MCRs help to meet the requirements of an ecologically sustainable process. As a result, scientists have turned this potent technology into one of the most efficient and cost-effective techniques for sequential and parallel synthesis of heterocyclic APIs [47].

The use of heterogeneous catalysts in boosting the efficiency of a wide variety of organic syntheses is one of the most appealing synthetic techniques favoured by organic chemists. Because of the necessity and desire for more environmentally friendly manufacturing techniques, heterogeneous catalysis is being applied in the fine chemicals sector. The availability of catalytic materials and new tools for generating and analysing particular active areas on catalyst surfaces are assisting this trend [48, 49]. One of the major applications of the nanomaterials in the synthesis of drugs is their catalytic ability. Researchers are now putting out significant effort to include nanomaterials into catalysts as a rewarding and promising technique in the development of nano- platforms. At nanoscale level, many properties such as electrical, magnetic and optical behaviour change significantly when compared to the bulk material [50]. This change in the behaviour at nanoscale is mainly conducive to the small scale, high surface area/volume ratio and the increased number of surface atoms and results in efficient catalytic properties of the nanomaterials. Essentially, as particles get smaller (nanoscale) in size, the proportion of surface atoms increases and this has a profound effect on the density of inconsistent interfaces or other lattice defects such as dislocations or vacancies resulting in physical instability [51]. As a result, these surface atoms have high surface energy and are extremely active making them susceptible to a variety of chemical reactions [52, 53]. Moreover, when compared to traditional chemicals, molecules generated in the presence of nanocatalysts are ideal in their morphology, chemistry and activity against drug targets [42]. Hence the synthesis of drugs employing nano-catalysts yields a sustainable and inexpensive route of production with benefits of brief reaction time, maximum throughput, facile catalyst recovery and a solvent-free milieu [54].

A huge number of physiologically active chemicals have the pyridine ring system as a structural component. The pyridine ring is found in all three forms of vitamin

B_3, including nicotinamide, niacin, and nicotinamide riboside, indicating the relevance of this heterocyclic molecule. Derivatives of pyridine moiety have long been known for their pharmacological properties such as anticancer, anti-bacterial, IKK-b inhibitors, potassium channel opening, potent inhibitor of HIV-1 integrase and antiprion [55, 56]. Omeprazol which is used to treat gastro esophageal reflux diseases and other diseases related to excessive stomach acid since 1998, Netupitant; an antiemetic drug that has been used since 2014 and Ciprofloxacin, Tetracycline, Nystatin, Amoxicillin, Ampicillin, and Gentamicin; which are used as antimicrobial drugs, are the most common pyridine-based derivatives (Fig. **2**) currently available in the medicine market to combat human ailments. In addition Abemaciclib (2015), Ivosidenib (2019), Apalutamide (2018) and Lorlatinib (2018) are FDA approved anticancer drugs with pyridine ring [56]. 2-amino-3,5-dicyano-6-sulfanyl pyridines are pyridine derivatives with a wide range of biological features, including therapy of Hepatitis B Foundation infections, asthma, hypoxia/ischemia, Parkinson's disease, renal illness, epilepsy and cancer [57 - 59].

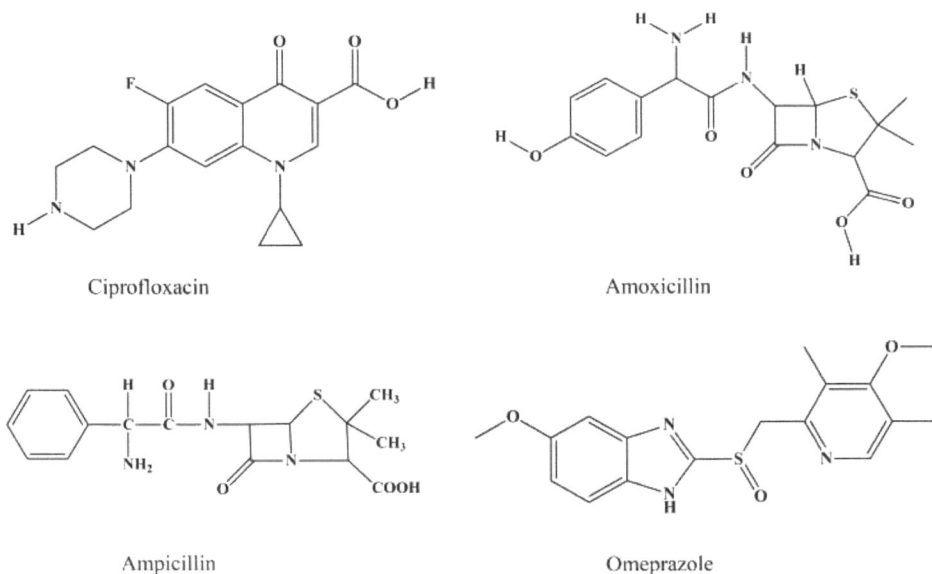

Ciprofloxacin

Amoxicillin

Ampicillin

Omeprazole

Fig. (2). Pyridine moiety-containing commercial drugs.

Copper iodide nanoparticles have been employed as the catalyst for the development of a simple, mild, and environmentally acceptable technique for producing high yield of 2-amino-3,5-dicyano-6-aryl(alkyl) thiopyridines, under reflux conditions [60]. Multicomponent reaction of thiols, aldehydes and malononitrile in water/ethanol medium has been carried out in this study with

10%mole of nanocatalysts resulting in 90% maximum yield. (Fig. **3**). They have also employed SnO nanoparticles for the synthesis of the same compound under reflux condition in ethanol and yielded 92% of the product with 9 mole% [55]. Condensation reactions are frequently more active when strong solid acids or bases are used. With the fact that a metal oxide surface composed of an ordered array of acid-base centres [61 - 63], cationic metal centre being the Lewis acid and the anionic oxygen centre being the Lewis base, they have proposed that the surface features of SnO NPs, which contain Sn^{2+} as an acid and O^{2-} as a base, and similarly in CuO which contains Cu^{2+} as an acid and O^{2-} as a base, enable them to have a very efficient catalytic behaviour. Moreover, the decrease in the SnO particle size has shown an increase of the catalytic activity due to the increased surface area offering extra accessibility to the active sites for the substrate molecules. The recyclability studies have shown that the catalyst can be reused with a minimal loss of activity, five times. Due to the extreme stability of the SnO nanoparticles they have exhibited no change in morphology before and after the catalytic activity.

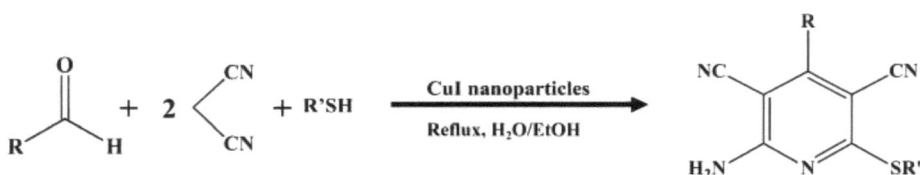

Fig. (3). The model reaction for the preparation of polyfunctionalized pyridines.

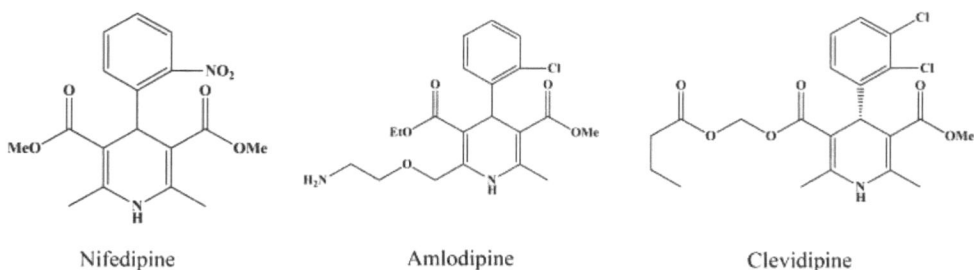

Nifedipine   Amlodipine   Clevidipine

Fig. (4). 1, 4-dihydropyridine moiety-containing commercial drugs.

Another commercially ubiquitous, reduced pyridine derivative is 1, 4-dihydropyridines, which is present in the efficacious drug molecules including amlodipine, nifedipine, diludine, felodipine, and oxodipine (Fig. **4**) which are used in the treatment of cardiovascular disorders [64, 65]. The prevalence of 1, 4-dihydropyridines is high in many medications, notably in ion channel blockers, due to the high transport tolerance in many active processes and the geometrical spacing. Nifedipine is one of the earliest dihydropyridine drugs in the market since the 1970s to treat hypertension and chest pain while Amlodipine is a more competent calcium channel blocker with less adverse side effects. In comparison to the previous substances, Clevidipine is a fast-acting calcium channel blocker that was approved by the FDA in 2008 and has a rapid therapeutic effect and clearance [66].

The conventional Hantzsch technique in which an aldehyde, β-ketoester and ammonia are cyclo condensed either in acetic acid or in refluxing ethanol is widely used to synthesise 1,4- dihydropyridines [67]. Neutral, mild, reusable and environmentally benign nanocatalysts are being used in the production of these dihydropyridine derivatives to overcome the issue of slow reaction efficiency suffered by the modified Hantzsch technique involving unsaturated and aliphatic aldehydes, emerged with time so far [68]. For instance nanocrystalline CuO has been employed as a catalyst in MCRs comprising aromatic amines, β-ketoesters and cinnamaldehyde under mild conditions for the synthesis of 1, 4-dihydropyridines and has yielded moderate to good yields [69]. The catalysts have been retrieved and reused four times with remarkably comparable activity.

In another study, a facile one-pot synthesis of two 1,4-dihydropyridine derivatives was described with high yields in short reaction times, employing 2 mol% copper iodide nanoparticles (CuI NPs) as a catalyst under reflux conditions at 80 ˚C with ethanol [70]. The two derivatives have been synthesised *via* four-component coupling reactions of aldehydes and ammonium acetate with either two equivalent of ethyl acetoacetate or one equivalent of ethyl acetoacetate and one equivalent of malononitrile. This approach featured various advantages, including the elimination of hazardous catalysts and elimination of tedious chromatographic methods for product purification. Moreover the reusability of the catalyst without any loss of activity and yield even after five cycles is outstanding.

A multicomponent synthesis of 1,4-dihydropyridines from ammonium acetate, ethyl acetoacetate and aldehydes in water is shown to be efficiently catalysed by the mixed metal oxide $ZnFe_2O_4$ nanopowder, a dual Lewis acid–base combination catalyst [71]. High yields, fast reaction times, a simple work-up method, and a low environmental impact are just a few of the benefits of this procedure. This approach takes advantage of the sheer fact that water, a green solvent, when combined with $ZnFe_2O_4$ nanoparticles as a catalyst, can be magnetically collected and reused for subsequent runs without any diminution in catalytic activity. Similarly, Cu doped ZnO nanocatalysts have exhibited a good catalysis with a yield of 90% under reflux conditions at 80 ˚C with water as a solvent]72]. The catalytic performance of $TiCl_2$/nano-g-Al_2O_3 nanoparticles in synthesising 1,4-

dihydropyridine derivatives has also been investigated as a simple, efficient green protocol, using a solvent-free multicomponent coupling reaction comprising aldehyde, 1,3-dicarbonyl compounds, and NH_4OAc, which generated the highest yield of 90% at 90 °C. Very recently, it has also been investigated that out of several Zirconia-based metal oxide catalysts in synthesising 1,4-dihydropyridine, CuO/ZrO_2, CeO_2/ZrO_2, and NiO/ZrO_2, NiO/ZrO_2 offered an exceptional yield of 98 percent in just 20 minutes at 25 °C in ethanol, whilst 2.5 percent CuO/ZrO_2 gave 73 percent yield in 60 minutes and 2.5 percent CeO_2/ZrO_2 gave 81 percent yield in 45 minutes [73]. The authors have attributed this efficient, economical, and pragmatic catalysis to the presence of a greater number of active NiO sites in the ZrO_2 blend, as well as the active material being uniformly dispersed throughout the support's surface, combining to selectively accelerate the reaction rate.

It was recently discovered that providing a stimulus such as ultrasound [74, 75] or light wave irradiation [76] to magnetic nanocatalysts might improve their catalytic performance in some situations. Ultrasonication prevents the demerit of agglomeration of the magnetic nanoparticles whilst small high-temperature bubbles created around the ultrasonic transducers, which heat the magnetic nanocatalysts' surfaces offer an extra local driving force for surface alteration and will synergistically accelerate the catalytic activity. This synergistic effect of the catalysts and the ultra-sonication has already been utilised in the synthesis of 1, 4-dihydropyridine APIs. The collaborative effect of ultrasound waves of frequency of 50 kHz, power density of 250 W L^{-1} and a pyrimidine-2,4-diami-e-functionalized Fe_3O_4/SiO_2 core/shell nanocatalyst achieve 89% conversion in just 10 minutes of ultra-sonication whilst the yield is 45% in the presence of the catalyst alone and less than 20% in the presence of ultra-sonication alone [77].

Multi-substituted Imidazoles and benzimidazoles are another extremely versatile pharmacological class. Both imidazole and benzimidazole rings have two nitrogen atoms that are amphoteric, meaning they have both acidic and basic properties. The hydrogen atom can be found on either of the two nitrogen atoms in these rings, which are comparable tautomeric forms. Furthermore, electron-rich nitrogen heterocycles were capable of not only accepting or donating protons, but also forming a variety of weak interactions. Because of the unique structural properties of imidazole and benzimidazole rings, which have the desired electron-rich characteristic, imidazole and benzimidazole derivatives may easily attach to a number of therapeutic targets, resulting in a wide range of pharmacological properties such as antifungal, antiparasitic, antiemetic, antihistaminic, antiulcer, antiviral, antibacterial, antihypertensive, anticancer, and other therapeutic agents with high therapeutic potency and market value [78 - 80]. Picoprazole, Lansoprazole, Losartan, Candesartan, Chlormidazole, Econazole and

Clotrimazole are some of the existing imidazole and benzimidazole derived drugs in the medicinal market (Fig. **5**).

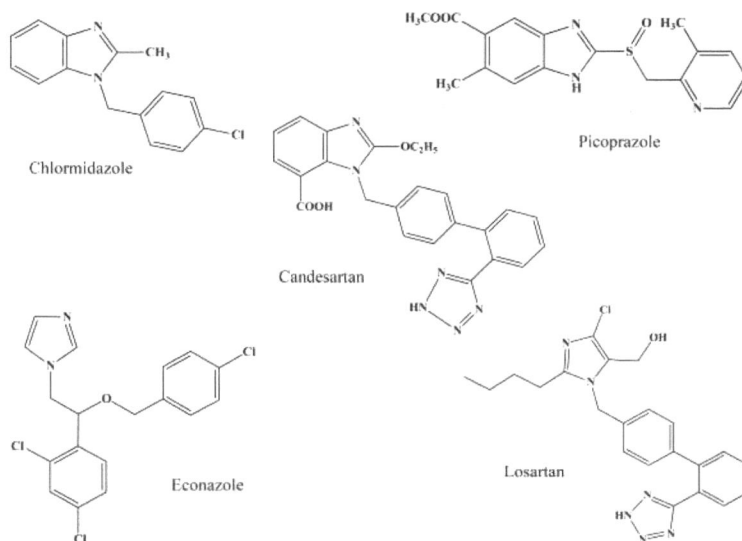

Fig. (5). Some imidazole and benzimidazole derived drugs.

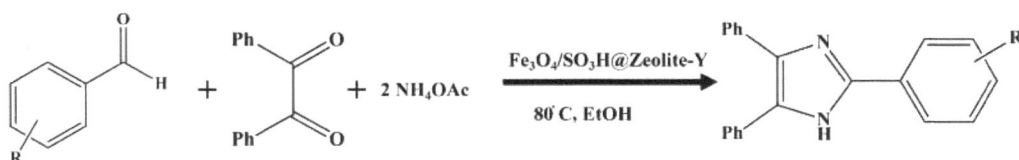

Fig. (6). Synthesis of 2,4,5-trisubstituted imidazoles catalyzed by Fe_3O_4/SO_3H@zeolite-Y.

Zeolosulforic acid supported Fe_3O_4 magnetic nanoparticles (Fe_3O_4/SO_3H@zeolite-Y) are used as a magnetic solid acid catalyst for synthesizing 2,4,5-trisubstituted imidazoles, offering excellent catalytic activities, high stability, ease of implementation, cost efficiency, better selectivity, facile preparation and reusability. (Fig. **6**) [81]. At optimized conditions, condensation of the 3 components; benzaldehyde (1 mmol), benzil (1 mmol) and ammonium acetate (2 mmol), a yield of 98% was achieved in just 45 minutes under reflux conditions with ethanol as the solvent with only 0.020 g of this efficient, economical, and pragmatic catalyst, whilst the catalyst-free condensation yielded only 50% even after 4 hours. An external permanent magnet was employed to easily recycle the nanocatalyst, which could be reused up to five times without a substantial loss of function.

Many organic solvents are noxious and volatile, especially chlorinated hydrocarbons, which are extensively utilized in large quantities for chemical processes and constitute a severe hazard to the environment. As a result, in the field of green synthesis, the design of solvent free catalytic reactions has acquired a great deal of interest recently. By employing a one-pot, three-component synthesis of benzils, aldehydes, and ammonium acetate at 80^0C in solvent-free conditions, a general and highly efficient method for making 2,4,5-triaryl modified imidazoles was developed using $NiO.5ZnO.5Fe_2O_4$ as the catalyst [82]. The catalyst retained the catalytic ability without a significant loss even after four runs of subsequent use.

Similarly Iron–diethylenetriamine Penta (methylene phosphonic acid) (Fe-DTPMP) organic–metal nanocatalysts has been employed in the synthesis of 2,4,5-Trisubstituted imidazoles with a 90% yield in 30 minutes with only 0.05 g of the catalyst under solvent free conditions [83]. A novel, green $NiFe_2O_4$/geopolymer nanocatalyst based on bentonite has been synthesized for the production of imidazole heterocycles [84]. They have employed the geopolymer based on bentonite as a substrate for the embedment of $NiFe_2O_4$ nanoparticles. The reaction yielded 80%-90% of 2,4,5-Trisubstituted imidazole derivatives in short reaction times in the presence of composite nanocatalysts and ultra-sonication. The synthesized nanocatalyst has a high recyclability, with no significant loss in catalytic activity after eight cycles.

Cobalt ferrite nanoparticles, fabricated with sulfonic acid, effectively synthesize biologically significant 2-substituted benzimidazole derivatives through green, facile synthesis using o-phenylenediamine and aliphatic, aromatic, and heterocyclic aldehydes [85]. Some of the distinguished characteristics of the current catalytic system is the extraordinary yield (up to 98%), simple work-up procedure, wide functional group tolerance, short reaction time (10-25 min), mild reaction conditions, and outstanding values of green chemistry metrics such as carbon efficiency (100%), lower E factor (0.126), high atom economy value (90.65 percent) and high RME value (88.83%). Facile retrieval of the catalyst from the reaction mixture using an external magnet, highly stable catalytic efficiency and reusability for at least seven serial runs has made this catalytic system more attractive.

4.2. Nanomaterials in API Formulation

Pure nanodrugs are a relatively new class of nanotherapeutics that consist primarily of active drug molecules in the form of nanoparticles along with a one or more excipients that are widely considered as safe [86]. In comparison to small-molecule medicines, which frequently have poor pharmacokinetic profiles and extensive secondary effects, nanotherapeutics have been proven to improve therapeutic effectiveness and decrease off-target toxicity by modifying drug biodistribution. Greater intracellular drug concentrations, higher therapeutic effectiveness, and reduced systemic toxicity result from enhanced absorption into target cells [86, 87]. In particular, for orally administered medications, the solubility of the pharmaceuticals is critical for drug absorption. The solubility rate, on the other hand, is directly proportional to the drug's surface area [88]. As a result, shrinking drug crystals to nanosize and increasing surface area has a significant influence on drug bioavailability.

The nanodrug formulation techniques range from basic self-assembly to chemical alterations including drug coupling or conjugation with diverse functional molecules such as carbohydrates, lipids, and photosensitizers. Inclusion of redox-responsive linkers and tumour targeting ligands during nanodrug production confers additional properties such as on-target delivery, and conjugation with immunotherapeutic reagents improves immune response as well as therapeutic effectiveness.

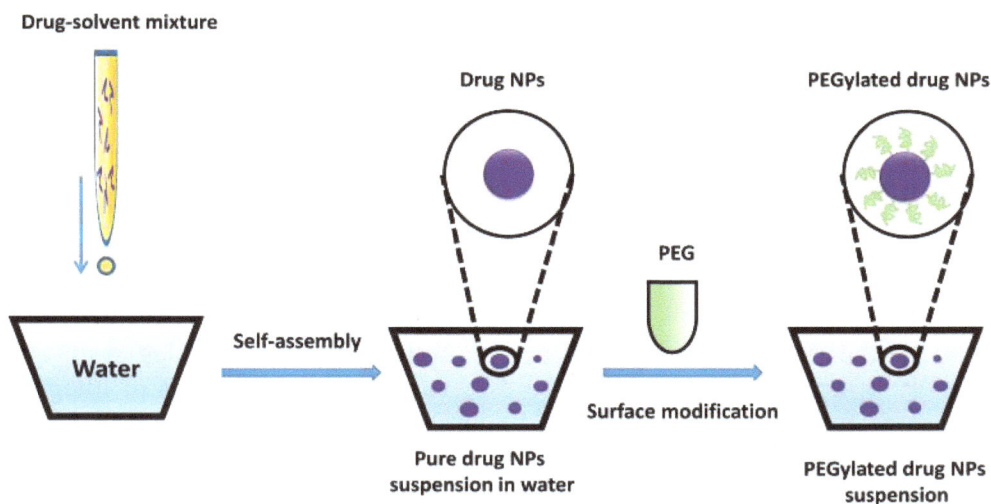

Fig. (7). Self-assembly of drug molecules and surface modification.

In the self-assembly technique (Fig. **7**), the drug molecules are first dissolved in a tiny amount of organic solvent before being introduced drop wise into an aqueous solution while vigorously stirring [89]. The interactions between hydrophobic small molecules result in the fast formation of uniform nanoparticles [90]. The generated nanoparticles can then be stabilized using small concentrations of surfactants. Self-assembled nanodrugs have larger drug loading capacities, better water solubility, longer blood circulation half-lives, higher drug delivery efficiency, and less adverse effects [91]. For instance pure Doxorubicin nanoparticles (DOX NPs) have been synthesized *via* self-assembly method with the consequent addition of PLGA-PEG as a surfactant and the synthesized NPs exhibited good biocompatibility and stability, and long blood circulation times [92]. DOX NPs had a faster release in an acidic environment, had a higher accumulation in tumours than free DOX and the tumour development in mice treated with free DOX and DOX NPs was 5.40 ± 0.30 -fold and 2.09 ± 0.25-fold, respectively. The inclusion of 10-Hydroxycamptothecin (HCPT) found to overcome multidrug resistance (MDR) in DOX-resistant breast cancer cell lines and shown stronger *in vivo* cytotoxicity and tumour inhibition than DOX NPs alone.

The same group combined three commonly used hydrophobic drugs, methotrexate (MTX), HCPT, and paclitaxel (PTX), into nanorods before conjugating them with PEG to improve bioenvironmental stability [93]. Solvent exchange method has been used for the synthesis. Initially the three anticancer drugs (MTX, HCPT and PTX) of equal weight were dissolved in the DMSO solution, and were dropped into 10 mL of aqueous solution by microsyringe under vigorous stirring. To obtain PEGylated multidrug nanocrystals (MDNC), poly(maleic anhydride-alt-1-octadecene)- poly(ethylene glycol) (C18PMH-PEG/H_2O) solution was added to the resulted MDNCs solution, and the mixture was then subjected to ultrasonic treatment and stored to obtain MDNCs-PEG solution. The study found that the particular nanodrug had nearly three times the therapeutic efficacy of free drugs at the same dose and effectively suppressed MDR. In a similar manner, Curcumin, Camptothecin, and HCPT pure nanodrug formulations have been prepared alone and in combinations as well [94 - 96].

To overcome the limitations of conventional small molecules and obtain extremely effective antitumour capability, various advancements in integrating two therapy modalities into a single system have been made in addition to the aforementioned pure chemotherapeutic medicines. Self-assembled chemotherapeutic drugs along with immunotherapeutic drugs, phototherapeutic drugs and other organic molecules have been synthesized. For instance, chemotherapeutic 7-ethyl-10-hydroxycamptothecin (SN-38) drug and photodynamic therapeutic drug chlorin e6 (Ce6) have been self-assembled into a nanodrug with a size of 154.87 ± 1.82 nm *via* π-π stacking and subsidiary hydrogen bonds [97].They have used the antisolvent precipitation method, in which drug components are dissolved in DMF and the solution is quickly injected into deionized water under continuous ultra-sonication followed by the dialyzing of the mixture against deionized water, to remove DMF and the free drug [98]. The nanodrug revealed improved cellular uptake by murine mammary carcinoma (4T1) cell lines and 85% tumour inhibition efficacy in the presence of laser which was substantially higher than those without laser (65%) and injected individual SN-38 and Ce6 (less than 20%), demonstrating the nanoparticles' excellent synergistic antitumour efficacy due to combined chemo-photodynamic therapy, higher cellular inculcation and enhanced tumour accumulation. In another study, Yan *et al.* described a chemo-photodynamic treatment using HCPT and Ce6, which were blended to self-assemble *via* reprecipitation method into nanorods in water [99]. Initially, they have prepared separate stock solutions of HCPT and Ce6 in DMSO. The two solutions were then mixed in different proportions and injected to a NaOH solution under ultrasonication to obtain the nano formulation. The nanorods with a uniform size of 360 nm in length and 135 nm in width, boosted both HCPT and Ce6 cell uptake and resulted in almost complete inhibition of the tumour growth, through synergistic therapy. Indocyanine green (ICG), the only FDA-approved photothermal therapeutic drug, has a high potential for self-assembly by virtue of its hydrophilic sulphate and hydrophobic indole skeletons [100]. The self-assembly of chemotherapeutic agent PTX with ICG has resulted in uniform NPs (140 ± 1.4 nm) delivering a combined system for chemo-photothermal therapy enhancing the solubility of PTX in the absence of any carriers [101]. The combined technique had a synergistic impact on cancer cell cytotoxicity *in vitro*, which was attributable to increased cellular uptake and prolonged release of PTX. Furthermore, an *in vivo* investigation revealed that PTX/ICG NDs accumulated more in the tumour site than free ICG and had a good synergistic chemo-photothermal treatment effectiveness against tumours in H22 tumour-bearing mice. Another study combining photodynamic treatment and chemotherapy used organic nanorods made from the rational co-assembly of the chemical anticancer medication PTX and the photosensitizer di-iodinated borondipyrromethene (BDP-I2) [102]. BDP-I2 was chosen because of its high singlet oxygen ($^1O_2$) quantum yields, which contribute to the production of deadly reactive oxygen species (ROS), which can enhance the permeability of cell membranes and eventually damage cells by interfering with their normal function. The photodynamic action hastened the endosomal escape of the nanorods, which increased the chemotherapeutic effectiveness of PTX.

Immunotherapy is another ground-breaking advancement in cancer treatment that seeks to activate immune cells to hunt for and eliminate cancerous cells [103]. Despite the fact that new immunomodulatory medicines have been approved by the FDA, their use is still hampered by limited patient response, dosage restrictions, and low stability [104]. NPs have been employed to improve the effectiveness of immunotherapeutic medications by releasing their payload at specific areas such as tumour tissues and lymph nodes. Pathophysiological hurdles such as tight extracellular matrix, renal clearance, and endonuclease degradation can be addressed by nanodrug formulations [105]. In this context, Indomethacin (IDM), a COX-2 inhibitor and nonsteroidal anti-inflammatory medication that inhibits the formation of prostaglandin E2 (PGE2), which promotes an immunosuppressive milieu in tumour cells, has been self-assembled with PTX to generate nanocrystal aggregates *via* π-π stackings and hydrogen bonding [106]. Feng *et al.* [107] established the self-assembly capabilities of the ICG templating technique by synthesizing stable NPs from a range of compounds, including PTX, Docetaxel Sorafenib, Vandetanib, and celecoxib *etc*, using ICG and investigated the immunotherapeutic effects of the combinational usage of PTX and ICG. The synthesis was carried out by adding PTX dissolved in DMSO drop wise to a solution of ICG, under continuous shaking. The mixture was centrifuged to collect nanodrug pellets and suspended again in water followed by ultracentrifugation to remove free drugs. The fluorescence imaging and PTX distribution confirmed that that ICG template self-assembled PTX facilitated the tumour accumulation of ICG and PTX *via* EPR effect. Under laser irradiation, modest dosages of PTX decreased the immunosuppressive tumour microenvironment by suppressing regulatory T lymphocytes, whilst ICG promoted immunogenic cell death. *In vitro* and *in vivo* testing with triple negative breast cancer cells, synergistic therapy increased intratumoural drug accumulation by 11.2-fold and increased the half-life by 3-fold when compared to free PTX.

Using the ultrasonic aided reprecipitation approach, Koseki *et al.* created pure drug nanocrystals that contain approximately 100% of the molecules of 7-ethy--10-hydroxycamptothecin (SN-38) [108]. The ultrasound-assisted reprecipitation approach was used to create rod-like nanocrystals with *ca.* 150 nm in a long axis, and the nanofibers were obtained without irradiation. Furthermore, the cytostatic efficacy of SN-38 nanocrystals against cancer cells was significantly stronger than that of irinotecan hydrochloride, a clinically utilized prodrug of SN-38. This research show that the ultrasound-assisted precipitation approach has the potential to be a strong method for fabricating nanoparticles integrated with just small molecule drugs. SN-38 is an anticancer drug that inhibits DNA topoisomerase I. Although SN-38 has significant anticancer action, its limited water solubility restricts its therapeutic applicability. Hence, water-soluble irinotecan hydrochloride has been developed as a prodrug of SN-38 [109, 110]. The cytostatic activity of SN-38 nanocrystals was tested on three types of cancer cells, including HepG2, KPL-4, and MCF-7, and the SN-38 nanocrystals shown much stronger activity than irinotecan hydrochloride.

The rising resistance of microbes to antibacterial drugs has resulted in major health consequences in recent years. Nanotechnology has demonstrated promising uses in pharmaceuticals and microbiological research to address the issue of antibiotic resistance. Researchers have examined many nanosized antibacterial agents in recent years, including non-metal, metallic and metal oxide nanoparticles, and polymeric nanoparticles as well [111 - 113].

Brain-eating amoebae produce catastrophic infections in the human central nervous system, with a 95% fatality rate [114, 115]. Areeba *et al.* has revealed for the first time that guanabenz conjugated to gold and silver nanoparticles exhibits strong antiamoebic action against both *Acanthamoeba castellanii* (*A. castellanii*) and *Naegleria fowleri* (*N. fowleri*) that causes granulomatous amoebic encephalitis and primary amoebic meningoencephalitis respectively [116]. The one-phase reduction process was used to synthesize gold and silver conjugated guanabenz nanoparticles. Notably, pretreatment of *A. castellanii* with guanabenz and its nanoconjugates reduced host cell cytopathogenicity from 65% to 38% and 2%, respectively, in the case of gold and silver nanoconjugates. Furthermore, the cytotoxicity of guanabenz and its nanoconjugates against human cells was shown to be minimal. Guanabenz is already licensed for hypertension and penetrates the blood brain barrier. With this recent finding the researchers have suggested that the guanabenz and its conjugated gold and silver nanoparticles might be repurposed as a possible treatment for brain-eating amoebic infections.

The same group have combined gold Nps with curcumin, the active ingredient in turmeric and a long-time anti-inflammatory medication used to treat a number of ailments [117]. Even at high doses, the hydrophobic molecule curcumin has been demonstrated to be highly safe in studies including both humans and animals, albeit its limited bioavailability in people is a result of their quick metabolism and poor absorption [118]. This problematic situation can be mitigated by overcoming low aqueous solubility of curcumin, using nanoparticles to enhance the bioavailability of curcumin. The conjugation of curcumin with gold Nps amoebicidal activities of the drugs has increased by up to 56% and 37% against *B. mandrillaris* and *N. fowleri*, respectively [119]. Hence a potential to cure infections caused by brain-eating amoebae using curcumin and gold-conjugated curcumin nanoparticles exist and it might also serve as a prototype for treatment of other diseases.

For improved anti-diabetic, anti-oxidant, and antibacterial action, another team created silver nanoparticles (GP-AgNPs) mediated by the fungus *Gynura procumbens* (GP) in chitosan (FCS) capsules [120]. The synthesized FCS-G--AgNPs has shown minimal inhibitory concentration for Bacillus cereus (8.12 ± 0.12 μg/mL), Staphylococcus aureus (4.08 ± 0.47 μg/mL), Listeria monocytogenes (4.95 ± 0.32 μg/mL), Escherichia coli (8.25 ± 0.18 μg/mL), and Salmonella enterica (4.12 ± 0.64 μg/mL). Furthermore, the biocompatibility of FCS-GP-AgNPs was tested in A549, LN229, and NIH3T3 cells. In conclusion,

FCS-GP-AgNPs demonstrated biocompatibility in terms of lower cytotoxicity and showed promise in antibacterial and enzyme inhibitory activities associated with diabetes.

The Table **1** summarizes the drugs described in the above context along with their uses.

Table 1. Drugs synthesized with the contribution of nanotechnology and their uses.

Use of Nanotechnology	Drug		Use
Use of nano catalysts in synthesis.	Pyridine derivatives	Omeprazol	Treat gastro esophageal reflux diseases and other diseases related with excessive stomach acid.
		Netupitant	Antiemetic drug
		Ciprofloxacin, Tetracycline, Nystatin, Amoxicillin, Ampicillin, Gentamicin	Antimicrobial drugs
		Abemaciclib Ivosidenib, Apalutamide Lorlatinib	Anticancer drugs
		Amlodipine, Nifedipine, Diludine, Felodipine, Oxodipine, Clevidipine	Treatment of cardiovascular disorders.
	Multisubstituted Imidazoles and benzimidazoles	Lansoprazole, Picoprazole	Treatment of duodenal and gastric ulcers.
		Losartan, Candesartan	Treat hypertension
		Chlormidazole, Econazole, Clotrimazole	Antifungal agent
Nanoformulations	Doxorubicin, Hydroxycamptothecin, methotrexate, paclitaxel, chlorin e6		Anticancer drugs
	Indocyanine green		Photothermal therapeutic drug

CONCLUSION

Nanotechnology is involved throughout the drug development process starting from lead identification to lead optimization and synthesis. Drug development using nanotechnology holds great promise for finding novel targets in disease sites or blood. Nanosensors that use single-molecule fluorescence (SMF) may identify proteins, nucleic acids, enzymes, viruses, and living organisms. For a clinical diagnosis, numerous microRNAs must be detected simultaneously as one disease is typically associated with the deregulation of numerous microRNAs and nanosensors have made it possible. In order to choose the best course of treatment, methods like protein corona and array analysis can assist to uncover biomarkers early in the course of illness progression.

Lead compounds are synthetic or natural substances with biological activity against a pharmacological target. Lead optimization involves chemical refinement to enhance biological activity, drug-like qualities, and reduce toxicity. Ultrasensitive dynamic light scattering (DLS)-based biosensors that employ gold NPs and allow the detection of protein activity and imaging of biological platforms using QDs based fluorescent materials through fluorescence anisotropy or fluorescence resonance energy transfer (FRET) have expanded live cell imaging applications in drug discovery, shortening preclinical lead optimization cycles and improving clinical predictability.

The pharmaceutical industry is also focusing on reducing development time and time to market by identifying and synthesizing desirable active pharmaceutical ingredients (APIs) to meet the growing demand for drugs. Optimizing the development process of APIs is promising to meet the increasing demand for drugs. Researchers are exploring the potential of nanomaterials in drug synthesis due to their catalytic ability, a promising technique in the development of nano-platforms. Pure nanodrugs, a new class of nanotherapeutics, consist of active drug molecules in nanoparticles and safe excipients, are also utilized for improving therapeutic effectiveness and decreasing off-target toxicity compared to small-molecule medicines.

PRACTICE QUESTIONS

1. Explain the steps to establish a new drug candidate for a disease briefly.
2. Define what a lead compound in medicinal chemistry is?
3. Describe how the use of nanotechnology and nanomaterials has facilitated the development of an improved lead compound starting with the target identification phase.
4. List out the special characteristics observed in nanoparticles when they are utilized as nanocatalysts during drug synthesis.
5. Compare and contrast the use of nanoparticles as catalysts in drug synthesis when compared to conventional bulk catalysts.
6. Explain the nanodrug formulation methods briefly.
7. Discuss the significance of nanodrugs when compared to the conventional drug formulations.

REFERENCES

[1] Wang, S.; Sim, T.B.; Kim, Y.S.; Chang, Y.T. Tools for target identification and validation. *Curr. Opin. Chem. Biol.,* **2004**, *8*(4), 371-377.
[http://dx.doi.org/10.1016/j.cbpa.2004.06.001] [PMID: 15288246]

[2] Liu, M.; Qiu, J.G.; Ma, F.; Zhang, C.Y. Advances in single molecule fluorescent nanosensors. *Wiley Interdiscip. Rev. Nanomed. Nanobiotechnol.,* **2021**, *13*(5), e1716.
[http://dx.doi.org/10.1002/wnan.1716] [PMID: 33779063]

[3] Wang, Z.; Wang, L.; Zhang, Q.; Tang, B.; Zhang, C. Single quantum dot-based nanosensor for sensitive detection of 5-methylcytosine at both CpG and non-CpG sites. *Chem. Sci.,* **2018**, *9*(5), 1330-1338.
[http://dx.doi.org/10.1039/C7SC04813K] [PMID: 29675180]

[4] Lin, S.; Gregory, R.I. MicroRNA biogenesis pathways in cancer. *Nat. Rev. Cancer,* **2015**, *15*(6), 321-333.
[http://dx.doi.org/10.1038/nrc3932] [PMID: 25998712]

[5] Ma, F.; Zhang, Q.; Zhang, C. Catalytic self-assembly of quantum-dot-based microRNA nanosensor directed by toehold-mediated strand displacement cascade. *Nano Lett.,* **2019**, *19*(9), 6370-6376.
[http://dx.doi.org/10.1021/acs.nanolett.9b02544] [PMID: 31460766]

[6] Li, B.; Liu, Y.; Liu, Y.; Tian, T.; Yang, B.; Huang, X.; Liu, J.; Liu, B. Construction of Dual-Color Probes with Target-Triggered Signal Amplification for *In Situ* Single-Molecule Imaging of MicroRNA. *ACS Nano,* **2020**, *14*(7), 8116-8125.
[http://dx.doi.org/10.1021/acsnano.0c01061] [PMID: 32568523]

[7] Porkka, K.P.; Pfeiffer, M.J.; Waltering, K.K.; Vessella, R.L.; Tammela, T.L.J.; Visakorpi, T. MicroRNA expression profiling in prostate cancer. *Cancer Res.,* **2007**, *67*(13), 6130-6135.
[http://dx.doi.org/10.1158/0008-5472.CAN-07-0533] [PMID: 17616669]

[8] Ma, F.; Jiang, S.; Zhang, C. SiRNA-directed self-assembled quantum dot biosensor for simultaneous detection of multiple microRNAs at the single-particle level. *Biosens. Bioelectron.,* **2020**, *157*, 112177.
[http://dx.doi.org/10.1016/j.bios.2020.112177] [PMID: 32250933]

[9] Sur, M.; AlArdati, H.; Ross, C.; Alowami, S. TdT expression in Merkel cell carcinoma: potential diagnostic pitfall with blastic hematological malignancies and expanded immunohistochemical analysis. *Mod. Pathol.,* **2007**, *20*(11), 1113-1120.
[http://dx.doi.org/10.1038/modpathol.3800936] [PMID: 17885674]

[10] Komori, T.; Okada, A.; Stewart, V.; Alt, F.W. Lack of N regions in antigen receptor variable region genes of TdT-deficient lymphocytes. *Science,* **1993**, *261*(5125), 1171-1175.
[http://dx.doi.org/10.1126/science.8356451] [PMID: 8356451]

[11] Wang, L.J.; Luo, M.L.; Zhang, Q.; Tang, B.; Zhang, C.Y. Single quantum dot-based nanosensor for rapid and sensitive detection of terminal deoxynucleotidyl transferase. *Chem. Commun.,* **2017**, *53*(80), 11016-11019.
[http://dx.doi.org/10.1039/C7CC05485H] [PMID: 28936504]

[12] Farka, Z.; Mickert, M.J.; Hlaváček, A.; Skládal, P.; Gorris, H.H. Single molecule upconversion-linked immunosorbent assay with extended dynamic range for the sensitive detection of diagnostic biomarkers. *Anal. Chem.,* **2017**, *89*(21), 11825-11830.
[http://dx.doi.org/10.1021/acs.analchem.7b03542] [PMID: 28949515]

[13] Li, W.; Jiang, W.; Dai, S.; Wang, L. Multiplexed detection of cytokines based on dual bar-code strategy and single-molecule counting. *Anal. Chem.,* **2016**, *88*(3), 1578-1584.
[http://dx.doi.org/10.1021/acs.analchem.5b03043] [PMID: 26721199]

[14] Hu, J.; Li, Y.; Li, Y.; Tang, B.; Zhang, C. Single quantum dot-based nanosensor for sensitive detection of O-GlcNAc transferase activity. *Anal. Chem.,* **2017**, *89*(23), 12992-12999.

[http://dx.doi.org/10.1021/acs.analchem.7b04065] [PMID: 29115822]

[15]   Han, Y.; Ye, Z.; Wang, F.; Chen, T.; Wei, L.; Chen, L.; Xiao, L. Single-particle enumeration-based ultrasensitive enzyme activity quantification with fluorescent polymer nanoparticles. *Nanoscale,* **2019**, *11*(31), 14793-14801.
[http://dx.doi.org/10.1039/C9NR01817D] [PMID: 31353389]

[16]   Dvir, H.; Silman, I.; Harel, M.; Rosenberry, T.L.; Sussman, J.L. Acetylcholinesterase: From 3D structure to function. *Chem. Biol. Interact.,* **2010**, *187*(1-3), 10-22.
[http://dx.doi.org/10.1016/j.cbi.2010.01.042] [PMID: 20138030]

[17]   Zhang, X.; Zhang, X.; Luo, C.; Liu, Z.; Chen, Y.; Dong, S.; Jiang, C.; Yang, S.; Wang, F.; Xiao, X. Volume-enhanced raman scattering detection of viruses. *Small,* **2019**, *15*(11), 1805516.
[http://dx.doi.org/10.1002/smll.201805516] [PMID: 30706645]

[18]   Wu, Z.; Zeng, T.; Guo, W.J.; Bai, Y.Y.; Pang, D.W.; Zhang, Z.L. Digital single virus immunoassay for ultrasensitive multiplex avian influenza virus detection based on fluorescent magnetic multifunctional nanospheres. *ACS Appl. Mater. Interfaces,* **2019**, *11*(6), 5762-5770.
[http://dx.doi.org/10.1021/acsami.8b18898] [PMID: 30688060]

[19]   You, C.C.; Miranda, O.R.; Gider, B.; Ghosh, P.S.; Kim, I.B.; Erdogan, B.; Krovi, S.A.; Bunz, U.H.F.; Rotello, V.M. Detection and identification of proteins using nanoparticle–fluorescent polymer 'chemical nose' sensors. *Nat. Nanotechnol.,* **2007**, *2*(5), 318-323.
[http://dx.doi.org/10.1038/nnano.2007.99] [PMID: 18654291]

[20]   Arvizo, R.R.; Giri, K.; Moyano, D.; Miranda, O.R.; Madden, B.; McCormick, D.J.; Bhattacharya, R.; Rotello, V.M.; Kocher, J.P.; Mukherjee, P. Identifying new therapeutic targets *via* modulation of protein corona formation by engineered nanoparticles. *PLoS One,* **2012**, *7*(3), e33650.
[http://dx.doi.org/10.1371/journal.pone.0033650] [PMID: 22442705]

[21]   Giri, K.; Shameer, K.; Zimmermann, M.T.; Saha, S.; Chakraborty, P.K.; Sharma, A.; Arvizo, R.R.; Madden, B.J.; Mccormick, D.J.; Kocher, J.P.A.; Bhattacharya, R.; Mukherjee, P. Understanding protein-nanoparticle interaction: a new gateway to disease therapeutics. *Bioconjug. Chem.,* **2014**, *25*(6), 1078-1090.
[http://dx.doi.org/10.1021/bc500084f] [PMID: 24831101]

[22]   Schrittwieser, S.; Pelaz, B.; Parak, W.J.; Lentijo-Mozo, S.; Soulantica, K.; Dieckhoff, J.; Ludwig, F.; Schotter, J. Direct protein quantification in complex sample solutions by surface-engineered nanorod probes. *Sci. Rep.,* **2017**, *7*(1), 4752.
[http://dx.doi.org/10.1038/s41598-017-04970-5] [PMID: 28684848]

[23]   Hajipour, M.J.; Ghasemi, F.; Aghaverdi, H.; Raoufi, M.; Linne, U.; Atyabi, F.; Nabipour, I.; Azhdarzadeh, M.; Derakhshankhah, H.; Lotfabadi, A.; Bargahi, A.; Alekhamis, Z.; Aghaie, A.; Hashemi, E.; Tafakhori, A.; Aghamollaii, V.; Mashhadi, M.M.; Sheibani, S.; Vali, H.; Mahmoudi, M. Sensing of Alzheimer's disease and multiple sclerosis using nano-bio interfaces. *J. Alzheimers Dis.,* **2017**, *59*(4), 1187-1202.
[http://dx.doi.org/10.3233/JAD-160206] [PMID: 28759965]

[24]   Zheng, X.T.; Goh, W.L.; Yeow, P.; Lane, D.P.; Ghadessy, F.J.; Tan, Y.N. Ultrasensitive dynamic light scattering based nanobiosensor for rapid anticancer drug screening. *Sens. Actuators B Chem.,* **2019**, *279*, 79-86.
[http://dx.doi.org/10.1016/j.snb.2018.09.088]

[25]   You, M.; Lyu, Y.; Han, D.; Qiu, L.; Liu, Q.; Chen, T.; Sam Wu, C.; Peng, L.; Zhang, L.; Bao, G.; Tan, W. DNA probes for monitoring dynamic and transient molecular encounters on live cell membranes. *Nat. Nanotechnol.,* **2017**, *12*(5), 453-459.
[http://dx.doi.org/10.1038/nnano.2017.23] [PMID: 28319616]

[26]   Isherwood, B.; Timpson, P.; McGhee, E.J.; Anderson, K.I.; Canel, M.; Serrels, A.; Brunton, V.G.; Carragher, N.O. Live cell *in vitro* and *in vivo* imaging applications: accelerating drug discovery. *Pharmaceutics,* **2011**, *3*(2), 141-170.

[http://dx.doi.org/10.3390/pharmaceutics3020141] [PMID: 24310493]

[27]   Bruchez, M.P. Turning all the lights on: quantum dots in cellular assays. *Curr. Opin. Chem. Biol.,* **2005,** *9*(5), 533-537.
[http://dx.doi.org/10.1016/j.cbpa.2005.08.019] [PMID: 16125995]

[28]   Bentolila, L.A.; Ebenstein, Y.; Weiss, S. Quantum dots for *in vivo* small-animal imaging. *J. Nucl. Med.,* **2009,** *50*(4), 493-496.
[http://dx.doi.org/10.2967/jnumed.108.053561] [PMID: 19289434]

[29]   Yu, Y.; Lee, W.D.; Tan, Y.N. Protein-protected gold/silver alloy nanoclusters in metal-enhanced singlet oxygen generation and their correlation with photoluminescence. *Mater. Sci. Eng. C,* **2020,** *109*, 110525.
[http://dx.doi.org/10.1016/j.msec.2019.110525] [PMID: 32228897]

[30]   Yu, Y.; Zheng, X.T.; Yee, B.W.; Tan, Y.N. Biomimicking synthesis of photoluminescent molecular lantern catalyzed by in-situ formation of nanogold catalysts. *Mater. Sci. Eng. C,* **2017,** *77*, 1111-1116.
[http://dx.doi.org/10.1016/j.msec.2017.04.029] [PMID: 28531986]

[31]   Yu, Y.; Mok, B.Y.L.; Loh, X.J.; Tan, Y.N. Rational design of biomolecular templates for synthesizing multifunctional noble metal nanoclusters toward personalized theranostic applications. *Adv. Healthc. Mater.,* **2016,** *5*(15), 1844-1859.
[http://dx.doi.org/10.1002/adhm.201600192] [PMID: 27377035]

[32]   Zheng, X.T.; Choi, Y.; Phua, D.G.G.; Tan, Y.N. Noncovalent fluorescent biodot–protein conjugates with well-preserved native functions for improved sweat glucose detection. *Bioconjug. Chem.,* **2020,** *31*(3), 754-763.
[http://dx.doi.org/10.1021/acs.bioconjchem.9b00856] [PMID: 31995367]

[33]   Choi, Y.; Zheng, X.T.; Tan, Y.N. Bioinspired carbon dots (biodots): emerging fluorophores with tailored multiple functionalities for biomedical, agricultural and environmental applications. *Mol. Syst. Des. Eng.,* **2020,** *5*(1), 67-90.
[http://dx.doi.org/10.1039/C9ME00086K]

[34]   Zheng, X.T.; Tan, Y.N. Development of Blood-Cell-Selective Fluorescent Biodots for Lysis☐Free Leukocyte Imaging and Differential Counting in Whole Blood. *Small,* **2020,** *16*(12), 1903328.
[http://dx.doi.org/10.1002/smll.201903328] [PMID: 31414726]

[35]   Zheng, X.T.; Lai, Y.C.; Tan, Y.N. Nucleotide-derived theranostic nanodots with intrinsic fluorescence and singlet oxygen generation for bioimaging and photodynamic therapy. *Nanoscale Adv.,* **2019,** *1*(6), 2250-2257.
[http://dx.doi.org/10.1039/C9NA00058E] [PMID: 36131960]

[36]   Xu, H.V.; Zheng, X.T.; Zhao, Y.; Tan, Y.N. Uncovering the Design Principle of Amino Acid-Derived Photoluminescent Biodots with Tailor-Made Structure–Properties and Applications for Cellular Bioimaging. *ACS Appl. Mater. Interfaces,* **2018,** *10*(23), 19881-19888.
[http://dx.doi.org/10.1021/acsami.8b04864] [PMID: 29786414]

[37]   Tavakkoli Yaraki, M.; Hu, F.; Daqiqeh Rezaei, S.; Liu, B.; Tan, Y.N. Metal-enhancement study of dual functional photosensitizers with aggregation-induced emission and singlet oxygen generation. *Nanoscale Adv.,* **2020,** *2*(7), 2859-2869.
[http://dx.doi.org/10.1039/D0NA00182A] [PMID: 36132415]

[38]   Geng, J.; Goh, W.L.; Zhang, C.; Lane, D.P.; Liu, B.; Ghadessy, F.; Tan, Y.N. A highly sensitive fluorescent light-up probe for real-time detection of the endogenous protein target and its antagonism in live cells. *J. Mater. Chem. B Mater. Biol. Med.,* **2015,** *3*(29), 5933-5937.
[http://dx.doi.org/10.1039/C5TB00819K] [PMID: 32262648]

[39]   Zheng, X.T.; Tan, Y.N. Recent development of nucleic acid nanosensors to detect sequence-specific binding interactions: From metal ions, small molecules to proteins and pathogens. *Sensors International,* **2020,** *1*, 100034.
[http://dx.doi.org/10.1016/j.sintl.2020.100034] [PMID: 34766041]

[40]   Fan, Y.; Liu, H.; Han, R.; Huang, L.; Shi, H.; Sha, Y.; Jiang, Y. Extremely high brightness from polymer-encapsulated quantum dots for two-photon cellular and deep-tissue imaging. *Sci. Rep.,* **2015**, *5*(1), 9908.
[http://dx.doi.org/10.1038/srep09908] [PMID: 25909393]

[41]   Zhao, D.; Li, J.; Yang, T.; He, Z. "Turn off–on" fluorescent sensor for platinum drugs-DNA interactions based on quantum dots. *Biosens. Bioelectron.,* **2014**, *52*, 29-35.
[http://dx.doi.org/10.1016/j.bios.2013.08.031] [PMID: 24016536]

[42]   Hajipour, A.R.; Khorsandi, Z.; Mortazavi, M.; Farrokhpour, H. Green, efficient and large-scale synthesis of benzimidazoles, benzoxazoles and benzothiazoles derivatives using ligand-free cobalt-nanoparticles: as potential anti-estrogen breast cancer agents, and study of their interactions with estrogen receptor by molecular docking. *RSC Advances,* **2015**, *5*(130), 107822-107828.
[http://dx.doi.org/10.1039/C5RA22207A]

[43]   Brahmachari, G.; Banerjee, B. Facile and One-Pot Access to Diverse and Densely Functionalized 2-Amino-3-cyano-4 *H* -pyrans and Pyran-Annulated Heterocyclic Scaffolds *via* an Eco-Friendly Multicomponent Reaction at Room Temperature Using Urea as a Novel Organo-Catalyst. *ACS Sustain. Chem.& Eng.,* **2014**, *2*(3), 411-422.
[http://dx.doi.org/10.1021/sc400312n]

[44]   Brahmachari, G.; Banerjee, B. Facile and Chemically Sustainable One-Pot Synthesis of a Wide Array of Fused *O* - and *N* -Heterocycles Catalyzed by Trisodium Citrate Dihydrate under Ambient Conditions. *Asian J. Org. Chem.,* **2016**, *5*(2), 271-286.
[http://dx.doi.org/10.1002/ajoc.201500465]

[45]   Kaur, G.; Devi, P.; Thakur, S.; Kumar, A.; Chandel, R.; Banerjee, B. Magnetically Separable Transition Metal Ferrites: Versatile Heterogeneous Nano-Catalysts for the Synthesis of Diverse Bioactive Heterocycles. *ChemistrySelect,* **2019**, *4*(7), 2181-2199.
[http://dx.doi.org/10.1002/slct.201803600]

[46]   Martins, P.; Jesus, J.; Santos, S.; Raposo, L.; Roma-Rodrigues, C.; Baptista, P.; Fernandes, A. Heterocyclic Anticancer Compounds: Recent advances and the paradigm shift towards the use of nanomedicine's tool box. *Molecules,* **2015**, *20*(9), 16852-16891.
[http://dx.doi.org/10.3390/molecules200916852] [PMID: 26389876]

[47]   Tewari, N.; Dwivedi, N.; Tripathi, R.P. Tetrabutylammonium hydrogen sulfate catalyzed eco-friendly and efficient synthesis of glycosyl 1,4-dihydropyridines. *Tetrahedron Lett.,* **2004**, *45*(49), 9011-9014.
[http://dx.doi.org/10.1016/j.tetlet.2004.10.057]

[48]   Sheldon, R.A.; Dakka, J. Heterogeneous catalytic oxidations in the manufacture of fine chemicals. *Catal. Today,* **1994**, *19*(2), 215-245.
[http://dx.doi.org/10.1016/0920-5861(94)80186-X]

[49]   Sheldon, R.A.; Downing, R.S. Heterogeneous catalytic transformations for environmentally friendly production. *Appl. Catal. A Gen.,* **1999**, *189*(2), 163-183.
[http://dx.doi.org/10.1016/S0926-860X(99)00274-4]

[50]   Alves, H.P.A.; Costa, A.C.S.; Correa, M.A.; Bohn, F.; Della Pace, R.D.; Acchar, W. Structural, magnetic and electric properties of ZrO2 tapes decorated with magnetic nanoparticles. *Ceram. Int.,* **2019**, *45*(12), 14500-14504.
[http://dx.doi.org/10.1016/j.ceramint.2019.04.123]

[51]   Kumar, N.; Kumbhat, S. Unique Properties.*Essentials in Nanoscience and Nanotechnology*; John Wiley & Sons: New Jersey, **2016**, pp. 326-356.
[http://dx.doi.org/10.1002/9781119096122.ch8]

[52]   Lopes, P.P.; Strmcnik, D.; Tripkovic, D.; Connell, J.G.; Stamenkovic, V.; Markovic, N.M. Relationships between Atomic Level Surface Structure and Stability/Activity of Platinum Surface Atoms in Aqueous Environments. *ACS Catal.,* **2016**, *6*(4), 2536-2544.
[http://dx.doi.org/10.1021/acscatal.5b02920]

[53]   Liu, P.; Guan, P.; Hirata, A.; Zhang, L.; Chen, L.; Wen, Y.; Ding, Y.; Fujita, T.; Erlebacher, J.; Chen, M. Visualizing Under-Coordinated Surface Atoms on 3D Nanoporous Gold Catalysts. *Adv. Mater.,* **2016**, *28*(9), 1753-1759.
[http://dx.doi.org/10.1002/adma.201504032] [PMID: 26676880]

[54]   Maleki, A.; Paydar, R. Graphene oxide–chitosan bionanocomposite: a highly efficient nanocatalyst for the one-pot three-component synthesis of trisubstituted imidazoles under solvent-free conditions. *RSC Advances,* **2015**, *5*(42), 33177-33184.
[http://dx.doi.org/10.1039/C5RA03355A]

[55]   Safaei-Ghomi, J.; Shahbazi-Alavi, H.; Heidari-Baghbahadorani, E. SnO nanoparticles as an efficient catalyst for the one-pot synthesis of chromeno[2,3-b]pyridines and 2-amino-3,5-dicyano-6-sulfanyl pyridines. *RSC Advances,* **2014**, *4*(92), 50668-50677.
[http://dx.doi.org/10.1039/C4RA04769A]

[56]   Khan, E. Pyridine derivatives as biologically active precursors; organics and selected coordination complexes. *ChemistrySelect,* **2021**, *6*(13), 3041-3064.
[http://dx.doi.org/10.1002/slct.202100332]

[57]   Beukers, M.W.; Chang, L.C.W.; von Frijtag Drabbe Künzel, J.K.; Mulder-Krieger, T.; Spanjersberg, R.F.; Brussee, J.; IJzerman, A.P. New, non-adenosine, high-potency agonists for the human adenosine A_{2B} receptor with an improved selectivity profile compared to the reference agonist N-ethylcarboxamidoadenosine. *J. Med. Chem.,* **2004**, *47*(15), 3707-3709.
[http://dx.doi.org/10.1021/jm049947s] [PMID: 15239649]

[58]   Chang, L.C.W.; von Frijtag Drabbe Künzel, J.K.; Mulder-Krieger, T.; Spanjersberg, R.F.; Roerink, S.F.; van den Hout, G.; Beukers, M.W.; Brussee, J.; IJzerman, A.P. A series of ligands displaying a remarkable agonistic-antagonistic profile at the adenosine A1 receptor. *J. Med. Chem.,* **2005**, *48*(6), 2045-2053.
[http://dx.doi.org/10.1021/jm049597+] [PMID: 15771447]

[59]   Fredholm, B.B.; IJzerman, A.P.; Jacobson, K.A.; Klotz, K-N.; Linden, J. International Union of Pharmacology. XXV. Nomenclature and classification of adenosine receptors. *Pharmacol. Rev.,* **2001**, *53*(4), 527-552.
[PMID: 11734617]

[60]   Safaei-Ghomi, J.; Ghasemzadeh, M.A. CuI nanoparticles: a highly active and easily recyclable catalyst for the synthesis of 2-amino-3,5-dicyano-6-sulfanyl pyridines. *J. Sulfur Chem.,* **2013**, *34*(3), 233-241.
[http://dx.doi.org/10.1080/17415993.2012.728220]

[61]   Dandia, A.; Parewa, V.; Jain, A.K.; Rathore, K.S. Step-economic, efficient, ZnS nanoparticle-catalyzed synthesis of spirooxindole derivatives in aqueous medium *via* Knoevenagel condensation followed by Michael addition. *Green Chem.,* **2011**, *13*(8), 2135-2145.
[http://dx.doi.org/10.1039/c1gc15244k]

[62]   Tanabe, K.; Hölderich, W.F. Industrial application of solid acid–base catalysts. *Appl. Catal. A Gen.,* **1999**, *181*(2), 399-434.
[http://dx.doi.org/10.1016/S0926-860X(98)00397-4]

[63]   Nasir Baig, R.B.; Varma, R.S. Organic synthesis *via* magnetic attraction: benign and sustainable protocols using magnetic nanoferrites. *Green Chem.,* **2013**, *15*(2), 398-417.
[http://dx.doi.org/10.1039/C2GC36455G]

[64]   Bossert, F.; Meyer, H.; Wehinger, E. 4-Aryldihydropyridines, a New Class of Highly Active Calcium Antagonists. *Angew. Chem. Int. Ed. Engl.,* **1981**, *20*(9), 762-769.
[http://dx.doi.org/10.1002/anie.198107621]

[65]   Gilpin, R.K.; Pachla, L.A. Pharmaceuticals and related drugs. *Anal. Chem.,* **1999**, *71*(12), 217-234.
[http://dx.doi.org/10.1021/a1990008k] [PMID: 10384784]

[66]   Baumann, M.; Baxendale, I.R. An overview of the synthetic routes to the best selling drugs containing

6-membered heterocycles. *Beilstein J. Org. Chem.*, **2013**, *9*, 2265-2319.
[http://dx.doi.org/10.3762/bjoc.9.265] [PMID: 24204439]

[67]   Hantzsch, A. Ueber die synthese pyridinartiger verbindungen aus acetessigäther und aldehydammoniak. *Justus Liebigs Ann. Chem.*, **1882**, *215*(1), 1-82.
[http://dx.doi.org/10.1002/jlac.18822150102]

[68]   Mathur, R.; Negi, K.S.; Shrivastava, R.; Nair, R. Recent developments in the nanomaterial-catalyzed green synthesis of structurally diverse 1,4-dihydropyridines. *RSC Advances*, **2021**, *11*(3), 1376-1393.
[http://dx.doi.org/10.1039/D0RA07807G] [PMID: 35424131]

[69]   Kantam, M.L.; Ramani, T.; Chakrapani, L.; Choudary, B.M. Synthesis of 1,4-dihydropyridine derivatives using nanocrystalline copper(II) oxide catalyst. *Catal. Commun.*, **2009**, *10*(4), 370-372.
[http://dx.doi.org/10.1016/j.catcom.2008.09.023]

[70]   Safaei-Ghomi, J.; Ziarati, A.; Teymuri, R. CuI nanoparticles as new, efficient and reusable catalyst for the one-pot synthesis of 1, 4-dihydropyridines. *Bull. Korean Chem. Soc.*, **2012**, *33*(8), 2679-2682.
[http://dx.doi.org/10.5012/bkcs.2012.33.8.2679]

[71]   Ravikumar Naik, T.R.; Shivashankar, S.A. Heterogeneous bimetallic ZnFe2O4 nanopowder catalyzed synthesis of Hantzsch 1,4-dihydropyridines in water. *Tetrahedron Lett.*, **2016**, *57*(36), 4046-4049.
[http://dx.doi.org/10.1016/j.tetlet.2016.07.071]

[72]   Alinezhad, H.; Mohseni Tavakkoli, S. Cu-doped ZnO nanocrystalline powder as a catalyst for green and convenient multi-component synthesis of 1,4-dihydropyridine. *Res. Chem. Intermed.*, **2015**, *41*(9), 5931-5940.
[http://dx.doi.org/10.1007/s11164-014-1712-8]

[73]   Bhaskaruni, S.V.H.S.; Maddila, S.; van Zyl, W.E.; Jonnalagadda, S.B. Four-Component Fusion Protocol with NiO/ZrO $_2$ as a Robust Recyclable Catalyst for Novel 1,4-Dihydropyridines. *ACS Omega*, **2019**, *4*(25), 21187-21196.
[http://dx.doi.org/10.1021/acsomega.9b02608] [PMID: 31867512]

[74]   Taheri-Ledari, R.; Rahimi, J.; Maleki, A.; Shalan, A.E. Ultrasound-assisted diversion of nitrobenzene derivatives to their aniline equivalents through a heterogeneous magnetic Ag/Fe$_3$O$_4$-IT nanocomposite catalyst. *New J. Chem.*, **2020**, *44*(45), 19827-19835.
[http://dx.doi.org/10.1039/D0NJ05147K]

[75]   Taheri-Ledari, R.; Hashemi, S.M.; Maleki, A. High-performance sono/nano-catalytic system: CTSN/Fe$_3$O$_4$–Cu nanocomposite, a promising heterogeneous catalyst for the synthesis of *N* - arylimidazoles. *RSC Advances*, **2019**, *9*(69), 40348-40356.
[http://dx.doi.org/10.1039/C9RA08062G] [PMID: 35542689]

[76]   Liang, Q.; Yu, L.; Jiang, W.; Zhou, S.; Zhong, S.; Jiang, W. One-pot synthesis of magnetic graphitic carbon nitride photocatalyst with synergistic catalytic performance under visible-light irradiation. *J. Photochem. Photobiol. Chem.*, **2017**, *335*, 165-173.
[http://dx.doi.org/10.1016/j.jphotochem.2016.11.012]

[77]   Taheri-Ledari, R.; Rahimi, J.; Maleki, A. Synergistic catalytic effect between ultrasound waves and pyrimidine-2,4-diamine-functionalized magnetic nanoparticles: Applied for synthesis of 1,4-dihydropyridine pharmaceutical derivatives. *Ultrason. Sonochem.*, **2019**, *59*, 104737.
[http://dx.doi.org/10.1016/j.ultsonch.2019.104737] [PMID: 31473427]

[78]   Gaba, M.; Singh, S.; Mohan, C. Benzimidazole: An emerging scaffold for analgesic and anti-inflammatory agents. *Eur. J. Med. Chem.*, **2014**, *76*, 494-505.
[http://dx.doi.org/10.1016/j.ejmech.2014.01.030] [PMID: 24602792]

[79]   Bhatnagar, A.; Sharma, P.; Kumar, N. A review on "Imidazoles": Their chemistry and pharmacological potentials. *Int. J. Pharm. Tech. Res.*, **2011**, *3*(1), 268-282.

[80]   Gaba, M.; Mohan, C. Development of drugs based on imidazole and benzimidazole bioactive heterocycles: recent advances and future directions. *Med. Chem. Res.*, **2016**, *25*(2), 173-210.

[http://dx.doi.org/10.1007/s00044-015-1495-5]

[81]   Kalhor, M.; Zarnegar, Z. Fe_3O_4/SO_3 H@zeolite-Y as a novel multi-functional and magnetic nanocatalyst for clean and soft synthesis of imidazole and perimidine derivatives. *RSC Advances,* **2019,** *9*(34), 19333-19346.
       [http://dx.doi.org/10.1039/C9RA02910A] [PMID: 35519374]

[82]   Khazaei, A.; Alavi Nik, H.A.; Ranjbaran, A.; Moosavi-Zare, A.R. Synthesis, characterization and application of $Ni_{0.5} Zn_{0.5} Fe_2 O_4$ nanoparticles for the one pot synthesis of triaryl-1H-imidazoles. *RSC Advances,* **2016,** *6*(82), 78881-78886.
       [http://dx.doi.org/10.1039/C6RA05158H]

[83]   Arpanahi, F.; Mombeni Goodajdar, B. Iron–Phosphonate Nanomaterial: As a Novel and Efficient Organic–Inorganic Hybrid Catalyst for Solvent-Free Synthesis of Tri-Substituted Imidazole Derivatives. *J. Inorg. Organomet. Polym. Mater.,* **2020,** *30*(7), 2572-2581.
       [http://dx.doi.org/10.1007/s10904-020-01530-9]

[84]   Hajizadeh, Z.; Radinekiyan, F.; Eivazzadeh-keihan, R.; Maleki, A. Development of novel and green $NiFe_2O_4$/geopolymer nanocatalyst based on bentonite for synthesis of imidazole heterocycles by ultrasonic irradiations. *Sci. Rep.,* **2020,** *10*(1), 11671.
       [http://dx.doi.org/10.1038/s41598-020-68426-z] [PMID: 32669578]

[85]   Yadav, P.; Kakati, P.; Singh, P.; Awasthi, S.K. Application of sulfonic acid fabricated cobalt ferrite nanoparticles as effective magnetic nanocatalyst for green and facile synthesis of benzimidazoles. *Appl. Catal. A Gen.,* **2021,** *612*, 118005.
       [http://dx.doi.org/10.1016/j.apcata.2021.118005]

[86]   Merisko-Liversidge, E.M.; Liversidge, G.G. Drug nanoparticles: formulating poorly water-soluble compounds. *Toxicol. Pathol.,* **2008,** *36*(1), 43-48.
       [http://dx.doi.org/10.1177/0192623307310946] [PMID: 18337220]

[87]   Xie, S.; Manuguri, S.; Proietti, G.; Romson, J.; Fu, Y.; Inge, A.K.; Wu, B.; Zhang, Y.; Häll, D.; Ramström, O.; Yan, M. Design and synthesis of theranostic antibiotic nanodrugs that display enhanced antibacterial activity and luminescence. *Proc. Natl. Acad. Sci. USA,* **2017,** *114*(32), 8464-8469.
       [http://dx.doi.org/10.1073/pnas.1708556114] [PMID: 28743748]

[88]   Noyes, A.A.; Whitney, W.R. The rate of solution of solid substances in their own solutions. *J. Am. Chem. Soc.,* **1897,** *19*(12), 930-934.
       [http://dx.doi.org/10.1021/ja02086a003]

[89]   Gao, Z.; He, T.; Zhang, P.; Li, X.; Zhang, Y.; Lin, J.; Hao, J.; Huang, P.; Cui, J. Polypeptide-Based Theranostics with Tumor-Microenvironment-Activatable Cascade Reaction for Chemo-ferroptosis Combination Therapy. *ACS Appl. Mater. Interfaces,* **2020,** *12*(18), 20271-20280.
       [http://dx.doi.org/10.1021/acsami.0c03748] [PMID: 32283924]

[90]   Zhu, R.; Su, L.; Dai, J.; Li, Z.W.; Bai, S.; Li, Q.; Chen, X.; Song, J.; Yang, H. Biologically Responsive Plasmonic Assemblies for Second Near-Infrared Window Photoacoustic Imaging-Guided Concurrent Chemo-Immunotherapy. *ACS Nano,* **2020,** *14*(4), 3991-4006.
       [http://dx.doi.org/10.1021/acsnano.9b07984] [PMID: 32208667]

[91]   Qin, S.Y.; Zhang, A.Q.; Cheng, S.X.; Rong, L.; Zhang, X.Z. Drug self-delivery systems for cancer therapy. *Biomaterials,* **2017,** *112*, 234-247.
       [http://dx.doi.org/10.1016/j.biomaterials.2016.10.016] [PMID: 27768976]

[92]   Yu, C.; Zhou, M.; Zhang, X.; Wei, W.; Chen, X.; Zhang, X. Smart doxorubicin nanoparticles with high drug payload for enhanced chemotherapy against drug resistance and cancer diagnosis. *Nanoscale,* **2015,** *7*(13), 5683-5690.
       [http://dx.doi.org/10.1039/C5NR00290G] [PMID: 25740312]

[93]   Zhou, M.; Zhang, X.; Yang, Y.; Liu, Z.; Tian, B.; Jie, J.; Zhang, X. Carrier-free functionalized multidrug nanorods for synergistic cancer therapy. *Biomaterials,* **2013,** *34*(35), 8960-8967.
       [http://dx.doi.org/10.1016/j.biomaterials.2013.07.080] [PMID: 23958027]

[94] Zhang, J.; Li, S.; An, F.F.; Liu, J.; Jin, S.; Zhang, J.C.; Wang, P.C.; Zhang, X.; Lee, C.S.; Liang, X.J. Self-carried curcumin nanoparticles for *in vitro* and *in vivo* cancer therapy with real-time monitoring of drug release. *Nanoscale,* **2015,** *7*(32), 13503-13510.
[http://dx.doi.org/10.1039/C5NR03259H] [PMID: 26199064]

[95] Qin, S.Y.; Peng, M.Y.; Rong, L.; Li, B.; Wang, S.B.; Cheng, S.X.; Zhuo, R.X.; Zhang, X.Z. Self-defensive nano-assemblies from camptothecin-based antitumor drugs. *Regen. Biomater.,* **2015,** *2*(3), 159-166.
[http://dx.doi.org/10.1093/rb/rbv011] [PMID: 26816639]

[96] Li, W.; Zhang, X.; Hao, X.; Jie, J.; Tian, B.; Zhang, X. Shape design of high drug payload nanoparticles for more effective cancer therapy. *Chem. Commun.,* **2013,** *49*(93), 10989-10991.
[http://dx.doi.org/10.1039/c3cc46718j] [PMID: 24136236]

[97] Zhao, Y.; Zhao, Y.; Ma, Q.; Zhang, H.; Liu, Y.; Hong, J.; Ding, Z.; Liu, M.; Han, J. Novel carrier-free nanoparticles composed of 7-ethyl-10-hydroxycamptothecin and chlorin e6: Self-assembly mechanism investigation and *in vitro/in vivo* evaluation. *Colloids Surf. B Biointerfaces,* **2020,** *188*, 110722.
[http://dx.doi.org/10.1016/j.colsurfb.2019.110722] [PMID: 31887649]

[98] Guo, Y.; Zhao, S.; Qiu, H.; Wang, T.; Zhao, Y.; Han, M.; Dong, Z.; Wang, X. Shape of nanoparticles as a design parameter to improve docetaxel antitumor efficacy. *Bioconjug. Chem.,* **2018,** *29*(4), 1302-1311.
[http://dx.doi.org/10.1021/acs.bioconjchem.8b00059] [PMID: 29426226]

[99] Wen, Y.; Zhang, W.; Gong, N.; Wang, Y.F.; Guo, H.B.; Guo, W.; Wang, P.C.; Liang, X.J. Carrier-free, self-assembled pure drug nanorods composed of 10-hydroxycamptothecin and chlorin e6 for combinatorial chemo-photodynamic antitumor therapy *in vivo*. *Nanoscale,* **2017,** *9*(38), 14347-14356.
[http://dx.doi.org/10.1039/C7NR03129G] [PMID: 28731112]

[100] Zhang, X.; Li, N.; Zhang, S.; Sun, B.; Chen, Q.; He, Z.; Luo, C.; Sun, J. Emerging carrier□free nanosystems based on molecular self□assembly of pure drugs for cancer therapy. *Med. Res. Rev.,* **2020,** *40*(5), 1754-1775.
[http://dx.doi.org/10.1002/med.21669] [PMID: 32266734]

[101] Lin, J.; Li, C.; Guo, Y.; Zou, J.; Wu, P.; Liao, Y.; Zhang, B.; Le, J.; Zhao, R.; Shao, J.W. Carrier-free nanodrugs for *in vivo* NIR bioimaging and chemo-photothermal synergistic therapy. *J. Mater. Chem. B Mater. Biol. Med.,* **2019,** *7*(44), 6914-6923.
[http://dx.doi.org/10.1039/C9TB00687G] [PMID: 31482166]

[102] Li, Y.; Hu, X.; Zheng, X.; Liu, Y.; Liu, S.; Yue, Y.; Xie, Z. Self-assembled organic nanorods for dual chemo-photodynamic therapies. *RSC Advances,* **2018,** *8*(10), 5493-5499.
[http://dx.doi.org/10.1039/C8RA00067K] [PMID: 35542427]

[103] Li, Y.; Ayala-Orozco, C.; Rauta, P.R.; Krishnan, S. The application of nanotechnology in enhancing immunotherapy for cancer treatment: current effects and perspective. *Nanoscale,* **2019,** *11*(37), 17157-17178.
[http://dx.doi.org/10.1039/C9NR05371A] [PMID: 31531445]

[104] Zhu, Y.; Xing, L.; Zheng, X.; Yang, C.X.; He, Y.J.; Zhou, T.J.; Jin, Q.R.; Jiang, H.L. Amplification of tumor antigen presentation by NLGplatin to improve chemoimmunotherapy. *Int. J. Pharm.,* **2020,** *573*, 118736.
[http://dx.doi.org/10.1016/j.ijpharm.2019.118736] [PMID: 31756442]

[105] Saeed, M.; Gao, J.; Shi, Y.; Lammers, T.; Yu, H. Engineering Nanoparticles to Reprogram the Tumor Immune Microenvironment for Improved Cancer Immunotherapy. *Theranostics,* **2019,** *9*(26), 7981-8000.
[http://dx.doi.org/10.7150/thno.37568] [PMID: 31754376]

[106] Zhang, C.; Long, L.; Xiong, Y.; Wang, C.; Peng, C.; Yuan, Y.; Liu, Z.; Lin, Y.; Jia, Y.; Zhou, X.; Li, X. Facile engineering of indomethacin-induced paclitaxel nanocrystal aggregates as carrier-free nanomedicine with improved synergetic antitumor activity. *ACS Appl. Mater. Interfaces,* **2019,** *11*(10),

9872-9883.
[http://dx.doi.org/10.1021/acsami.8b22336] [PMID: 30767506]

[107] Feng, B.; Niu, Z.; Hou, B.; Zhou, L.; Li, Y.; Yu, H. Enhancing Triple Negative Breast Cancer Immunotherapy by ICG-Templated Self-Assembly of Paclitaxel Nanoparticles. *Adv. Funct. Mater.*, **2020**, *30*(6), 1906605.
[http://dx.doi.org/10.1002/adfm.201906605]

[108] Koseki, Y.; Ikuta, Y.; Taemaitree, F.; Saito, N.; Suzuki, R.; Dao, A.T.N.; Onodera, T.; Oikawa, H.; Kasai, H. Fabrication of size-controlled SN-38 pure drug nanocrystals through an ultrasound-assisted reprecipitation method toward efficient drug delivery for cancer treatment. *J. Cryst. Growth*, **2021**, *572*, 126265.
[http://dx.doi.org/10.1016/j.jcrysgro.2021.126265]

[109] Noda, K.; Nishiwaki, Y.; Kawahara, M.; Negoro, S.; Sugiura, T.; Yokoyama, A.; Fukuoka, M.; Mori, K.; Watanabe, K.; Tamura, T.; Yamamoto, S.; Saijo, N. Irinotecan plus cisplatin compared with etoposide plus cisplatin for extensive small-cell lung cancer. *N. Engl. J. Med.*, **2002**, *346*(2), 85-91.
[http://dx.doi.org/10.1056/NEJMoa003034] [PMID: 11784874]

[110] Kunimoto, T.; Nitta, K.; Tanaka, T.; Uehara, N.; Baba, H.; Takeuchi, M.; Yokokura, T.; Sawada, S.; Miyasaka, T.; Mutai, M. Antitumor activity of 7-ethyl-10-[4-(1-piperidino)-1-piperidino]carb-nyloxy-camptothec in, a novel water-soluble derivative of camptothecin, against murine tumors. *Cancer Res.*, **1987**, *47*(22), 5944-5947.
[PMID: 3664496]

[111] Azam, A.; Ahmed, A.S.; Oves, M.; Khan, M.S.; Habib, S.S.; Memic, A. Antimicrobial activity of metal oxide nanoparticles against Gram-positive and Gram-negative bacteria: a comparative study. *Int. J. Nanomedicine*, **2012**, *7*, 6003-6009.
[http://dx.doi.org/10.2147/IJN.S35347] [PMID: 23233805]

[112] Besinis, A.; De Peralta, T.; Handy, R.D. The antibacterial effects of silver, titanium dioxide and silica dioxide nanoparticles compared to the dental disinfectant chlorhexidine on *Streptococcus mutans* using a suite of bioassays. *Nanotoxicology*, **2014**, *8*(1), 1-16.
[http://dx.doi.org/10.3109/17435390.2012.742935] [PMID: 23092443]

[113] Zarrindokht, E-K.; Pegah, C. Antibacterial activity of ZnO nanoparticle on gram-positive and gram-negative bacteria. *Afr. J. Microbiol. Res.*, **2011**, *5*(12), 1368-1373.

[114] Martinez, A.J.; Visvesvara, G.S. Free-living, amphizoic and opportunistic amebas. *Brain Pathol.*, **1997**, *7*(1), 583-598.
[http://dx.doi.org/10.1111/j.1750-3639.1997.tb01076.x] [PMID: 9034567]

[115] Schuster, F.; Visvesvara, G.S. Opportunistic amoebae: challenges in prophylaxis and treatment. *Drug Resist. Updat.*, **2004**, *7*(1), 41-51.
[http://dx.doi.org/10.1016/j.drup.2004.01.002] [PMID: 15072770]

[116] Anwar, A.; Mungroo, M.R.; Anwar, A.; Sullivan, W.J., Jr; Khan, N.A.; Siddiqui, R. Repositioning of Guanabenz in Conjugation with Gold and Silver Nanoparticles against Pathogenic Amoebae *Acanthamoeba castellanii* and *Naegleria fowleri*. *ACS Infect. Dis.*, **2019**, *5*(12), 2039-2046.
[http://dx.doi.org/10.1021/acsinfecdis.9b00263] [PMID: 31612700]

[117] Aggarwal, B. B.; Kumar, A.; Bharti, A. C. *Anticancer potential of curcumin: Preclinical and clinical studies.*, *Anticancer research*, **2003**, *23*(1/A), 363-398.

[118] Anand, P.; Kunnumakkara, A.B.; Newman, R.A.; Aggarwal, B.B. Bioavailability of curcumin: Problems and promises. *Mol. Pharm.*, **2007**, *4*(6), 807-818.
[http://dx.doi.org/10.1021/mp700113r] [PMID: 17999464]

[119] Mungroo, M.R.; Anwar, A.; Khan, N.A.; Siddiqui, R. Gold-Conjugated Curcumin as a Novel Therapeutic Agent against Brain-Eating Amoebae. *ACS Omega*, **2020**, *5*(21), 12467-12475.
[http://dx.doi.org/10.1021/acsomega.0c01305] [PMID: 32548431]

[120] Sathiyaseelan, A.; Saravanakumar, K.; Mariadoss, A.V.A.; Wang, M.H. Biocompatible fungal chitosan encapsulated phytogenic silver nanoparticles enhanced antidiabetic, antioxidant and antibacterial activity. *Int. J. Biol. Macromol.,* **2020**, *153*, 63-71.
[http://dx.doi.org/10.1016/j.ijbiomac.2020.02.291] [PMID: 32112842]

CHAPTER 3

Development of Nanomaterials as Drug Candidates

Abstract: Nanomaterials, with their unique therapeutic traits such as antioxidant, anti-inflammatory, antibacterial, antiviral, and anticancer properties, can be used as drug candidates to treat a wide range of diseases. Nano complexes like dendrimers, carbon nanotubes, fullerenes, graphene-based nanomaterials, carbon quantum dots, nanohydrogels, peptide nanostructures, MXenes, Silicene, and Antimonene have been distinguished by researchers, among the many nanomaterials because of their lower toxicity, ease of tuning to the desired end use, complex interactions with biological macromolecules, and solubility properties. This chapter will present the most recent research details on nanomaterials that have been developed as therapeutic candidates to treat a number of illnesses.

Keywords: Dendrimers, Fullerenes, Graphene based nanomaterials, Peptide nanostructures, Nano-drug candidates, Nanohydrogels.

1. INTRODUCTION

Contemporary processes of discovering and developing drugs encompass a progression of consecutive steps, commencing with fundamental research and advancing towards targeted activities, ultimately resulting in the creation of novel medications for addressing human ailments. A potential drug must fulfil precise requirements, such as selectively binding to the intended receptor site, triggering the desired functional response, ensuring proper bioavailability and distribution in the body, and exhibiting the desired effects in animal models of human diseases without causing toxicity. Additionally, a molecule must meet fundamental criteria for future production and storage to be considered a viable drug candidate.

Nanomaterials fulfilling most of the above criteria can be employed as medication candidates to treat a variety of diseases and ailments due to their special intrinsic therapeutic capabilities, such as antioxidant, anti-inflammatory, antibacterial, antiviral, and anticancer properties. The physicochemical properties of these nanodrug candidates, such as size, hydrophobicity, and surface charge, have proven to increase the cellular uptake than larger ones.

Nano complexes like dendrimers, carbon nanotubes, fullerenes, graphene-based nanomaterials, carbon quantum dots, nanohydrogels, peptide nanostructures,

Laksiri Weerasinghe, Imalka Munaweera and Senuri Kumarage

MXenes, silicene, and antimonene have been distinguished by researchers, among the many nanomaterials because of their lower toxicity, ease of tuning to the desired end use, complex interactions with biological macromolecules, and solubility properties. This chapter will focus on the most recent research details on nanomaterials that have been developed as therapeutic candidates to treat a number of illnesses.

2. DENDRIMERS

Multidrug-resistant bacterial infections have the potential to become the leading cause of mortality by 2050 [1]. A potential alternative infection control method is the development of antibacterial dendritic polymers. Development of antibacterial dendritic polymers is the potential alternative infection control method. The class of synthetic polymers known as dendrimers is notable for its typical symmetry, high branching, and monodispersed nature. There is an enormous potential of their usage in medicinal applications because of their distinctive characteristics, which include condensed branching structures with exact control of the size, form, and various functional groups on their outer layer. It has been demonstrated that the quantity of ligands on their outer shell has a considerable impact on inhibiting the multivalent adhesion activities of viruses, bacteria, cells, proteins, and combinations. Their branching architecture appears to be crucial to their use. Dendrimers can be used as medications because of their extensive and multifaceted interactions with biological macromolecules as well as their higher binding affinities. Multivalent substitutions in dendrimers are a powerful alternative for single molecular drugs [2].

Dendrimers offer a platform for antibacterial agents and antiviral agents. The permeabilization of bacterial membranes over the time and rupturing their lipid bilayer *via* the electrostatic attraction between the positively charged dendrimer and the negative surface of the bacterium could be the reason for the underlying antibacterial activity. This means that, like other antimicrobial materials, the positive charge multivalency of high-generation cationic dendrimers is a critical factor in determining their antibacterial efficacy [3]. The most extensively studied antibacterial dendrimer is poly(amidoamine) (PAMAM) (Fig. **1**). For instance, a recent study evaluated the connection between dendrimer formation and dendrimer charge type when used against *S. aureus* [4]. Here, antibacterial experiments were performed on three different types of polyanionic dendrimers, including those with the terminal groups; succinamic acid, sodium carboxylate, and hydroxyl, as well as polycationic dendrimers with primary amine ended PMAM, to assess their inhibitory zone and antibacterial activity. Anionic dendrimers were weaker than cationic dendrimers in terms of potency. Primary amine dendrimers with the formula $G(5)-128NH_2$ and $G(4)-64NH_2$ had the greatest inhibition, respectively. The effects of succinamic acid carboxylate, and hydroxyl dendrimers were weaker.

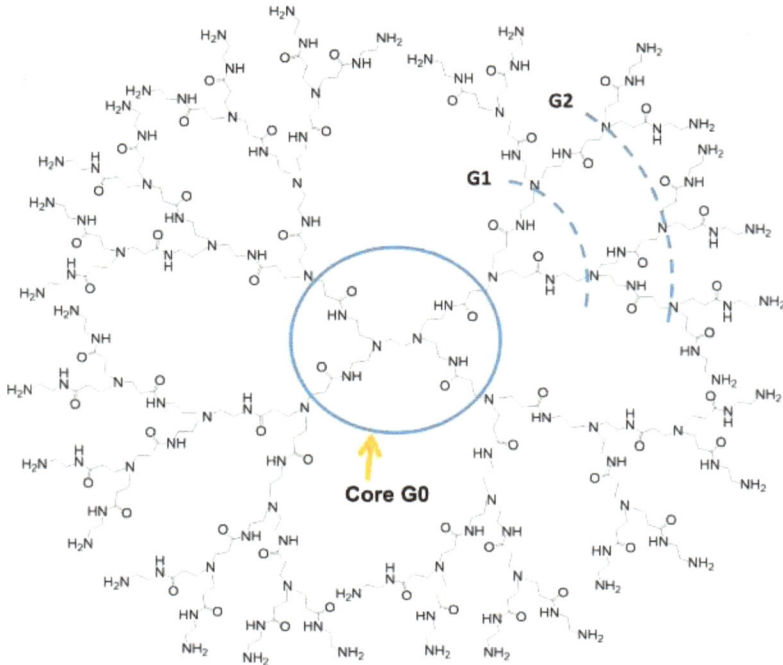

Fig. (1). Generation 2 (G2) PAMAM dendrimer.

In a recent study, the role of several peripheral groups in dendrimer penetration into *P. aeruginosa* biofilms was examined [1]. At the beginning, the penetration of the dendrimers with NH_3^+ groups at their periphery to the acidic environment of *P. aeruginosa* biofilms was faster than those with OH^- or COO^- groups. Additionally, the negatively charged biofilm components and the peripherally charged dendrimers with NH_3^+ developed an electrostatic attraction that allowed the dendrimer to accumulate close to the top of the biofilm. Dendrimers containing peripheral OH- and COO- groups, however, accumulate more strongly and uniformly throughout the biofilm depth, compared to NH_3^+ based dendrimers. The surface composition of dendrimers regulates the depth of penetration and accumulation in biofilms. This finding will have significant implications for the ongoing development of new antibacterial or antimicrobial-carrying polymers [1].

Since cationic dendrimers are harmful to mammalian cells, nitric oxide (NO)-releasing dendrimers were developed in order to lower the concentration of cationic dendrimers while maintaining enough antibacterial activity. This preserved the antibacterial effect while significantly reducing toxicity on eukaryotic cells [5]. With PEGylation, the cationic dendrimers undergo a significant reduction in toxicity but with a decrease in their antimicrobial effectiveness. For instance PEGylated PAMAM exhibited a reduction in the antibacterial activity against *P. aeruginosa* [6]. This was explained with a decline in the charge density due to the reduction of cationic amine groups and masking of positive charges by the PEG chains, resulting in the decrease of the electrostatic interactions with the negatively charged bacterial surfaces. Similarly PEGylated carbosilane dendrimers also showed a decrease in antimicrobial activity against *P. aeruginosa,* when compared to non-functionalized carbosilane dendrimers [7].

Recently, the antibacterial efficacy of poly (aryl ether) PAMAM-based amphiphilic dendrimers was examined against *E. coli* and *S. aureus.* These dendrimers had various terminal spacers (including amines, esters, and hydrazine units), varying hydrophobicity, and a strong tendency to self-assemble. In terms of antibacterial potency, the amine-terminated dendrimer performed better than the other three dendrimers under investigation. Furthermore, the complete mechanistic investigation shows that the correct tuning of the hydrophobicity of amphiphilic dendrimers considerably facilitates bacterial membrane breakdown. Increased surface cationic charges showed a higher minimum inhibitory concentration (MIC), and the ratio of surface cationic charge to hydrophobicity significantly affected the antibacterial activity [8]. Anionic dendrimers have less potent antibacterial effects, but they have been used in conjunction with cationic dendrimers and in synergy with antibiotics to minimize the dosage of the medication [9].

Additionally, a number of dendrimer-based systems demonstrated antiviral activities by blocking the interaction between gp120, CD4 and CCR5 to prevent viral entry and replication or by specifically targeting late stages of viral replication [10]. Dendrimers are the only nano tool that has proceeded to human clinical trials as topical microbicides to combat HIV-1 transmission [11]. Astodrimer sodium (SPL7013), a generation-four lysine dendrimer with a polyanionic surface charge, has demonstrated activity against enveloped and non-enveloped viruses such as human immunodeficiency virus-1 (HIV-1), herpes simplex virus (HSV)-1 and 2, H1N1 and H3N2 influenza viruses, human respiratory syncytial virus (HRSV), and human papillomavirus (HPV) [12]. Antibacterial characteristics are likewise possessed by astodrimer sodium. In phase 2 and large phase 3 studies for the treatment and prevention of bacterial vaginosis (BV), Astodrimer 1% Gel (10 mg/mL astodrimer sodium) administered vaginally was demonstrated to be safe and effective [13 - 15] and is marketed in Europe, Australia, New Zealand and several countries in Asia. Antiviral efficacy of SPL7013 against SARS-CoV-2 has also recently been assessed [12].

Another study synthesized novel dendrimers with various amino acids (aromatic and non-aromatic), tryptamine (a "decarboxylated" analogue of Trp), and N-methyl Trp on the exterior in order to examine the relationship between the amino acid structure and antiviral activity [16]. While dendrimers with tyrosine had the strongest antiviral activity against EV71, dendrimers with N-Methyl Trp were the most effective against HIV-1 and HIV-2. Human cytomegalovirus (HCMV) and herpes simplex virus 2 (HSV-2) infections are both inhibited by PEGylated cationic carbosilane dendrimers, which have also demonstrated a significant level of antiviral efficacy [17].

3. CARBON BASED NANOPARTICLES

Carbon nanomaterials(CNMs) such as carbon nanotubes, graphene/graphene oxide, fullerenes, and carbon quantum dots (QDs) as an emerging class of novel materials, can exhibit considerable antimicrobial, anti-inflammatory and anticancer properties. These nanomaterials have attracted a great deal of interest due to their broad efficiency and novel features. The most important factor affecting the antimicrobial activity of CNMs is their size. Smaller particles with a higher surface to volume ratio can easily attach onto microbial cells and affect their cell membrane integrity, metabolic procedures, and structural components. As these unique characteristics are found in CNMs, a wide range of possibilities have been raised in terms of antimicrobial applications. In addition, CNMs such as QDs have shown their potential in tumour treatments as well.

3.1. Carbon Nanotubes

Three categories—single-walled carbon nanotubes (SWCNTs), double-walled carbon nanotubes (DWCNTs), and multi-walled carbon nanotubes (MWCNTs)—are distinguished by the structures of carbon nanotubes, which are made up of single, double, and multiple layers of graphene cylinders, respectively (Fig. **2**) [18].

Several studies indicate that SWCNTs can have outstanding antimicrobial activity. In reality, the size of these compounds plays a significant role in the deactivation of microbes. The bacteriostatic properties of carbon nanotubes have been explained as arising from direct contact-induced damage to microorganisms' cell membranes, leading to the fatality of the bacteria. Microorganisms that were incubated with carbon nanotubes underwent morphological changes that were linked to a loss of cellular integrity. Furthermore, it has been noted that exposure to small CNTs increases the efflux of plasmid DNA by five times, RNA by two times, and cytoplasmic material by two times [20]. An expanding field of research is examining the bacteriostatic properties of carbon nanotubes (CNTs), which are attributed to their large inner volume and high surface/volume ratio.

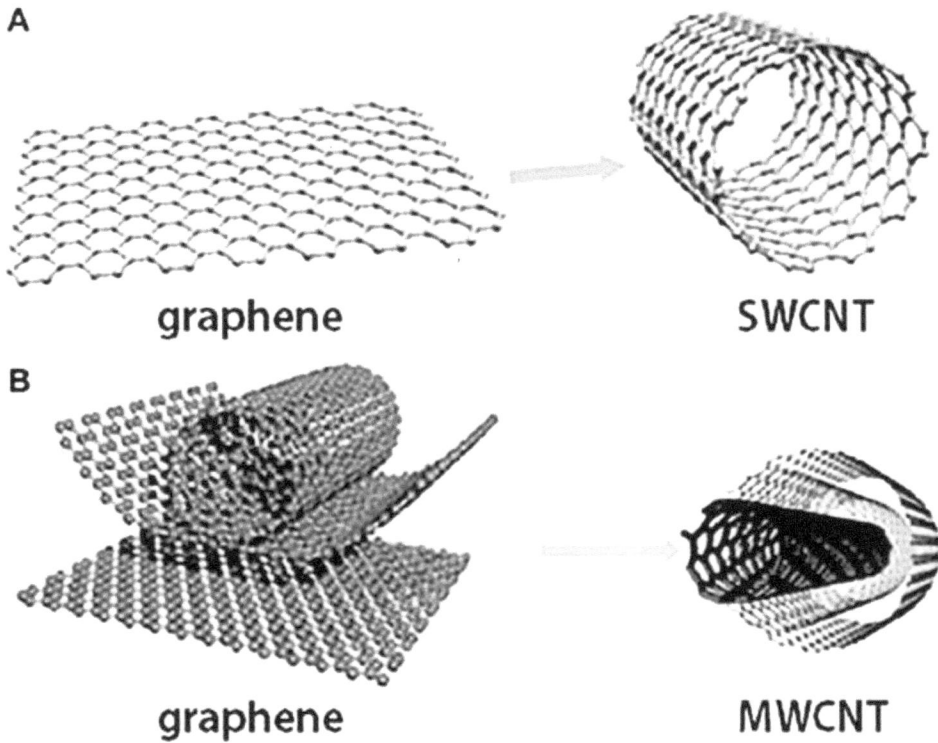

Fig. (2). Graphene and carbon nanotubes as (A) single wall carbon nanotube (SWCNT) and (B) multi-wall carbon nanotube (MWCNT) structures. Reprinted with permission from [19] **Copyright** © 2014 of Vidu *et al*. published by Frontiers Media SA and distributed under the terms of the Creative Commons Attribution License (CC BY).

When MWCNTs and SWCNTs were compared to *E. coli* for their antimicrobial qualities, it was discovered that SWCNTs were significantly more toxic to the microorganisms and that their surface was more active against them [21]. Thus, the diameter of the CNTs plays a significant role in the direct contact deactivation of microbial cells. The significantly increased cytotoxicity of SWCNTs was interconnected with changes in stress-related gene expression in addition to cell damage. The greater surface area that SWCNTs can contact with a cell surface, their improved penetration into the cell wall due to their smaller diameter, and their distinct chemical and electrical properties, all contribute to their enhanced cytotoxicity [21]. The activity of MWCNTs and SWNTs against bacilli and cocci differs despite having the same surface functionalities (-OH and -COOH). Although MWCNTs lack bacteriostatic qualities, SWCNTs with the same functional groups have potent antimicrobial capabilities against both Gram-positive and Gram-negative bacteria [22]. In addition to their size, the CNTs' surface charge greatly influences their antibacterial capabilities. Their ability to compromise the integrity of the cell membrane is the basis for this process. Reactive oxygen species (ROS), such as hydroxyl radicals, were produced by the negatively and positively charged CNTs, giving them superior antibacterial properties [18].

Because of their physicochemical properties and morphology, MWCNTs have also demonstrated intrinsic anti-proliferative, cytotoxic, and anti-migratory effects *in vitro*, conferring MWCNTs remarkable biomimicry, which allows them to associate with a number of the natural intracellular nano filaments such as actin or microtubules that can be used to destroy cancer [23]. These properties along with the ability to generate oxidative stress in cells can be exploited to defeat cancer. Numerous studies have shown that MWCNTs cause a variety of mitotic abnormalities, including aberrant spindles, chromosomal mal-segregation, and clastogenic effects. They also hinder cell migration and ultimately cause cell death in a variety of cell types, including cancer cells [24 - 26]. According to García-Hevia *et al.*, MWCNTs can cause strong anti-tumoural effects *in vivo* in solid malignant melanomas that are created by allograft transplantation, and these effects can persist even in solid melanomas that are created from cells resistant to paclitaxel [23]. These filaments have the ability to migrate within cultured cells and combine with the cytoskeleton's protein nanofibers to disrupt the biomechanics of cell division, simulating the action of conventional anti-cancer medications that bind to microtubules, like paclitaxel.

Benko *et al.*, also accessed the cytocompatibility, anticancer, antibacterial and ant-inflammatory properties of four types of highly dispersible MWCNTs of similar dimensions, but slightly different chemical compositions compared with unmodified MWCNTs [27]. They synthesized HO (highly oxidized CNTs with a high share of –C=O bonds), LO (low oxidized CNTs with a high share of –C–O bonds), HNH (highly oxidized and ammonia-modified CNTs) and LNH (low oxidized and ammonia-modified CNTs). It was discovered that even slight alterations in the chemical makeup had a significant impact on the CNTs' biological activity. In particular, CNTs with a high carbon atom count and a +2 coordination number caused cytotoxicity in melanoma and macrophage cells. They also demonstrated a moderate antibacterial effect against strains of both Gram-positive (*S. aureus*) and Gram-negative (*E. coli*) bacteria, but remained cytocompatible with human dermal fibroblasts. However, ammonia substitution of some OH groups reduced the cytotoxicity against macrophages without compromising any other beneficial properties. In addition, CNTs with a high +3 coordination number of carbon atoms exhibited high intrinsic cytocompatibility towards normal healthy cells but exhibited toxicity towards bacteria and cancer cells.

3.2. Fullerenes

Fullerene, the third allotropic form of carbon, is composed of closed-cavity molecules with an even number of carbon atoms in the sp2 hybridised state [1]. In addition to the most known fullerenes with 60 and 70 carbon atoms, there are more "higher" fullerenes with more atoms. Due to their abundance, the physicochemical characteristics of C_{60} fullerene and its derivatives, as well as their influence on biological processes, have received the greatest attention. Fullerene has the lowest toxicity among carbon nanomaterials, including graphene, MWCNTs, SWCNTs, and carbon dots [28]. After oral exposure, fullerenes showed very low toxicity, and *in vitro* tests revealed no mutagenic or genotoxic potential. Since pristine fullerenes are only partially absorbed from the gut, no toxicity is anticipated even after repeated exposure. Application of C_{60} in biological processes is constrained by the fact that it is insoluble in water [29]. But functionalized fullerenes with higher solubility might exhibit distinct features when used *in vivo* [30]. According to the reported literature, fullerene and its derivatives have medicinal properties such as antioxidant [31, 32], anti-inflammatory [33], antibacterial [18], and antiviral [34] properties. It is feasible to accurately "tune" the structure of fullerene derivatives in drug discovery in order to produce a therapeutic compound with a specific biological function.

Six categories have been established by Yang Xu *et al.* for fullerene derivatives: (1) amino acid, peptide, and primary amine derivatives; (2) piperazine and pyrrolidine derivatives; (3) carboxyl derivatives; (4) hydroxyl derivatives; (5) glycofullerene derivatives; and (6) fullerene complexes [35]. Most research focuses exclusively on chemically modified fullerenes that are extremely water-soluble (dendrofullerenes and fullerenols) (Fig. **3**), despite the fact that polyhydroxylation, in particular, is known to limit the capacity of fullerenes to interact with free radicals [36, 37].

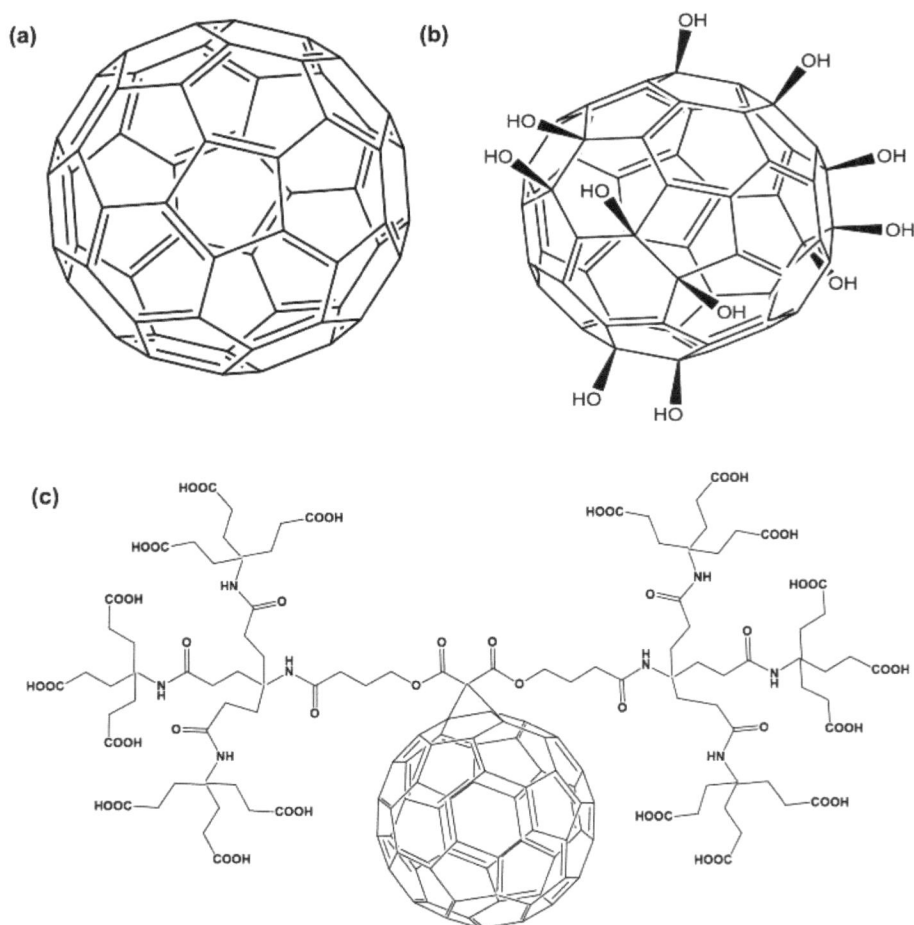

Fig. (3). (a) Fullerene, (b) fullerenol and (c) dendrofullerene.

The antioxidant activity of fullerenes is based on their abundance of conjugated double bonds and their low-lying, lowest unoccupied molecular orbital (LUMO), which is easily accessible to an electron and highly conducive to attack by radical species. One C_{60} molecule has reportedly acquired up to 34 methyl radical additions. It appears that this quenching procedure is catalytic. To put it another way, fullerene may interact with a variety of superoxides without being consumed. Due to this characteristic, fullerenes are known as radical sponges and are speculated to be the most effective radical scavenger in the world [38]. The capacity of fullerenes to localize inside the cell to mitochondria and other cell compartment locations, where the formation of free radicals occurs in diseased states, is its main benefit as a medicinal antioxidant. Namdar *et al.* discovered that fullerene C_{60} nanoparticles boost the antioxidant capacity of the brain and liver *via* increasing catalase activity [39]. As a result, fullerene C_{60} can be employed to protect the brain and liver from ROS buildup and oxidative stress in a variety of clinical circumstances.

When exposed to ionizing radiation, unmodified hydrated C_{60} fullerene molecules (C_{60}UHFM) were shown to inhibit the generation of ROS in water and 8-oxoguanine in DNA [40]. Long-lived protein radicals that form after irradiation are effectively eliminated by C_{60}UHFM. In a study, it was discovered that administering C_{60}UHFM intravenously 1 hour prior to exposure to ionizing radiation significantly lessened the severity of radiation-induced leukopenia and thrombocytopenia, decreased the amount of visceral haemorrhages, and protected small intestine of mice from radiation damage. Consequently, C_{60}UHFM is a strong antiradical, a potential radioprotector, and a proactive treatment for radiation-induced leuko and thrombocytopenia. It was discovered that the radioprotective qualities of C_{60}UHFM significantly outperformed those of fullerenol ($C_{60}(OH)_{24}$) and dendrofullerene.

ROS and oxidative stress are responsible for the emergence of insulin resistance, the dysfunction of pancreatic cells, and an increase in the production and utilisation of glucose in the liver [41, 42]. Therefore, water-soluble penta amino-acid derivatives of fullerene C_{60} (PDF) are being researched as potential drugs for the treatment of type-2 diabetes mellitus, and Soldatova *et al.* provided the first evidence of the antioxidant and antiglycation activity of PDFS [43]. The fullerenylpenta-N-pentaamino-acid derivatives of fullerene C_{60} that include amino succinic acid and the potassium salt of fullerenylpenta-N-3-hydroxy-L-tyrosine are the most potent antioxidants.

In hydrophilic environments, traces of hydrophobic C_{60} have been found to induce powerful anti-inflammatory and antioxidant effects in cells and animals. A novel anti-inflammatory and antioxidant medication candidate is C_{60} dissolved in grape seed oil. In freshly isolated human neutrophils, it prevented the production of tumour necrosis factor-α (TNF-α), cell migration, phagocytosis, and respiratory burst. Additionally, superoxide and 1,1-diphenyl-2-trinitrophenylhydrazine free radicals were significantly scavenged by the trace amount of C_{60} dissolved in grape seed oil. CRP, a blood inflammatory marker, was significantly lowered in beagle dogs after the oral administration of C_{60} dissolved in the grape seed oil [33].

Aqueous dispersion of unmodified C_{60} and its amine derivatives were tested for their antiviral efficacy against human cytomegalovirus (HCMV) and herpes simplex virus type 1 (HSV-1) infections [44]. In every test, C_{60} outperformed both

C_{60} derivatives and even Acyclovir in terms of *in vivo* antiviral effectiveness, with significantly reduced cytotoxicity that prevented HSV-1 and HCMV infections *in vitro* and suppressed HSV-1 activity through the virucidal impact. Fullerenes and their derivatives have potent HIV-inhibitory actions against [45] influenza virus [46], Ebola virus [47] and other viruses *in vitro* and *in vivo*. As a novel family of broad-spectrum antiviral medications, fullerenes and their derivatives have drawn considerable interest as a possible treatment for SARS-CoV-2 [48 - 50].

3.3. Graphene Oxide and Derivatives

The remarkable mechanical, electrical, and piezoelectric properties of GO have drawn considerable attention from researchers of many fields. GO is made up of a thin sheet of carbon atoms arranged in a beautiful six-sided hexagonal pattern. Large exact floor area, high electric mobility, and great conductivity are all characteristics of GO. In order to be effective against bacteria and viruses, GO displays a number of functional clusters on its edges and functional groups that include oxygen [51, 52].

By producing ROS and inducing physical and chemical oxidation in microorganism cell walls and membranes, graphene oxide (GO) and its derivatives reduce microbial resistance and cause microbial mortality [53, 54]. The literature has outlined three key antibacterial mechanisms of GO (Fig. **4**). The most frequent process is membrane stress, which occurs when microbes come into contact with GO sheets and their sharp edges. This physical damage results in cellular components leaking into the environment and microbial death. This phenomenon is also known as the nanoknife or nanoblade effect [55 - 57]. In other instances, GO results in oxidative stress that may be brought on by reactive oxygen species (ROS), which can damage microbial DNA and induce mitochondrial malfunction, both of which restrict bacterial growth [58]. The process for wrapping or trapping bacteria is dependent on separating them from their natural surroundings. These GO flakes cover the bacteria, preventing them from interacting with their surroundings and preventing bacterial growth and nutrition uptake [59]. The antibacterial patterns of GO against gram positive bacteria and gram negative bacteria were notably different: gram-positive *S. Aureus* was generally captured, whereas gram-negative *E. coli* and *Pseudomonas aeruginosa* were predominantly terminated by direct contact [60].

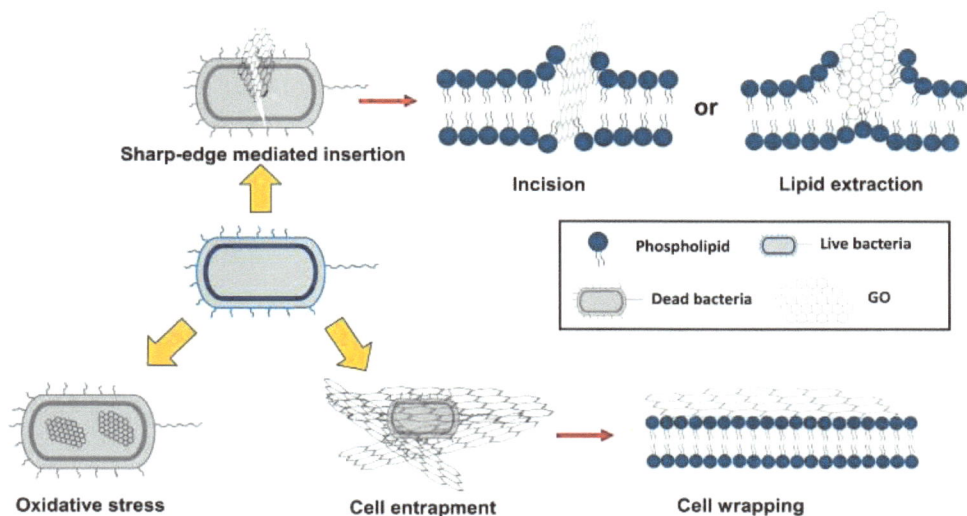

Fig. (4). Different antibacterial mechanisms of graphene derivatives.

A significant quantity of phospholipids may be extracted from the *Escherichia coli* (*E. coli*) cell membrane by insertion of graphene nanosheets into or cutting through the cell membrane. This procedure causes the *E. coli* membrane to degrade, which lowers the viability of bacteria [61]. The antibacterial activity of both GO and rGO is time and concentration-dependent [62]. Liu *et al.* performed a comparison of the antibacterial properties of GO and rGO [63]. They investigated the influence of concentration and incubation duration on microbiological viability loss and discovered that GO had a greater antibacterial action than rGO. Higher concentrations and incubation time increased antibacterial activity of GO more than rGO. They also examined the electron micrograph patterns for GO and rGO against *E. coli* and discovered that a thin coating of GO can disrupt cell integrity, whereas *E. coli* cells get trapped in the rGO.

By using the superficial bioreduction of graphene oxide (GO), viruses may be successfully captured, their surface proteins destroyed, and viral RNA extracted in an aqueous environment. These events show that GO has enormous promise for preventing environmental infections and that it is an effective nanomaterial for high-throughput viral detection and disinfection [64]. A variety of graphene derivatives with specified polyglycerol sulfate and fatty amine functionalities were produced in another study, and their interactions with HSV-1 were studied [65]. This research demonstrated that antiviral drugs against HSV-1 may be generated by controlled and stepwise functionalization of graphene sheets, which might lead to the development of antiviral medicines for future biological uses. Graphene binds to viruses by electrostatic interactions with polyglycerol sulfate, and hydrophobic interactions between alkyl chains further enhance antiviral effectiveness. There have been multiple reviews on the potential of graphene, GO, and graphene oxide compounds (Fig. **5**) to combat SARS-CoV-2 due to their antiviral capabilities [51, 66].

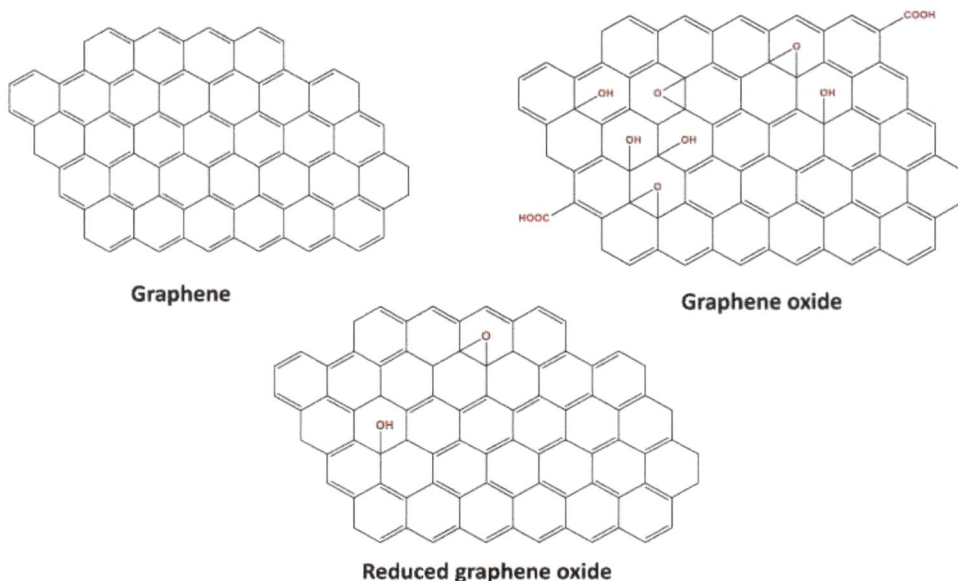

Graphene

Graphene oxide

Reduced graphene oxide

Fig. (5). Graphene and its derivatives including graphene oxide and reduced graphene oxide.

3.4. Carbon Quantum Dots

Carbon quantum dots (CQDs) are recognized as an essential nanomaterial and have drawn a lot of interest because of their special qualities, which include good solubility, favourable biocompatibility, and flexibility in surface modification [67].

Since CQDs are not likely to cause bacterial resistance, they are among the NPs with membrane-disruptive activity through a variety of mechanisms, including the oxidation of reactive oxygen species (ROS) and the effects of cations on membrane destruction. These combined mechanisms of action may even enhance their antimicrobial activity [68]. Recent studies have revealed that the hydrophilic CQDs have a large number of hydroxyl groups on their surface, which facilitate their coupling with bacteria and biofilm [69]. It has also been demonstrated that some hydrophobic CQDs have apparent antibiofilm action, which is attributed to the adherence of long surface alkyl chains to bacteria and strong, positively-charged quaternary ammonium groups [70]. Amphipathic CQDs generated from antibacterial peptides have been produced to provide CQDs with superior antibacterial efficacy and cytocompatibility for bacterial infections. CQDs with amphipathic properties, derived from hydrophilic lysine or arginine and hydrophobic tryptophan (Lys/Trp-CQDs and Arg/Trp-CQDs), have demonstrated effective bacterial membrane destruction without developing resistance, antibiofilm properties against *Staphylococcus aureus*, and good *in vitro* biocompatibility [68]. According to a study, the bactericidal activity of CQDs has been suggested to be caused by a combination of processes, including the oxidation of excess intracellular ROS, the fusing of hydrophobic groups, and the electrostatic contact of cationic residues. Furthermore, the *in vitro* cytotoxicity assessment has shown that the produced CQDs exhibit high hemocompatibility and cytocompatibility.

The inherent antitumor properties of as-prepared 1,7′-Dimethyl-2′-propyl-1H-3′H-[2,5′]bibenzoimidazolyl based CQDs have been tested, and the results indicated that CQDs have a significant anti-cancer effect against breast cancer cell lines *in vitro* and also demonstrate specificity of action against tumour cells in *ex ovo* chick chorioallantoic membrane (CAM), which was used as an *in vivo* model to investigate the differential action of CQDs. The results of this study indicated that CQDs have the least amount of cytotoxicity toward normal cells, which is consistent with the *in vitro* study that was conducted to examine their activity on red blood cells (RBCs) and white blood cells (WBCs) [71]. As-prepared CQDs have distinct cell behaviour, exhibiting minimal cytotoxicity on normal host cells such as RBCs, WBCs, and embryonic cells and a high specificity of action against tumour cells. This work demonstrates unequivocally that carbon dots can treat tumours using an *ex ovo* model. CQDs are, therefore, viable substitutes for cancer treatment. Accordingly they have postulated that CQDs may interact with cell membrane receptors found on tumour cells, such as nuclear antigens, tumour markers expressed only on the membrane of the tumour cell. Consequently, in both *in vitro* and *ex ovo* procedures, this might be the cause of cell disruption in tumour cells without having a negative impact on healthy cells. Comparing CQDs with Aspirin, the latter drug caused 12.45% hemolysis in RBCs and 11.25% toxicity in WBCs at the highest concentration of 150 μg/mL, while CQDs showed the least amount of toxicity on both RBCs and WBCs cells, exhibiting a toxicity of 11.32% and 6.83% on RBCs and WBCs, respectively. These results suggest that CQDs are safe for use against regular eukaryotic cells. Additionally, despite their restricted capacity to produce $^1O_2$, it has been demonstrated that certain CQDs can be employed as photosensitizers (PSs) in photodynamic therapy (PDT), in which PSs are able to transmit light energy to nearby oxygen, thereby inducing the production of reactive oxygen ($^1O_2$), including singlet oxygen, which is used to eradicate tumours [67]. Porphyrin-Based Carbon Dots, for example, have demonstrated strong cytotoxicity upon irradiation, high photostability, biocompatibility, and cellular uptake. The efficacious *in vivo* treatment outcomes confirm that Porphyrin-Based CDs may effectively inhibit the growth of solid tumours [72].

4. NANOHYDROGEL

Hydrogels are three-dimensional (3D) polymeric networks that can contain a high quantity of water yet, they will not dissolve in aqueous environments owing to fundamental crosslinks in their structures. Pharmaceutical industry is seeing an increase in the use of nanohydrogels, which combine hydrogel qualities such as hydrophilicity and flexibility (which may be cast into any shape or form), versatility, rapid water absorption, and prolonged holding capacity with nanoparticulate properties. Nanohydrogels have been created using a variety of natural, synthetic, and hybrid polymers [73].

Hydrogels are commonly used in wound healing as advanced moisture donor dressings, enhancing collagenase synthesis and autolytic debridement [74 - 76]. They improve oxygen delivery to the wounds and allow exudate absorption and retention within the gel mass [77]. Furthermore, hydrogels can provide antimicrobial properties, preventing or reducing the formation of microbial infections, which are one of the key issues associated with wound healing [78].

Natural hydrogels are regarded as beneficial biomaterials because they effectively prevent bacterial infections. Chitosan, which is a natural polymer derived from chitin, is one of the most prominent and most frequently studied natural polysaccharide hydrogels. Although there are several antimicrobial mechanisms suggested for chitosan, electrostatic interactions with microbial surfaces and consequent cell rupture are the most frequently cited and suggested mechanisms. At pHs below 6, chitosan polymers possess a positive charge with the presence of amine groups. Hence it can electrostatically interact with negatively charged regions on the microbial membrane [79], thereby binding and interfering with the bacterial membrane's normal processes by causing the leakage of internal components and impeding the transfer of nutrients into the cells [80, 81]. As indicated by several research, some antibacterial and antifungal actions of chitosan are dependent on both of its inherent physicochemical qualities (such as molecular weight, degree of deacetylation, and hydrophobicity) and external variables (such as the pH of the medium, concentration, and species of bacteria) [82 - 84]. It was proposed that chitosan may impact the permeability of the outer membrane in Gram-negative bacteria by generating ionic connections that stop nutrients from entering the cell and raise internal osmotic pressure [85]. Another suggested antibacterial mechanism is the chelation of amino groups with Ca^{2+} or Mg^{2+} present in the cell walls. The bonds formed will impede the toxin production, inhibiting the microbial growth [86].

An injectable hydrogel with effective antibacterial properties against Gram-positive and Gram-negative bacteria was made from two natural polymers, chitosan and konjac glucomannan, which were linked together by Schiff base connections by Chen *et al.* [87]. The hydrogel exhibited a killing efficiency of 96% and 98% was exhibited against Gram-positive *Staphylococcus aureus* and Gram-negative *Escherichia coli* bacteria, respectively. A semi interpenetrating hydrogel was synthesised by mixing chitosan and bacterial cellulose and their subsequent cross-linking with glutaraldehyde. The hydrogel showed antibacterial activity which was dependent on the chitosan-to-cellulose ratio and was effective towards both gram negative and gram positive bacteria [88].

Plant-based bioactive compounds have been utilised to treat diseases brought on by pathogenic bacteria, as well as to replace chemically produced medications and decrease their side effects. In this case, researchers have employed essential oil nanohydrogels as an alternative source of the antimicrobial substance. An *Azadirachta indica* oil nanohydrogel was created by Kaur *et al.*, and it demonstrated promising antibacterial action against *S. aureus*, *E. coli*, and *C. albicans* with minimum inhibitory, bactericidal, and fungicidal concentrations ranging from 6.25 to 3.125 (g/mL) [89]. The albumin protein denaturation assay using the nanohydrogel demonstrated 50.23-82.57% inhibition compared to standard diclofenac sodium (59.47-92.32%), demonstrating its anti-inflammatory effectiveness. In another study, nanofiber hydrogels have been produced using ginger residue from juice production [90].To sustain low energy needs, to simplify the components required for sustainable manufacturing, and to eliminate the potential of introducing hazardous side effects, the hydrogels were made using simple vacuum-assisted filtering using just ginger nanofibers and without cross-linker. The hydrogels using ginger fibers were prepared to sustain low energy needs, simplify the components required for sustainable manufacturing, and eliminate the potential of introducing hazardous side effects. The Ginger essential oil was employed to functionalize hydrogels to provide antibacterial action.

5. PEPTIDE NANOSTRUCTURES

Peptides are defined as chains of polypeptides with 50 or less amino acids with a molecular weight of 5000 Da, exhibiting a significant secondary structure but no tertiary structure. Traditionally, bioactive peptides, or naturally occurring peptide hormones, have been used as the source of therapeutic peptides [91, 92]. Peptides can form nanostructures, such as micelles, vesicles, nanotubes, nanoparticles, nanobelt, nanofibers and nanotubes [93] and have been used as antimicrobial agents and anticancer agents. CG_3R_6TAT, an amphiphilic peptide with potent antimicrobial activity against a variety of bacteria, yeasts, and fungi, has been synthesized as cationic self-assembled core-shell nanoparticles, and it has shown to have a high therapeutic index against *S. aureus* infection in mice [94]. In comparison to their unassembled counterparts, the self-assembled peptide nanostructure has demonstrated a better therapeutic index. Furthermore these peptide nanoparticles were able suppress the bacterial growth of *S. aureus* in the brain, by crossing the blood-brain barrier in rabbits with meningitis. The 12-residue peptide KLD-12 (KLD) is well-known for its capacity to adopt nanostructures and for having tissue-engineering characteristics [95]. In order to incorporate antimicrobial properties, the N-terminus of KLD-12 was decorated with two (KLD-2R) and three (KLD-3R) arginine residues. And these derivatives maintained β- sheet structures and self-assembled into nanostructures similar to KLD-12. These variants of KLD demonstrated extremely strong antibacterial activity against the studied microorganisms and may be able to stop secondary infections, which typically happen when such tissue engineering materials are applied externally. A recent study has developed a transformable peptide nanoparticle as an anticancer drug. This peptide will self-assemble as micelles in aqueous conditions and once it is attached to HER2 in cancer cells, it will transform into nanofibrils, resulting in the disruption of HER2 dimerization and associated signalling pathways, consequently leading to cancer cell apoptosis [96].

Peptides can also form nanogels. These biocompatible, low-molecular-mass building blocks have the capacity to self-assemble into an organized hydrogel that may be used for medicinal purposes. Peptide-based nanohydrogels are of great interest because they can self-assemble into hydrogels without the use of noxious compounds like crosslinkers, exhibit nontoxic *in vivo* degradation because the building blocks are naturally occurring amino acids, and are simple to synthesize on a large scale and to functionalize [97].

Antibacterial peptides, a class of tiny natural polypeptide molecules generated by multicellular animals, have been used to create nanohydrogels with intrinsic antibacterial characteristics. They function as direct antimicrobial agents as well as effectors and regulators of the innate immune systems of many species. At least a few hundred of these proteins have currently been identified as promising drug candidates for clinical use because of multiple advantages such as biocompatibility, biodegradability, and simplicity of production and modification [98, 99]. Consequently, they provide an outstanding basis for the development of natural hydrogels with antimicrobial properties.

Sallick *et al.* have demonstrated the high inherent antibacterial activity of a β-hairpin based peptide hydrogel [100]. A variety of pathogens, including Gram-positive (*Staphylococcus epidermidis, Staphylococcus aureus, and Streptococcus pyogenes*) and Gram-negative (*Klebsiella pneumoniae* and *Escherichia coli*) bacteria, were demonstrated to be successfully eradicated by gels during the studies. The postulated antibacterial action mechanism is based on membrane rupture causing cell mortality upon cellular contact with the gel surface [101]. Diphenylalanine peptide with strong antibacterial activity when self-assembled against Escherichia coli was produced by Schnaider *et al.* [102]. It was demonstrated that nano-assemblies entirely prevented bacterial growth, prompted stress-response regulons to become more active, significantly altered the shape of bacteria, and caused membrane penetration and depolarization. Later, different ultrashort fluorenyl-9-methoxycarbony (Fmoc)-peptide hydrogelators and peptides capable of forming soft hydrogels were created by McCloskey *et al.* The majority of the created supramolecular hydrogels showed selective action against Gram-positive (*Staphylococcus aureus, Staphylococcus epidermidis*), Gram-negative (*Escherichia coli, Pseudomonas aeruginosa*), and Gram-neutral (*Escherichia coli, Pseudomonas aeruginosa*) pathogen biofilms, demonstrating a high potential for their use as antibacterial agents [103]. With further studies it was proposed that altering the amino, carboxylic, or both terminal functional groups might change the antibacterial selectivity against *Staphylococcus aureus* [104].

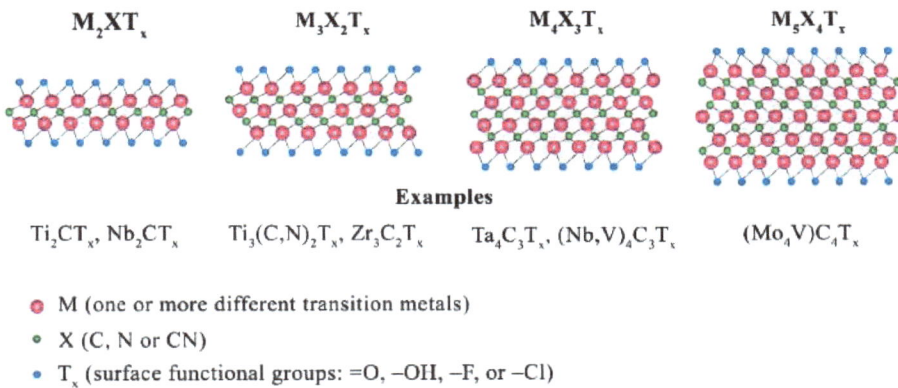

M_2XT_x $M_3X_2T_x$ $M_4X_3T_x$ $M_5X_4T_x$

Examples

Ti_2CT_x, Nb_2CT_x $Ti_3(C,N)_2T_x$, $Zr_3C_2T_x$ $Ta_4C_3T_x$, $(Nb,V)_4C_3T_x$ $(Mo_4V)C_4T_x$

- M (one or more different transition metals)
- X (C, N or CN)
- T_x (surface functional groups: =O, –OH, –F, or –Cl)

Fig. (6). Schematic representation of the structure of MXene with n = 1–4 and some examples. Reprinted with permission from [107] Copyright (© 2021) of Pogorielov *et al.*, published by MDPI and distributed under the terms and conditions of the Creative Commons Attribution (CC BY) license (https://creativecommons.org/licenses/by/4.0/).

6. MXENES

MXene, the most recent 2D nanostructure, excelled in the therapeutic domain because of its better chemical structures and physicochemical properties. The typical formula for MXenes, which are 2D transition metal carbides and nitrides, is $M_{n+1}X_nT_x$, where M is for transition metal (such as Ti, V, Nb, and Mo), X is for carbon and/or nitrogen, n is 1-4, and T_x is the terminal groups of the MXenes (F, OH, O, *etc.*) (Fig. **6**) [105]. Since the compound's discovery, Ti_3C_2 and Ti_2C linkages have been the most widely used MXene in medicinal and biological applications [106].

2D MXene's superior conductivity and tensile strength allowed for improved bone tissue and neural regeneration. The first known sample of MXene has an exceptional electrical conductivity of around 10,000 S cm^{-1} and a volumetric capacitance of 1500 F cm^{-3}. MXene's volumetric capacitance is significantly greater than that of graphene, which is between 60 and 100 F cm^{-3} .With its exceptional qualities, MXene presents a viable alternative for the regeneration of electrically active tissues, such as those found in the heart and brain. Dopaminergic neurons were grown on Ti_3C_2 nanosheets due to their biocompatibility, ability to promote neurite growth, and their role in synaptic initiation. These films successfully encourage the proliferation and migration of progenitor neurons [108].

Intriguing physicochemical characteristics and a planar nanostructure have made 2D MXenes useful in theranostic nanomedicine as well. In case of photoacoustic imaging and photothermal therapy (PTT), certain MXenes, for example, exhibit high photothermal-conversion performance and intense absorption in the near-infrared (NIR) region (750–1000 nm for the first NIR biological window and 1000–1350 nm for the second NIR biological window) [109]. For effective photothermal tumour eradication in NIR I bio window, Wang *et al.* developed 2D ultrathin Ti_3C_2 and Ta_4C_3 (MXene) nanosheets [110, 111]. However, tissue absorption and laser scattering have a significant impact on the photothermal conversion efficiency of 2D MXenes for efficient tumour hyperthermia ablation. The NIR II bio window offers significant benefits in phototherapy due to its greater maximum permitted exposure (MPE) and increased penetration depth when compared to the conventional NIR I bio window. Based on this foundation, researchers have made noteworthy progress in creating photothermal nano agents based on MXene inside the NIR II biological window. Ultrathin 2D Nb_2C and Mo_2C MXenes for effective photothermal tumour ablation in NIR II bio window have been successfully fabricated recently [112, 113].

The antibacterial mechanism of MXene is attributed to several reasons, including its hydrophilic nature, high electrical conductivity, oxygen-containing functional groups on the surface, atomic layer thickness, and optical features such as the localized surface plasmon resonance effect. Based on studies by Rasool *et al.*, Ti_3C_2 MXenes have up to 99% antibacterial activity against strains of Gram-positive *Bacillus subtilis* and Gram-negative *Escherichia coli* bacteria. Comparable outcomes (up to 100%) were seen when antibacterial capabilities of double transition-metal $TiVCT_x$ MXene were investigated [114, 115]. As the primary mode of action, the authors propose mechanical destruction of the cell membrane [116]. Because of the increased MXene electroconductivity, the scientists claim that the antibacterial impact of the examined MXene is even stronger than that of graphene oxide. The colony count approach yielded results which indicated stoichiometry determined the decreasing order of antibacterial activity against both bacterial strains. The results indicate a strong positive association between the antibacterial activity of MXenes and their thickness: single layer $Ti_3C_2T_x$ > multilayer $Ti_3C_2T_x$ > Ti_3AlC_2. The number of *B. subtilis* and *E. coli* colonies decreased significantly with higher dosages of $Ti_3C_2T_x$.

The principal destructive mechanism associated with the antibacterial process of $Ti_3C_2T_x$ MXene nanoparticles was found between $Ti_3C_2T_x$ MXene and the cell membrane, resulting in mechanical damage to cell walls. One possibility is that $Ti_3C_2T_x$ nanomaterials, which have the lowest size, a reactive surface, and significant reducing activity, were directly or indirectly taken up by microbial cells by endocytosis. Then $Ti_3C_2T_x$ and specific compounds in microbial cell walls and cytoplasm may have interacted to break the cells, which in turn may have led to the destruction of microorganisms [115]. The negatively charged Ti_3C_2 nanosheet's surface anionic properties will also provide a conductive link across the lipid bilayer insulation, facilitating the passage of electrons from bacterial cell components to the surrounding environment and ultimately causing cell death. Similar to GO nanomaterials, it is plausible that the lipopolysaccharide chain in the cell membrane and the oxygen-containing groups on the surface of $Ti_3C_2T_x$ MXene form hydrogen bonds, which might inhibit the development of bacteria [115]. Subsequent research by Arabi Shamsabadi *et al.* verified the relationship between antibacterial capabilities of MXene nanosheets and their size and exposure duration. Quantitative studies using fluorescence imaging, complementary technologies, and flow cytometry revealed that the smallest nanomaterials also possess the strongest antibacterial qualities against both Gram-positive and Gram-negative bacteria [117]. The growth kinetics measuring methodologies indicate that the direct physical contact between the sharp edges of the nanoparticles and the bacterial membrane surface is critical for the nanomaterials' antibacterial activity [117]. MXene influences the degree of oxidative stress that cells experience by generating reactive oxygen species. The ability to produce ROS has been extensively investigated for a number of MXenes, including $Ti_3C_2T_x$, Ti_2CT_x, and Ti_2NT_x [118 - 120]. $Ti_3C_2T_x$ MXene surfaces often have a negative zeta potential due to functional groups such as Ti-OH, Ti-F, and Ti-O, which contribute to MXene's strong affinity to the cell surface and ease of chemical reactions leading to ROS generation. In microorganisms, ROS are generated and consumed in regulated amounts by various species; nevertheless, excessive ROS can cause oxidative damage to cell membranes and biomacromolecules (lipids, proteins, and DNA) in microbes, potentially resulting in mitochondrial malfunction and cell death. The impact of MXene type and dosage on the amount of ROS inside E. coli cells suggests that MXenes limit the function of antioxidant enzymes in bacteria, which causes ROS to build up inside the cells [121]. A variety of cell segments experience oxidative damage as a result of the excess ROS. The greater oxidation levels at higher MXene concentrations were validated by measuring the levels of protein oxidation in *E. Coli* cultured with varying doses of $Ti_3C_2T_x$. Furthermore, the oxidative damage to the bacterial membrane caused by ROS creation from MXenes is confirmed by the increased synthesis of malondialdehyde, a byproduct of membrane lipid peroxidation. Upon incubation with MXenes, the vital antioxidant enzyme in bacteria; superoxide dismutase activity declines, indicating that ROS production has deactivated this enzyme. The scientists have identified that oxidative stress and mechanical damage to the cell membrane caused by the sharp edges of the nanosheets as two of the main processes of MXenes' toxicity against animal and bacterial cells as seen in *in vitro* testing.

7. SILICENE

The multifaceted properties of silicene, including its high specific surface area, good optical properties, distinct electronic properties, and desirable biocompatibility and biodegradability, offer a promising avenue for applications in biomedicine. The remarkable potential of silicene in biomedical applications, such as tumour treatments, bioimaging, and antimicrobial materials, has been brought to light by the intriguing results to date and the obvious advancement. Silicene is a novel topological structure of monoelemental silicon materials, which extends the conventional 0D silicon nanoparticles to a new 2D layered graphene-like structure. Silicene is obtained by the ultimate scaling of silicon monatomic sheet in a buckled honeycomb lattice. The silicene sheet's unusual low-buckled structure gives it a more amazing quantum spin hall effect than graphene given that its silicon atoms are not all on the same plane as graphene [122].

Rich in hydroxyl groups and hydrophilic, silicene lends itself easily to modification. Under physiological circumstances, it breaks down into harmless, non-toxic components that are expelled through the urine or feces. The biocompatibility of silicene reduces health risks and harmful responses in the body. With its potent light absorption capacity and excellent photothermal conversion efficiency, it is a prime contender for near-infrared photothermal treatment that induces tumour hyperthermia ablation [122]. Lin and colleagues (2019) created few-layered silicene nanosheets by a wet-chemistry method and methodically investigated their photothermal therapeutic use [123]. As synthesized, the single-/few-layered silicene nanosheets revealed a freestanding, graphene-like shape with a thickness of 0.6 nm. According to optical physics investigations, the photothermal conversion efficiency (η) of silicene reached 36.09% under NIR-II (l ¼ 1,064 nm) irradiation, which is much better than 30.6% of typical 2D photothermal conversion nanomaterials such as Ti_3C_2 [111], and 21% of representative PTT agent Au nanorods [124]. Ultra-deep tissue phototherapy has been made possible by NIR-II area irradiation, which has a deeper tissue penetration than light at the first NIR window (NIR-I) [125]. In light of this, researchers have examined silicene's quantitative photothermal action in more detail. When exposed to laser light at 1,064 nm with a power density of 1.0 W/cm2, the temperature of the silicene suspension rose to 47 ˚C, which is the highest acceptable standard for skin exposure [125]. It is evident that silicene-based nanomedicine can cause tumour overheating to eliminate cancerous cells without endangering healthy cells. A considerable increase in the therapeutic temperature might be achieved by the accumulation of silicene in the tumour location, as determined by tracking the infrared thermal fluctuations of mice with tumours under NIR-II irradiation. This study developed a novel paradigm for photothermal nanoagents, by introducing silicene, which efficiently suppresses the growth of cancer cells in tumour-bearing mice. It also inventively created nanomaterials based on silicene for use in biomedical applications and provided fresh insight into the wide range of applications of silicene.

Silicene may be used as an efficient antibacterial agent to destroy harmful bacteria, just as other 2D nanomaterials including LDHs, Graphene, and MXenes. The antibacterial ability of graphene-like silicon nanosheets (GS NSs) to prevent the development of Gram (+) *Staphylococcus aureus* and Gram (-) *Escherichia coli* was recently studied by Luo *et al*. [126]. In this instance, the bulk silicene was exfoliated with the use of ultrasound to create novel 2D GS NSs. A series of concentrations of GS NSs were cultured with *E. Coli* and *S. aureus* for 4 hours in order to assess their antibacterial activity. A concentration-dependent bacterial growth suppression by GS NSs was observed during the experiment. Additionally, they postulated that the fundamental antibacterial mechanism of GS NSs is based on a robust contact between the nanosheet and bacterial biofilm, which facilitates the rupture of cell membranes and the release of cytoplasmic material, ultimately leading to the induction of cell death. The Cell Counting Kit-

8 (CCK-8) assay was used to investigate the *in vitro* cytotoxicity of GS NSs on normal cells. The results showed that GS NSs do not appear to have any discernible negative effects on the survival of NIH/3T3. Subcutaneous implant therapy was used to create animal models of S. aureus infection in order to observe the antibacterial efficacy of GS NSs *in vivo*. The application of a 20 mg/kg dosage of GS NSs demonstrated a notable bactericidal effectiveness against implant-caused infection models, as well as a desirable wound repair without the development of a significant skin lesion. These GS NSs may be viewed as a novel 2D NM with the potential use in the efficient removal of harmful bacteria, in contrast to standard treatments including antibiotics or metal nanoparticles for antibacterial uses.

8. ANTIMONENE

Antimonene (AM) was first experimentally separated by Zamora *et al.* [127] and Abellan *et al.* [128] in 2016. The remarkable capacity of AM to effectively absorb light in the near-infrared (NIR) range brought it to prominence. Compared to many other nanomaterials equipped with photothermal agents, such as graphene oxide, silver nanorods, nanoshells, and quantum dots, antimonene has the remarkable attribute of having an exceptionally high photothermal conversion efficiency [129]. In theory, AM has remarkable features such as strain-induced band transition, strong stability, great carrier mobility, and exceptional spin electron properties [130]. The photothermal conversion efficiency (η) of AM QDs value, as evaluated by Tao *et al.*, was 45.5%, much greater than photothermal agents (PTA) such as graphene oxide (25%), Au nanoshell (13%), $Cu_{2-x}Se$ nanoparticles (22%), MoS2 PEG nanosheets (27.6%), which is only surpassed by Ti nanosheets (61.5%) [131, 132]. This intriguing outcome further demonstrates AM's enormous potential as a PTA in PTT and PDT.

Nevertheless, the direct use of antimonene (AM) nanomaterial is severely limited due to its rapid breakdown in physiological fluids. To address this problem, AM have been modified by a variety of techniques, including dimension optimization, PEGylation, size control, and cell membrane (CM) camouflage. When cloaked with CM, the resultant AM nanoparticles (55 nm) demonstrated enhanced photothermal efficacy and significantly better stability than traditional AM nanosheets. This qualified them for use as an effective PTT/PDT combined with anticancer treatment with minimal side effects and enhanced tumour targeting capability [133]. In contrast, a clearly reduced absorbance at 808 nm and temperature following irradiation was noted for the smaller AM NPs (2 nm) with increased specific surface area, which ruled out the possibility of effective phototherapy. On the other hand, large AM NPs (295 nm) showed a considerable improvement in photothermal effects and stability due to their decreased specific surface area. The restricted fenestration space of newly created tumour vasculature may, however, significantly weaken the EPR effect due to the oversize of the large NPs [134].

The potential of AMQD-based nanomaterials as PTAs was investigated by Tao *et al.* [132]. AM QDs were coated with 1,2-Distearoyl-sn-glyce-o-3-phosphoethanolamine-N-[methoxy(poly ethylene glycol)] (DSPE-PEG) in this work. Different broad and high absorption from UV to NIR was observed in AM QDs coated with PEG. During *in vivo* investigation, PEG-AM QDs were administered into subcutaneous transplanted tumour of MCF-7 nude mice, and the tumour was exposed to an 808 nm laser at 1 Wcm^{-2} for 10 minutes. Following PTT, the tumour was eliminated with negligible growth and no regeneration.

Zhang *et al.* created a novel technique for treating tumours with AM as a radiosensitizer [26]. Here, AM NPs, such as AM QDs and AM nanosheets (AMNSs), were produced and coated with polylactic acid glycolic acid (PLGA) as an amphiphilic carrier to enhance the biological stability. AMNPs were converted into Sb_2O_5 and Sb_2O_3, which had distinct cytotoxicity for cancer cells, when exposed to X-ray radiation. By causing excessive ROS production and mitochondrial disruption, Sb_2O_3 has a severe cytotoxic impact. ROS mostly consist of peroxy and singlet oxygen radicals. AMNPs@PLGA in conjunction with X-ray in A375 nude mice model for melanoma, hindered the activity of VEGF/VEGFR2 and DNA repair related protein, causing S phase arrest and apoptosis, which in turn prevented the tumour growth. Although AM has shown potential biomedical application, as Sb is not a necessary component of the human body, more research is needed to determine if AM is biocompatible.

CONCLUSION

Nanomaterials can be employed as medication candidates to treat a variety of diseases due to their special therapeutic capabilities, such as antioxidant, anti-inflammatory, antibacterial, antiviral, and anticancer properties. Nano complexes like dendrimers, carbon nanotubes, fullerenes, graphene-based nanomaterials, carbon quantum dots, nanohydrogels, peptide nanostructures, MXenes, Silicene, and Antimonene have been distinguished by researchers as nano-drug candidates due to their intrinsic properties.

Dendrimers are a subclass of synthetic polymers distinguished by their typical symmetry, strong branching, and monodispersed nature. Due to their unique qualities, which include condensed branching structures with precise control over size, form, and numerous functional groups on their outer layer, they have a significant potential for use in medical applications. It has been shown that multivalent adhesion activities of cells, viruses, proteins, bacteria, and combinations are significantly inhibited by the number of ligands on their outer shell. Due to their broad and complex interactions with biological macromolecules as well as their higher binding affinities, dendrimers can be employed as drugs. Dendrimer multivalent replacements are a potent substitute for single-molecule medicines.

Carbon nanomaterials (CNMs), including carbon nanotubes, graphene oxide, fullerenes, and carbon quantum dots (QDs), have antimicrobial, anti-inflammatory, and anticancer properties. Their unique characteristics have sparked interest in these materials. CNTs are classified as SWCNTs and MWCNTs. Exposure to CNTs increases plasmid DNA, RNA, and cytoplasmic material efflux of microbes resulting in antimicrobial activity. The high surface area, their improved penetration into the cell wall, and distinct chemical and electrical properties contribute to their enhanced cytotoxicity. MWCNTs have intrinsic anti-proliferative, cytotoxic, and anti-migratory effects *in vitro*, allowing them to associate with natural intracellular nano filaments like actin or microtubules. These properties, along with the ability to generate oxidative stress in cells, can be exploited to defeat cancer. The physicochemical properties of C60 fullerene and its derivatives, as well as their impact on biological processes, have drawn great interest due to their abundance. The insoluble nature of C60 in water limits its use in biological processes. Fullerenes and their derivatives have therapeutic qualities like antioxidant, anti-inflammatory, antibacterial, and antiviral capabilities. In drug discovery, it is possible to precisely "tune" the structure of fullerene derivatives to create a medicinal substance with a particular biological activity. Graphene oxide (GO) is a thin carbon sheet with highly effective mechanical, electrical, and piezoelectric capabilities against bacteria and viruses. It decreases microbiological resistance and results in mortality by producing reactive oxygen species (ROS) and oxidation in microbial cell walls and membranes. Membrane stress, oxidative stress, and separating bacteria from their environment are the three main antibacterial mechanisms of GO. These pathways ultimately increase the efficiency of GO in battling microbial infections by preventing microbial development and harm. Carbon quantum dots (CQDs) are a popular nanomaterial due to their solubility, biocompatibility, and surface modification flexibility. They exhibit membrane-disruptive activity through ROS oxidation and cation effects, potentially enhancing their antimicrobial properties. CQDs show minimal cytotoxicity on normal host cells and high specificity against tumour cells.

Hydrogels are three-dimensional polymeric networks that can hold water but do not dissolve in water. Nanohydrogels, which combine hydrogel properties such as hydrophilicity, flexibility, and quick water absorption, are rapidly being used in the pharmaceutical industry. These nanohydrogels are applied to wounds as sophisticated moisture donor dressings to speed up the production of collagenase and autolytic debridement. Additionally, they have an antibacterial effect that delays or prevents microbial infections. Natural hydrogels are regarded as advantageous biomaterials for preventing bacterial infections.

Peptides have been utilized as antibacterial and anticancer treatments and can produce nanostructures such as micelles, vesicles, nanotubes, nanoparticles, nanobelts, and nanotubes. Bioactive peptides, or naturally occurring peptide hormones, have traditionally been employed as a source of therapeutic peptides. Nanogels can also be created by peptides. Since the building blocks of peptide-based nanohydrogels are naturally occurring amino acids, they exhibit nontoxic *in vivo* degradation, can self-assemble into hydrogels without the use of harmful substances like crosslinkers, and are easy to synthesize and functionalize on a large scale.

2D MXene's superior conductivity and tensile strength allow for improved bone tissue and neural regeneration. Intriguing physicochemical characteristics and a planar nanostructure have made 2D MXenes useful in theranostic nanomedicine as well. MXenes exhibit high photothermal-conversion performance and intense absorption in the near-infrared (NIR) region. MXene's antibacterial mechanism is attributed to its hydrophilic nature, high electrical conductivity, oxygen-containing functional groups, atomic layer thickness, and optical features.

Silicene's high specific surface area, optical properties, electronic properties, and biocompatibility make it promising for biomedicine, including tumour treatments, bioimaging, and antimicrobial materials. With its potent light absorption capacity and excellent photothermal conversion efficiency, it is a prime contender for near-infrared photothermal treatment that induces tumour hyperthermia ablation. Silicene may be used as an efficient antibacterial agent to destroy harmful bacteria as well.

The remarkable capacity of antimonene (AM) to effectively absorb light in the near-infrared (NIR) range brought it to prominence. Compared to many other nanomaterials equipped with photothermal agents, such as graphene oxide, silver nanorods, nanoshells, and quantum dots, antimonene has the remarkable attribute of having an exceptionally high photothermal conversion efficiency demonstrating enormous potential as a PTA in PTT and PDT. Nevertheless, the direct use of antimonene (AM) nanomaterial is severely limited due to its rapid breakdown in physiological fluids. To address this problem, AM materials have been modified by a variety of techniques, including dimension optimization, PEGylation, size control, and cell membrane (CM) camouflage.

Table **1** summarizes the drug candidates with their biomedical applications, mode of actions and special features described so far in this chapter.

Table 1. Summary of the drug candidates with their applications, mode of actions and special features.

Nano Drug Candidate	Biomedical Application	Mode of Action	Special Features	Refs.
Dendrimers	Antibacterial	Lipid bilayer rupture *via* the electrostatic attraction between the positively charged dendrimer and the negatively charged surface of the bacterium.	Surface composition of dendrimers regulates the depth of penetration and accumulation in biofilms.	[1, 3]
	Antiviral	Blocking the interaction between gp120, CD4 and CCR5 to prevent viral entry and replication or by specifically targeting the late stages of viral replication.		[10]
CNTs	Antimicrobial	Direct contact-induced damage to microorganisms' cell membranes, leading to the fatality of the bacteria. Increases efflux of plasmid DNA, RNA, and cytoplasmic material. SWCNTs were interconnected with changes in stress-related gene expression. Reactive oxygen species (ROS) production.	SWCNTs were more toxic towards microorganisms.	[18, 20, 21]
	Anticancer	ROS production Causes mitotic abnormalities, including aberrant spindles, chromosomal mal-segregation, and clastogenic effects. They also hinder cell migration.	MWCNTs show remarkable biomimicry, which allows them to associate with a number of natural intracellular nano filaments such as actin or microtubules disrupting the biomechanics of cell division.	[23 - 26]

(Table 1) cont.....

Nano Drug Candidate	Biomedical Application	Mode of Action	Special Features	Refs.
Fullerenes	Antioxidant	Abundance of conjugated double bonds and their low-lying, lowest unoccupied molecular orbital (LUMO), which is easily accessible to an electron and highly conducive to attack by radical species.	The lowest toxicity among carbon nanomaterials, including graphene, MWCNTs, SWCNTs, and carbon dots.	[28, 38]
	Anti-inflammatory	Inhibited the ROS production induced by the PMA which is the inflammatory cell activator (Human). Decrease of inflammatory Marker CRP in Canine Blood.		[33]
	Antiviral	Interact with molecules on the cell surface, thereby preventing the virus from interacting with the cellular receptor, and hence blocking its entry into the cells.		[44]
Graphene oxide and derivatives	Antimicrobial	ROS generation and inducing physical and chemical oxidation in microorganism cell walls and membranes. Membrane stress- Physical damage to the cell membrane by the sharp edges of GO leaking the cellular by direct contact components. Wrapping or trapping bacteria is dependent on separating them from their natural surroundings.	The antibacterial activity of both GO and rGO are time and concentration-dependent.	[54 - 56, 59, 60]
	Antiviral	Viruses may be successfully captured, their surface proteins destroyed, and viral RNA extracted.	High-throughput viral detection and disinfection.	[64]

(Table 1) cont.....

Nano Drug Candidate	Biomedical Application	Mode of Action	Special Features	Refs.
CQDs	Antibacterial/antibiofilm	Membrane disruption through the production of ROS and the effects of cations on membrane destruction.	Not likely to cause bacterial resistance. CQDs exhibit high hemocompatibility and cytocompatibility.	[68]
	Anticancer	Interact with cell membrane receptors found on tumour cells, such as nuclear antigens, tumour markers expressed only on the membrane of the tumour cells. Act as photosensitizers in photodynamic therapy.	Minimal cytotoxicity on normal host cells such as RBCs, WBCs, and embryonic cells and a high specificity of action against tumour cells. Less haemolysis than that of Aspirin.	[71]
Nanohydrogel	Moisture donor dressings for wound healing.	Improves oxygen delivery to the wounds and allows exudate absorption and retention within the gel mass.		[77]
	Antibacterial/Antifungal	Electrostatic interactions with microbial surfaces and consequent cell rupture, causing the leaking of internal components and impeding the transfer of nutrients into the cells. Chelation of amino groups with Ca^{2+} or Mg^{2+} present in the cell walls. The bonds formed will impede toxin production, inhibiting the microbial growth.	Antimicrobial activity depends on inherent physicochemical qualities and external variables (such as the pH of the medium, concentration, and species of bacteria).	[80, 81, 86]

(Table 1) cont.....

Nano Drug Candidate	Biomedical Application	Mode of Action	Special Features	Refs.
Peptide nanostructures	Antimicrobial	Membrane rupture causing cell mortality upon cellular contact. Cause stress-response regulons to become more active, significantly altered the shape of bacteria, and caused membrane penetration and depolarization.	Peptides can form nanostructures, such as micelles, vesicles, nanotubes, nanoparticles, nanobelt, nanofibers and nanotubes, nanogels.	[101, 102]
	Anticancer	Peptides will self-assemble as micelles in aqueous conditions and once it is attached to cancer cells, it will transform into nanofibrils, resulting in the disruption of cancer cells, dimerization and associated signalling pathways, consequently leading to cancer cell apoptosis.		[96]

(Table 1) cont.....

Nano Drug Candidate	Biomedical Application	Mode of Action	Special Features	Refs.
MXenes	Regeneration of electrically active tissues.	The ability to promote neurite growth, and initiate synaptic growth. Encourage the proliferation and migration of progenitor neurons.	Superior conductivity and tensile strength.	[108]
	Anticancer	Photothermal therapy	High photothermal-conversion performance and intense absorption in the near-infrared (NIR).	[109]
	Antibacterial	Specific compounds in microbial cell walls and cytoplasm interact to break the cells, which in turn led to the destruction of microorganisms. Oxidative stress damages cell membranes and biomacromolecules (lipids, proteins, and DNA) in microbes, potentially resulting in mitochondrial malfunction and cell death. Limit the function of antioxidant enzymes in bacteria, which causes ROS build up inside the cells.	High antibacterial even stronger than that of GO. Antibacterial ability depends on size and exposure duration.	[115 - 117]

Nano Drug Candidate	Biomedical Application	Mode of Action	Special Features	Refs.
Silicene	Anticancer	Photothermal therapy	Has light absorption capacity and excellent photothermal conversion efficiency. Highly biocompatible. Under physiological circumstances, it breaks down into harmless, non-toxic components that are expelled through the urine or faeces.	[122]
	Antibacterial	Mechanical contact with bacterial biofilm, which facilitates the rupture of cell membranes and the release of cytoplasmic material, ultimately leading to the induction of cell death.		[126]
Antimonene	Anticancer	Photo thermal therapy and Photo dynamic therapy	Exceptionally high photothermal conversion efficiency, even higher than GO, Au NPs, $Cu_{2-x}Se$.	[131, 132]

PRACTICE QUESTIONS

1. Discuss the key factors for a compound to be a drug candidate.
2. Discuss the different mechanisms of antimicrobial activity of drug candidates.
3. Discuss which features of a drug candidate and how these feature affect its therapeutic ability.

REFERENCES

[1]   Rozenbaum, R.T.; Andrén, O.C.J.; van der Mei, H.C.; Woudstra, W.; Busscher, H.J.; Malkoch, M.; Sharma, P.K. Penetration and Accumulation of Dendrons with Different Peripheral Composition in *Pseudomonas aeruginosa* Biofilms. *Nano Lett.,* **2019**, *19*(7), 4327-4333.
[http://dx.doi.org/10.1021/acs.nanolett.9b00838] [PMID: 31142116]

[2]   Falanga, A.; Del Genio, V.; Galdiero, S. Peptides and Dendrimers: How to Combat Viral and Bacterial Infections. *Pharmaceutics,* **2021**, *13*(1), 101.
[http://dx.doi.org/10.3390/pharmaceutics13010101] [PMID: 33466852]

[3]   Gholami, M.; Mohammadi, R.; Arzanlou, M.; Akbari Dourbash, F.; Kouhsari, E.; Majidi, G.; Mohseni, S.M.; Nazari, S. *In vitro* antibacterial activity of poly (amidoamine)-G7 dendrimer. *BMC Infect. Dis.,* **2017**, *17*(1), 395.
[http://dx.doi.org/10.1186/s12879-017-2513-7] [PMID: 28583153]

[4]   Altaher, Y.; Kandeel, M. Structure-Activity Relationship of Anionic and Cationic Polyamidoamine (PAMAM) Dendrimers against *Staphylococcus aureus*. *J. Nanomater.,* **2022**, *2022*, 1-5.
[http://dx.doi.org/10.1155/2022/4013016]

[5]   Worley, B.V.; Slomberg, D.L.; Schoenfisch, M.H. Nitric oxide-releasing quaternary ammonium-modified poly(amidoamine) dendrimers as dual action antibacterial agents. *Bioconjug. Chem.,* **2014,** *25*(5), 918-927.
[http://dx.doi.org/10.1021/bc5000719] [PMID: 24797526]

[6]   Lopez, A.I.; Reins, R.Y.; McDermott, A.M.; Trautner, B.W.; Cai, C. Antibacterial activity and cytotoxicity of PEGylated poly(amidoamine) dendrimers. *Mol. Biosyst.,* **2009,** *5*(10), 1148-1156.
[http://dx.doi.org/10.1039/b904746h] [PMID: 19756304]

[7]   Quintana-Sanchez, S.; Gómez-Casanova, N.; Sánchez-Nieves, J.; Gómez, R.; Rachuna, J.; Wąsik, S.; Semaniak, J.; Maciejewska, B.; Drulis-Kawa, Z.; Ciepluch, K.; Mata, F.J.; Arabski, M. The Antibacterial Effect of PEGylated Carbosilane Dendrimers on *P. aeruginosa* Alone and in Combination with Phage-Derived Endolysin. *Int. J. Mol. Sci.,* **2022,** *23*(3), 1873.
[http://dx.doi.org/10.3390/ijms23031873] [PMID: 35163794]

[8]   Kannan, R.; Prabakaran, P.; Basu, R.; Pindi, C.; Senapati, S.; Muthuvijayan, V.; Prasad, E. Mechanistic Study on the Antibacterial Activity of Self-Assembled Poly(aryl ether)-Based Amphiphilic Dendrimers. *ACS Appl. Bio Mater.,* **2019,** *2*(8), 3212-3224.
[http://dx.doi.org/10.1021/acsabm.9b00140] [PMID: 35030765]

[9]   Wrońska, N.; Majoral, J.P.; Appelhans, D.; Bryszewska, M.; Lisowska, K. Synergistic effects of anionic/cationic dendrimers and levofloxacin on antibacterial activities. *Molecules,* **2019,** *24*(16), 2894.
[http://dx.doi.org/10.3390/molecules24162894] [PMID: 31395831]

[10]   Akbari, A.; Bigham, A.; Rahimkhoei, V.; Sharifi, S.; Jabbari, E. Antiviral polymers: A Review. *Polymers,* **2022,** *14*(9), 1634.
[http://dx.doi.org/10.3390/polym14091634] [PMID: 35566804]

[11]   Rodríguez-Izquierdo, I.; Sepúlveda-Crespo, D.; Lasso, J.M.; Resino, S.; Muñoz-Fernández, M.Á. Baseline and time-updated factors in preclinical development of anionic dendrimers as successful anti-HIV 1 vaginal microbicides. *Wiley Interdiscip. Rev. Nanomed. Nanobiotechnol.,* **2022,** *14*(3), e1774.
[http://dx.doi.org/10.1002/wnan.1774] [PMID: 35018739]

[12]   Paull, J.R.A.; Heery, G.P.; Bobardt, M.D.; Castellarnau, A.; Luscombe, C.A.; Fairley, J.K.; Gallay, P.A. Virucidal and antiviral activity of astodrimer sodium against SARS-CoV-2 *in vitro*. *Antiviral Res.,* **2021,** *191*, 105089.
[http://dx.doi.org/10.1016/j.antiviral.2021.105089] [PMID: 34010661]

[13]   Chavoustie, S.E.; Carter, B.A.; Waldbaum, A.S.; Donders, G.G.G.; Peters, K.H.; Schwebke, J.R.; Paull, J.R.A.; Price, C.F.; Castellarnau, A.; McCloud, P.; Kinghorn, G.R. Two phase 3, double-blind, placebo-controlled studies of the efficacy and safety of Astodrimer 1% Gel for the treatment of bacterial vaginosis. *Eur. J. Obstet. Gynecol. Reprod. Biol.,* **2020,** *245*, 13-18.
[http://dx.doi.org/10.1016/j.ejogrb.2019.11.032] [PMID: 31812702]

[14]   Waldbaum, A.S.; Schwebke, J.R.; Paull, J.R.A.; Price, C.F.; Edmondson, S.R.; Castellarnau, A.; McCloud, P.; Kinghorn, G.R. A phase 2, double-blind, multicenter, randomized, placebo-controlled, dose-ranging study of the efficacy and safety of Astodrimer Gel for the treatment of bacterial vaginosis. *PLoS One,* **2020,** *15*(5), e0232394.
[http://dx.doi.org/10.1371/journal.pone.0232394] [PMID: 32365097]

[15]   Schwebke, J.R.; Carter, B.A.; Waldbaum, A.S.; Agnew, K.J.; Paull, J.R.A.; Price, C.F.; Castellarnau, A.; McCloud, P.; Kinghorn, G.R. A phase 3, randomized, controlled trial of Astodrimer 1% Gel for preventing recurrent bacterial vaginosis. *Eur. J. Obstet. Gynecol. Reprod. Biol. X,* **2021,** *10*, 100121.
[http://dx.doi.org/10.1016/j.eurox.2021.100121] [PMID: 33537666]

[16]   Martínez-Gualda, B.; Sun, L.; Rivero-Buceta, E.; Flores, A.; Quesada, E.; Balzarini, J.; Noppen, S.; Liekens, S.; Schols, D.; Neyts, J.; Leyssen, P.; Mirabelli, C.; Camarasa, M.J.; San-Félix, A. Structure-activity relationship studies on a Trp dendrimer with dual activities against HIV and enterovirus A71. Modifications on the amino acid. *Antiviral Res.,* **2017,** *139*, 32-40.

[http://dx.doi.org/10.1016/j.antiviral.2016.12.010] [PMID: 28017762]

[17] Royo-Rubio, E.; Martín-Cañadilla, V.; Rusnati, M.; Milanesi, M.; Lozano-Cruz, T.; Gómez, R.; Jiménez, J.L.; Muñoz-Fernández, M.Á. Prevention of Herpesviridae infections by cationic PEGylated carbosilane dendrimers. *Pharmaceutics,* **2022**, *14*(3), 536.
[http://dx.doi.org/10.3390/pharmaceutics14030536] [PMID: 35335912]

[18] Azizi-Lalabadi, M.; Hashemi, H.; Feng, J.; Jafari, S.M. Carbon nanomaterials against pathogens; the antimicrobial activity of carbon nanotubes, graphene/graphene oxide, fullerenes, and their nanocomposites. *Adv. Colloid Interface Sci.,* **2020**, *284*, 102250.
[http://dx.doi.org/10.1016/j.cis.2020.102250] [PMID: 32966964]

[19] Vidu, R.; Rahman, M.; Mahmoudi, M.; Enachescu, M.; Poteca, T.D.; Opris, I. Nanostructures: A platform for brain repair and augmentation. *Front. Syst. Neurosci.,* **2014**, *8*, 91.
[http://dx.doi.org/10.3389/fnsys.2014.00091] [PMID: 24999319]

[20] Maksimova, Y.G. Microorganisms and Carbon Nanotubes: Interaction and Applications (Review). *Appl. Biochem. Microbiol.,* **2019**, *55*(1), 1-12. [Review].
[http://dx.doi.org/10.1134/S0003683819010101]

[21] Kang, S.; Herzberg, M.; Rodrigues, D.F.; Elimelech, M. Antibacterial effects of carbon nanotubes: size does matter! *Langmuir,* **2008**, *24*(13), 6409-6413.
[http://dx.doi.org/10.1021/la800951v] [PMID: 18512881]

[22] Arias, L.R.; Yang, L. Inactivation of bacterial pathogens by carbon nanotubes in suspensions. *Langmuir,* **2009**, *25*(5), 3003-3012.
[http://dx.doi.org/10.1021/la802769m] [PMID: 19437709]

[23] García-Hevia, L.; Villegas, J.C.; Fernández, F.; Casafont, Í.; González, J.; Valiente, R.; Fanarraga, M.L. Multiwalled Carbon Nanotubes Inhibit Tumor Progression in a Mouse Model. *Adv. Healthc. Mater.,* **2016**, *5*(9), 1080-1087.
[http://dx.doi.org/10.1002/adhm.201500753] [PMID: 26866927]

[24] Gonzalez, L.; Decordier, I.; Kirsch-Volders, M. Induction of chromosome malsegregation by nanomaterials. *Biochem. Soc. Trans.,* **2010**, *38*(6), 1691-1697.
[http://dx.doi.org/10.1042/BST0381691] [PMID: 21118149]

[25] Siegrist, K.J.; Reynolds, S.H.; Kashon, M.L.; Lowry, D.T.; Dong, C.; Hubbs, A.F.; Young, S.H.; Salisbury, J.L.; Porter, D.W.; Benkovic, S.A.; McCawley, M.; Keane, M.J.; Mastovich, J.T.; Bunker, K.L.; Cena, L.G.; Sparrow, M.C.; Sturgeon, J.L.; Dinu, C.Z.; Sargent, L.M. Genotoxicity of multiwalled carbon nanotubes at occupationally relevant doses. *Part. Fibre Toxicol.,* **2014**, *11*(1), 6.
[http://dx.doi.org/10.1186/1743-8977-11-6] [PMID: 24479647]

[26] Rodriguez-Fernandez, L.; Valiente, R.; Gonzalez, J.; Villegas, J.C.; Fanarraga, M.L. Multiwalled carbon nanotubes display microtubule biomimetic properties *in vivo*, enhancing microtubule assembly and stabilization. *ACS Nano,* **2012**, *6*(8), 6614-6625.
[http://dx.doi.org/10.1021/nn302222m] [PMID: 22769231]

[27] Benko, A.; Medina-Cruz, D.; Wilk, S.; Ziąbka, M.; Zagrajczuk, B.; Menaszek, E.; Barczyk-Woźnicka, O.; Guisbiers, G.; Webster, T.J. Anticancer and antibacterial properties of carbon nanotubes are governed by their functional groups. *Nanoscale,* **2023**, *15*(45), 18265-18282.
[http://dx.doi.org/10.1039/D3NR02923A] [PMID: 37795813]

[28] Khorsandi, Z.; Borjian-Boroujeni, M.; Yekani, R.; Varma, R.S. Carbon nanomaterials with chitosan: A winning combination for drug delivery systems. *J. Drug Deliv. Sci. Technol.,* **2021**, *66*, 102847.
[http://dx.doi.org/10.1016/j.jddst.2021.102847]

[29] Tabata, Y.; Ikada, Y. Biological functions of fullerene. *Pure Appl. Chem.,* **1999**, *71*(11), 2047-2053.
[http://dx.doi.org/10.1351/pac199971112047]

[30] Aschberger, K.; Johnston, H.J.; Stone, V.; Aitken, R.J.; Tran, C.L.; Hankin, S.M.; Peters, S.A.K.; Christensen, F.M. Review of fullerene toxicity and exposure : Appraisal of a human health risk

assessment, based on open literature. *Regul. Toxicol. Pharmacol.,* **2010**, *58*(3), 455-473.
[http://dx.doi.org/10.1016/j.yrtph.2010.08.017] [PMID: 20800639]

[31]   Injac, R.; Prijatelj, M.; Strukelj, B. Fullerenol nanoparticles: toxicity and antioxidant activity. *Oxidative Stress and Nanotechnology: Methods and Protocols,* **2013**, 75-100.

[32]   Zhou, Y.; Li, J.; Ma, H.; Zhen, M.; Guo, J.; Wang, L.; Jiang, L.; Shu, C.; Wang, C. Biocompatible [60]/[70] Fullerenols: Potent defense against oxidative injury induced by reduplicative chemotherapy. *ACS Appl. Mater. Interfaces,* **2017**, *9*(41), 35539-35547.
[http://dx.doi.org/10.1021/acsami.7b08348] [PMID: 28945341]

[33]   Hui, M.; Jia, X.; Li, X.; Lazcano-Silveira, R.; Shi, M. Anti-inflammatory and antioxidant effects of liposoluble c60 at the cellular, molecular, and whole-animal Levels. *J. Inflamm. Res.,* **2023**, *16*, 83-93.
[http://dx.doi.org/10.2147/JIR.S386381] [PMID: 36643955]

[34]   Szunerits, S.; Barras, A.; Khanal, M.; Pagneux, Q.; Boukherroub, R. Nanostructures for the Inhibition of Viral Infections. *Molecules,* **2015**, *20*(8), 14051-14081.
[http://dx.doi.org/10.3390/molecules200814051] [PMID: 26247927]

[35]   Xu, P.Y.; Li, X.Q.; Chen, W.G.; Deng, L.L.; Tan, Y.Z.; Zhang, Q.; Xie, S.Y.; Zheng, L.S. Progress in antiviral fullerene research. *Nanomaterials,* **2022**, *12*(15), 2547.
[http://dx.doi.org/10.3390/nano12152547] [PMID: 35893515]

[36]   Chiang, L.Y.; Swirczewski, J.W.; Hsu, C.S.; Chowdhury, S.K.; Cameron, S.; Creegan, K. Multi-hydroxy additions onto C60 fullerene molecules. *J. Chem. Soc. Chem. Commun.,* **1992**, (24), 1791-1793.
[http://dx.doi.org/10.1039/c39920001791]

[37]   Guldi, D.M.; Asmus, K.D. Activity of water-soluble fullerenes towards OH-radicals and molecular oxygen. *Radiat. Phys. Chem.,* **1999**, *56*(4), 449-456.
[http://dx.doi.org/10.1016/S0969-806X(99)00325-4]

[38]   Krusic, P.J.; Wasserman, E.; Keizer, P.N.; Morton, J.R.; Preston, K.F. Radical Reactions of C $_{60}$. *Science,* **1991**, *254*(5035), 1183-1185.
[http://dx.doi.org/10.1126/science.254.5035.1183] [PMID: 17776407]

[39]   Namdar, F.; Shahyad, S.; Mohammadi, M.T. Fullerene C60 nanoparticles potentiate the antioxidant defense system of brain and liver by increment of catalase activity in normal rats. *Novelty in Clinical Medicine,* **2023**, *2*(1), 32-38.

[40]   Gudkov, S.V.; Guryev, E.L.; Gapeyev, A.B.; Sharapov, M.G.; Bunkin, N.F.; Shkirin, A.V.; Zabelina, T.S.; Glinushkin, A.P.; Sevost'yanov, M.A.; Belosludtsev, K.N.; Chernikov, A.V.; Bruskov, V.I.; Zvyagin, A.V. Unmodified hydrated C_{60} fullerene molecules exhibit antioxidant properties, prevent damage to DNA and proteins induced by reactive oxygen species and protect mice against injuries caused by radiation-induced oxidative stress. *Nanomedicine,* **2019**, *15*(1), 37-46.
[http://dx.doi.org/10.1016/j.nano.2018.09.001] [PMID: 30240826]

[41]   Evans, J.L.; Goldfine, I.D.; Maddux, B.A.; Grodsky, G.M. Oxidative stress and stress-activated signaling pathways: a unifying hypothesis of type 2 diabetes. *Endocr. Rev.,* **2002**, *23*(5), 599-622.
[http://dx.doi.org/10.1210/er.2001-0039] [PMID: 12372842]

[42]   Rehman, K.; Akash, M.S.H. Mechanism of generation of oxidative stress and pathophysiology of type 2 diabetes mellitus: how are they interlinked? *J. Cell. Biochem.,* **2017**, *118*(11), 3577-3585.
[http://dx.doi.org/10.1002/jcb.26097] [PMID: 28460155]

[43]   Soldatova, Y.V.; Zhilenkov, A.V.; Kraevaya, O.A.; Troshin, P.A.; Faingold, I.I.; Kotelnikova, R.A. Antioxidant and Antiglycation Activity of Pentaamine Acid Derivatives of Fullerene C60. *Nanobiotechnology Reports,* **2022**, *17*(6), 840-845.
[http://dx.doi.org/10.1134/S2635167622060118]

[44]   Klimova, R.; Andreev, S.; Momotyuk, E.; Demidova, N.; Fedorova, N.; Chernoryzh, Y.; Yurlov, K.; Turetskiy, E.; Baraboshkina, E.; Shershakova, N.; Simonov, R.; Kushch, A.; Khaitov, M.; Gintsburg,

A. Aqueous fullerene C $_{60}$ solution suppresses herpes simplex virus and cytomegalovirus infections. *Fuller. Nanotub. Carbon Nanostruct.,* **2020**, *28*(6), 487-499.
[http://dx.doi.org/10.1080/1536383X.2019.1706495]

[45] Yasuno, T.; Ohe, T.; Kataoka, H.; Hashimoto, K.; Ishikawa, Y.; Furukawa, K.; Tateishi, Y.; Kobayashi, T.; Takahashi, K.; Nakamura, S.; Mashino, T. Fullerene derivatives as dual inhibitors of HIV-1 reverse transcriptase and protease. *Bioorg. Med. Chem. Lett.,* **2021**, *31*, 127675.
[http://dx.doi.org/10.1016/j.bmcl.2020.127675] [PMID: 33161121]

[46] Sinegubova, E.O.; Kraevaya, O.A.; Volobueva, A.S.; Zhilenkov, A.V.; Shestakov, A.F.; Baykov, S.V.; Troshin, P.A.; Zarubaev, V.V. Water-Soluble Fullerene C$_{60}$ Derivatives Are Effective Inhibitors of Influenza Virus Replication. *Microorganisms,* **2023**, *11*(3), 681.
[http://dx.doi.org/10.3390/microorganisms11030681] [PMID: 36985255]

[47] Muñoz, A.; Sigwalt, D.; Illescas, B.M.; Luczkowiak, J.; Rodríguez-Pérez, L.; Nierengarten, I.; Holler, M.; Remy, J.S.; Buffet, K.; Vincent, S.P.; Rojo, J.; Delgado, R.; Nierengarten, J.F.; Martín, N. Synthesis of giant globular multivalent glycofullerenes as potent inhibitors in a model of Ebola virus infection. *Nat. Chem.,* **2016**, *8*(1), 50-57.
[http://dx.doi.org/10.1038/nchem.2387] [PMID: 27055288]

[48] Hurmach, V.V.; Platonov, M.O.; Prylutska, S.V.; Scharff, P.; Prylutskyy, Y.I.; Ritter, U. C$_{60}$ fullerene against SARS-CoV-2 coronavirus: an in silico insight. *Sci. Rep.,* **2021**, *11*(1), 17748.
[http://dx.doi.org/10.1038/s41598-021-97268-6] [PMID: 34493768]

[49] Marforio, T.D.; Mattioli, E.J.; Zerbetto, F.; Calvaresi, M. Fullerenes against COVID-19: Repurposing C60 and C70 to clog the active site of SARS-CoV-2 protease. *Molecules,* **2022**, *27*(6), 1916.
[http://dx.doi.org/10.3390/molecules27061916] [PMID: 35335283]

[50] Page, T.M.; Nie, C.; Neander, L.; Povolotsky, T.L.; Sahoo, A.K.; Nickl, P.; Adler, J.M.; Bawadkji, O.; Radnik, J.; Achazi, K.; Ludwig, K.; Lauster, D.; Netz, R.R.; Trimpert, J.; Kaufer, B.; Haag, R.; Donskyi, I.S. Functionalized Fullerene for Inhibition of SARS☐CoV☐2 Variants. *Small,* **2023**, *19*(15), 2206154.
[http://dx.doi.org/10.1002/smll.202206154] [PMID: 36651127]

[51] Palmieri, V.; Papi, M. Can graphene take part in the fight against COVID-19? *Nano Today,* **2020**, *33*, 100883.
[http://dx.doi.org/10.1016/j.nantod.2020.100883] [PMID: 32382315]

[52] Akhavan, O.; Choobtashani, M.; Ghaderi, E. Protein Degradation and RNA Efflux of Viruses Photocatalyzed by Graphene–Tungsten Oxide Composite Under Visible Light Irradiation. *J. Phys. Chem. C,* **2012**, *116*(17), 9653-9659.
[http://dx.doi.org/10.1021/jp301707m]

[53] Xie, Y.Y.; Hu, X.H.; Zhang, Y.W.; Wahid, F.; Chu, L.Q.; Jia, S.R.; Zhong, C. Development and antibacterial activities of bacterial cellulose/graphene oxide-CuO nanocomposite films. *Carbohydr. Polym.,* **2020**, *229*, 115456.
[http://dx.doi.org/10.1016/j.carbpol.2019.115456] [PMID: 31826434]

[54] Akhavan, O.; Ghaderi, E. Toxicity of graphene and graphene oxide nanowalls against bacteria. *ACS Nano,* **2010**, *4*(10), 5731-5736.
[http://dx.doi.org/10.1021/nn101390x] [PMID: 20925398]

[55] Zainal-Abidin, M.H.; Hayyan, M.; Ngoh, G.C.; Wong, W.F. From nanoengineering to nanomedicine: A facile route to enhance biocompatibility of graphene as a potential nano-carrier for targeted drug delivery using natural deep eutectic solvents. *Chem. Eng. Sci.,* **2019**, *195*, 95-106.
[http://dx.doi.org/10.1016/j.ces.2018.11.013]

[56] Nasirzadeh, N.; Azari, M.R.; Rasoulzadeh, Y.; Mohammadian, Y. An assessment of the cytotoxic effects of graphene nanoparticles on the epithelial cells of the human lung. *Toxicol. Ind. Health,* **2019**, *35*(1), 79-87.
[http://dx.doi.org/10.1177/0748233718817180] [PMID: 30803420]

[57] Pulingam, T.; Thong, K.L.; Appaturi, J.N.; Nordin, N.I.; Dinshaw, I.J.; Lai, C.W.; Leo, B.F. Synergistic antibacterial actions of graphene oxide and antibiotics towards bacteria and the toxicological effects of graphene oxide on human epidermal keratinocytes. *Eur. J. Pharm. Sci.,* **2020**, *142*, 105087.
[http://dx.doi.org/10.1016/j.ejps.2019.105087] [PMID: 31626968]

[58] Khan, B.; Adeleye, A.S.; Burgess, R.M.; Russo, S.M.; Ho, K.T. Effects of graphene oxide nanomaterial exposures on the marine bivalve, Crassostrea virginica. *Aquat. Toxicol.,* **2019**, *216*, 105297.
[http://dx.doi.org/10.1016/j.aquatox.2019.105297] [PMID: 31550666]

[59] Akhavan, O.; Ghaderi, E.; Esfandiar, A. Wrapping bacteria by graphene nanosheets for isolation from environment, reactivation by sonication, and inactivation by near-infrared irradiation. *J. Phys. Chem. B,* **2011**, *115*(19), 6279-6288.
[http://dx.doi.org/10.1021/jp200686k] [PMID: 21513335]

[60] Cao, G.; Yan, J.; Ning, X.; Zhang, Q.; Wu, Q.; Bi, L.; Zhang, Y.; Han, Y.; Guo, J. Antibacterial and antibiofilm properties of graphene and its derivatives. *Colloids Surf. B Biointerfaces,* **2021**, *200*, 111588.
[http://dx.doi.org/10.1016/j.colsurfb.2021.111588] [PMID: 33529928]

[61] Tu, Y.; Lv, M.; Xiu, P.; Huynh, T.; Zhang, M.; Castelli, M.; Liu, Z.; Huang, Q.; Fan, C.; Fang, H.; Zhou, R. Destructive extraction of phospholipids from Escherichia coli membranes by graphene nanosheets. *Nat. Nanotechnol.,* **2013**, *8*(8), 594-601.
[http://dx.doi.org/10.1038/nnano.2013.125] [PMID: 23832191]

[62] Cao, G.; Yan, J.; Ning, X.; Zhang, Q.; Wu, Q.; Bi, L.; Zhang, Y.; Han, Y.; Guo, J. Antibacterial and antibiofilm properties of graphene and its derivatives. *Colloids Surf. B Biointerfaces,* **2021**, *200*, 111588.
[http://dx.doi.org/10.1016/j.colsurfb.2021.111588] [PMID: 33529928]

[63] Liu, S.; Zeng, T.H.; Hofmann, M.; Burcombe, E.; Wei, J.; Jiang, R.; Kong, J.; Chen, Y. Antibacterial activity of graphite, graphite oxide, graphene oxide, and reduced graphene oxide: membrane and oxidative stress. *ACS Nano,* **2011**, *5*(9), 6971-6980.
[http://dx.doi.org/10.1021/nn202451x] [PMID: 21851105]

[64] Song, Z.; Wang, X.; Zhu, G.; Nian, Q.; Zhou, H.; Yang, D.; Qin, C.; Tang, R. Virus capture and destruction by label-free graphene oxide for detection and disinfection applications. *Small,* **2015**, *11*(9-10), 1171-1176.
[http://dx.doi.org/10.1002/smll.201401706] [PMID: 25285820]

[65] Donskyi, I.S.; Azab, W.; Cuellar-Camacho, J.L.; Guday, G.; Lippitz, A.; Unger, W.E.S.; Osterrieder, K.; Adeli, M.; Haag, R. Functionalized nanographene sheets with high antiviral activity through synergistic electrostatic and hydrophobic interactions. *Nanoscale,* **2019**, *11*(34), 15804-15809.
[http://dx.doi.org/10.1039/C9NR05273A] [PMID: 31433428]

[66] Hashmi, A.; Nayak, V.; Singh, K.R.B.; Jain, B.; Baid, M.; Alexis, F.; Singh, A.K. Potentialities of graphene and its allied derivatives to combat against SARS-CoV-2 infection. *Materials Today Advances,* **2022**, *13*, 100208.
[http://dx.doi.org/10.1016/j.mtadv.2022.100208] [PMID: 35039802]

[67] Lai, C.; Lin, S.; Huang, X.; Jin, Y. Synthesis and properties of carbon quantum dots and their research progress in cancer treatment. *Dyes Pigments,* **2021**, *196*, 109766.
[http://dx.doi.org/10.1016/j.dyepig.2021.109766]

[68] Li, P.; Yu, M.; Ke, X.; Gong, X.; Li, Z.; Xing, X. Cytocompatible amphipathic carbon quantum dots as potent membrane-active antibacterial agents with low drug resistance and effective inhibition of biofilm formation. *ACS Appl. Bio Mater.,* **2022**, *5*(7), 3290-3299.
[http://dx.doi.org/10.1021/acsabm.2c00292] [PMID: 35700313]

[69] Shaikh, A.F.; Tamboli, M.S.; Patil, R.H.; Bhan, A.; Ambekar, J.D.; Kale, B.B. Bioinspired carbon

quantum dots: An antibiofilm agents. *J. Nanosci. Nanotechnol.,* **2019**, *19*(4), 2339-2345.
[http://dx.doi.org/10.1166/jnn.2019.16537] [PMID: 30486995]

[70] Ran, H.H.; Cheng, X.; Bao, Y.W.; Hua, X.W.; Gao, G.; Zhang, X.; Jiang, Y.W.; Zhu, Y.X.; Wu, F.G. Multifunctional quaternized carbon dots with enhanced biofilm penetration and eradication efficiencies. *J. Mater. Chem. B Mater. Biol. Med.,* **2019**, *7*(33), 5104-5114.
[http://dx.doi.org/10.1039/C9TB00681H] [PMID: 31432881]

[71] Prasad, K.S.; Shruthi, G.; Shivamallu, C. One-pot synthesis of aqueous carbon quantum dots using bibenzoimidazolyl derivative and their antitumor activity against breast cancer cell lines. *Inorg. Chem. Commun.,* **2019**, *101*, 11-15.
[http://dx.doi.org/10.1016/j.inoche.2019.01.001]

[72] Li, Y.; Zheng, X.; Zhang, X.; Liu, S.; Pei, Q.; Zheng, M.; Xie, Z. Porphyrin-based carbon dots for photodynamic therapy of hepatoma. *Adv. Healthc. Mater.,* **2017**, *6*(1), 1600924.
[http://dx.doi.org/10.1002/adhm.201600924] [PMID: 27860468]

[73] Quazi, M.Z.; Park, N. Nanohydrogels: advanced polymeric nanomaterials in the era of nanotechnology for robust functionalization and cumulative applications. *Int. J. Mol. Sci.,* **2022**, *23*(4), 1943.
[http://dx.doi.org/10.3390/ijms23041943] [PMID: 35216058]

[74] Dimatteo, R.; Darling, N.J.; Segura, T. *In situ* forming injectable hydrogels for drug delivery and wound repair. *Adv. Drug Deliv. Rev.,* **2018**, *127*, 167-184.
[http://dx.doi.org/10.1016/j.addr.2018.03.007] [PMID: 29567395]

[75] Liu, S.; Guo, W. Anti☐Biofouling and Healable Materials: Preparation, Mechanisms, and Biomedical Applications. *Adv. Funct. Mater.,* **2018**, *28*(41), 1800596.
[http://dx.doi.org/10.1002/adfm.201800596]

[76] Stashak, T.S.; Farstvedt, E.; Othic, A. Update on wound dressings: Indications and best use. *Clinical Techniques in Equine Practice,* **2004**, *3*(2), 148-163.
[http://dx.doi.org/10.1053/j.ctep.2004.08.006]

[77] Caló, E.; Khutoryanskiy, V.V. Biomedical applications of hydrogels: A review of patents and commercial products. *Eur. Polym. J.,* **2015**, *65*, 252-267.
[http://dx.doi.org/10.1016/j.eurpolymj.2014.11.024]

[78] Davies, C.E.; Wilson, M.J.; Hill, K.E.; Stephens, P.; Hill, C.M.; Harding, K.G.; Thomas, D.W. Use of molecular techniques to study microbial diversity in the skin: Chronic wounds reevaluated. *Wound Repair Regen.,* **2001**, *9*(5), 332-340.
[http://dx.doi.org/10.1046/j.1524-475x.2001.00332.x] [PMID: 11896975]

[79] Sahariah, P.; Másson, M. Antimicrobial Chitosan and Chitosan Derivatives: A Review of the Structure–Activity Relationship. *Biomacromolecules,* **2017**, *18*(11), 3846-3868.
[http://dx.doi.org/10.1021/acs.biomac.7b01058] [PMID: 28933147]

[80] Khalil, A.M.; Abdel-Monem, R.A.; Darwesh, O.M.; Hashim, A.I.; Nada, A.A.; Rabie, S.T. Synthesis, Characterization, and Evaluation of Antimicrobial Activities of Chitosan and Carboxymethyl Chitosan Schiff-Base/Silver Nanoparticles. *J. Chem.,* **2017**, *2017*, 1-11.
[http://dx.doi.org/10.1155/2017/1434320]

[81] Chien, R.C.; Yen, M.T.; Mau, J.L. Antimicrobial and antitumor activities of chitosan from shiitake stipes, compared to commercial chitosan from crab shells. *Carbohydr. Polym.,* **2016**, *138*, 259-264.
[http://dx.doi.org/10.1016/j.carbpol.2015.11.061] [PMID: 26794761]

[82] Ardean, C.; Davidescu, C.M.; Nemeş, N.S.; Negrea, A.; Ciopec, M.; Duteanu, N.; Negrea, P.; Duda-Seiman, D.; Musta, V. Factors Influencing the Antibacterial Activity of Chitosan and Chitosan Modified by Functionalization. *Int. J. Mol. Sci.,* **2021**, *22*(14), 7449.
[http://dx.doi.org/10.3390/ijms22147449] [PMID: 34299068]

[83] Li, J.; Zhuang, S. Antibacterial activity of chitosan and its derivatives and their interaction mechanism with bacteria: Current state and perspectives. *Eur. Polym. J.,* **2020**, *138*, 109984.

[http://dx.doi.org/10.1016/j.eurpolymj.2020.109984]

[84] Kingkaew, J.; Kirdponpattara, S.; Sanchavanakit, N.; Pavasant, P.; Phisalaphong, M. Effect of molecular weight of chitosan on antimicrobial properties and tissue compatibility of chitosan-impregnated bacterial cellulose films. *Biotechnol. Bioprocess Eng.; BBE,* **2014**, *19*(3), 534-544.
[http://dx.doi.org/10.1007/s12257-014-0081-x]

[85] Vishu Kumar, A.B.; Varadaraj, M.C.; Gowda, L.R.; Tharanathan, R.N. Characterization of chito-oligosaccharides prepared by chitosanolysis with the aid of papain and Pronase, and their bactericidal action against *Bacillus cereus* and *Escherichia coli. Biochem. J.,* **2005**, *391*(2), 167-175.
[http://dx.doi.org/10.1042/BJ20050093] [PMID: 15932346]

[86] Kapusta, O.; Jarosz, A.; Stadnik, K.; Giannakoudakis, D.A.; Barczyński, B.; Barczak, M. Antimicrobial Natural Hydrogels in Biomedicine: Properties, Applications, and Challenges—A Concise Review. *Int. J. Mol. Sci.,* **2023**, *24*(3), 2191.
[http://dx.doi.org/10.3390/ijms24032191] [PMID: 36768513]

[87] Chen, H.; Cheng, J.; Ran, L.; Yu, K.; Lu, B.; Lan, G.; Dai, F.; Lu, F. An injectable self-healing hydrogel with adhesive and antibacterial properties effectively promotes wound healing. *Carbohydr. Polym.,* **2018**, *201*, 522-531.
[http://dx.doi.org/10.1016/j.carbpol.2018.08.090] [PMID: 30241849]

[88] Wahid, F.; Hu, X.H.; Chu, L.Q.; Jia, S.R.; Xie, Y.Y.; Zhong, C. Development of bacterial cellulose/chitosan based semi-interpenetrating hydrogels with improved mechanical and antibacterial properties. *Int. J. Biol. Macromol.,* **2019**, *122*, 380-387.
[http://dx.doi.org/10.1016/j.ijbiomac.2018.10.105] [PMID: 30342151]

[89] Kaur, S.; Sharma, P.; Bains, A.; Chawla, P.; Sridhar, K.; Sharma, M.; Inbaraj, B.S. Antimicrobial and Anti-Inflammatory Activity of Low-Energy Assisted Nanohydrogel of *Azadirachta indica* Oil. *Gels,* **2022**, *8*(7), 434.
[http://dx.doi.org/10.3390/gels8070434] [PMID: 35877519]

[90] Squinca, P.; Berglund, L.; Hanna, K.; Rakar, J.; Junker, J.; Khalaf, H.; Farinas, C.S.; Oksman, K. Multifunctional ginger nanofiber hydrogels with tunable absorption: the potential for advanced wound dressing applications. *Biomacromolecules,* **2021**, *22*(8), 3202-3215.
[http://dx.doi.org/10.1021/acs.biomac.1c00215] [PMID: 34254779]

[91] Haggag, Y.A.; Donia, A.A.; Osman, M.A.; El-Gizawy, S.A. Peptides as drug candidates: limitations and recent development perspectives. *Biomed. J.,* **2018**, *1*(3)

[92] Watt, P.M. Screening for peptide drugs from the natural repertoire of biodiverse protein folds. *Nat. Biotechnol.,* **2006**, *24*(2), 177-183.
[http://dx.doi.org/10.1038/nbt1190] [PMID: 16465163]

[93] Huan, Y.; Kong, Q.; Mou, H.; Yi, H. Antimicrobial peptides: classification, design, application and research progress in multiple fields. *Front. Microbiol.,* **2020**, *11*, 582779.
[http://dx.doi.org/10.3389/fmicb.2020.582779] [PMID: 33178164]

[94] Liu, L.; Xu, K.; Wang, H.; Jeremy Tan, P.K.; Fan, W.; Venkatraman, S.S.; Li, L.; Yang, Y.Y. Self-assembled cationic peptide nanoparticles as an efficient antimicrobial agent. *Nat. Nanotechnol.,* **2009**, *4*(7), 457-463.
[http://dx.doi.org/10.1038/nnano.2009.153] [PMID: 19581900]

[95] Tripathi, J.K.; Pal, S.; Awasthi, B.; Kumar, A.; Tandon, A.; Mitra, K.; Chattopadhyay, N.; Ghosh, J.K. Variants of self-assembling peptide, KLD-12 that show both rapid fracture healing and antimicrobial properties. *Biomaterials,* **2015**, *56*, 92-103.
[http://dx.doi.org/10.1016/j.biomaterials.2015.03.046] [PMID: 25934283]

[96] Zhang, L.; Jing, D.; Jiang, N.; Rojalin, T.; Baehr, C.M.; Zhang, D.; Xiao, W.; Wu, Y.; Cong, Z.; Li, J.J.; Li, Y.; Wang, L.; Lam, K.S. Transformable peptide nanoparticles arrest HER2 signalling and cause cancer cell death *in vivo. Nat. Nanotechnol.,* **2020**, *15*(2), 145-153.
[http://dx.doi.org/10.1038/s41565-019-0626-4] [PMID: 31988501]

[97]   Ischakov, R.; Adler-Abramovich, L.; Buzhansky, L.; Shekhter, T.; Gazit, E. Peptide-based hydrogel nanoparticles as effective drug delivery agents. *Bioorg. Med. Chem.,* **2013**, *21*(12), 3517-3522.
        [http://dx.doi.org/10.1016/j.bmc.2013.03.012] [PMID: 23566763]

[98]   Carratalá, J.V.; Serna, N.; Villaverde, A.; Vázquez, E.; Ferrer-Miralles, N. Nanostructured antimicrobial peptides: The last push towards clinics. *Biotechnol. Adv.,* **2020**, *44*, 107603.
        [http://dx.doi.org/10.1016/j.biotechadv.2020.107603] [PMID: 32738381]

[99]   Fjell, C.D.; Hiss, J.A.; Hancock, R.E.W.; Schneider, G. Designing antimicrobial peptides: form follows function. *Nat. Rev. Drug Discov.,* **2012**, *11*(1), 37-51.
        [http://dx.doi.org/10.1038/nrd3591] [PMID: 22173434]

[100] Salick, D.A.; Kretsinger, J.K.; Pochan, D.J.; Schneider, J.P. Inherent antibacterial activity of a peptide-based β-hairpin hydrogel. *J. Am. Chem. Soc.,* **2007**, *129*(47), 14793-14799.
        [http://dx.doi.org/10.1021/ja076300z] [PMID: 17985907]

[101] Bai, Q.; Zheng, C.; Chen, W.; Sun, N.; Gao, Q.; Liu, J.; Hu, F.; Pimpi, S.; Yan, X.; Zhang, Y.; Lu, T. Current challenges and future applications of antibacterial nanomaterials and chitosan hydrogel in burn wound healing. *Materials Advances,* **2022**, *3*(17), 6707-6727.
        [http://dx.doi.org/10.1039/D2MA00695B]

[102] Schnaider, L.; Brahmachari, S.; Schmidt, N.W.; Mensa, B.; Shaham-Niv, S.; Bychenko, D.; Adler-Abramovich, L.; Shimon, L.J.W.; Kolusheva, S.; DeGrado, W.F.; Gazit, E. Self-assembling dipeptide antibacterial nanostructures with membrane disrupting activity. *Nat. Commun.,* **2017**, *8*(1), 1365.
        [http://dx.doi.org/10.1038/s41467-017-01447-x] [PMID: 29118336]

[103] McCloskey, A.P.; Draper, E.R.; Gilmore, B.F.; Laverty, G. Ultrashort self□assembling Fmoc□peptide gelators for anti□infective biomaterial applications. *J. Pept. Sci.,* **2017**, *23*(2), 131-140.
        [http://dx.doi.org/10.1002/psc.2951] [PMID: 28066954]

[104] Porter, S.L.; Coulter, S.M.; Pentlavalli, S.; Thompson, T.P.; Laverty, G. Self-assembling diphenylalanine peptide nanotubes selectively eradicate bacterial biofilm infection. *Acta Biomater.,* **2018**, *77*, 96-105.
        [http://dx.doi.org/10.1016/j.actbio.2018.07.033] [PMID: 30031161]

[105] Seidi, F.; Arabi Shamsabadi, A.; Dadashi Firouzjaei, M.; Elliott, M.; Saeb, M.R.; Huang, Y.; Li, C.; Xiao, H.; Anasori, B. MXenes Antibacterial Properties and Applications: A Review and Perspective. *Small,* **2023**, *19*(14), 2206716.
        [http://dx.doi.org/10.1002/smll.202206716] [PMID: 36604987]

[106] Solangi, N.H.; Mazari, S.A.; Mubarak, N.M.; Karri, R.R.; Rajamohan, N.; Vo, D.V.N. Recent trends in MXene-based material for biomedical applications. *Environ. Res.,* **2023**, *222*, 115337.
        [http://dx.doi.org/10.1016/j.envres.2023.115337] [PMID: 36682442]

[107] Pogorielov, M.; Smyrnova, K.; Kyrylenko, S.; Gogotsi, O.; Zahorodna, V.; Pogrebnjak, A. MXenes : A new class of two-dimensional materials: Structure, properties and potential applications. *Nanomaterials,* **2021**, *11*(12), 3412.
        [http://dx.doi.org/10.3390/nano11123412] [PMID: 34947759]

[108] Driscoll, N.; Richardson, A.G.; Maleski, K.; Anasori, B.; Adewole, O.; Lelyukh, P.; Escobedo, L.; Cullen, D.K.; Lucas, T.H.; Gogotsi, Y.; Vitale, F. Two-Dimensional Ti $_3$ C $_2$ MXene for High-Resolution Neural Interfaces. *ACS Nano,* **2018**, *12*(10), 10419-10429.
        [http://dx.doi.org/10.1021/acsnano.8b06014] [PMID: 30207690]

[109] Wang, Y.; Feng, W.; Chen, Y. Chemistry of two-dimensional MXene nanosheets in theranostic nanomedicine. *Chin. Chem. Lett.,* **2020**, *31*(4), 937-946.
        [http://dx.doi.org/10.1016/j.cclet.2019.11.016]

[110] Lin, H.; Wang, X.; Yu, L.; Chen, Y.; Shi, J. Two-dimensional ultrathin MXene ceramic nanosheets for photothermal conversion. *Nano Lett.,* **2017**, *17*(1), 384-391.
        [http://dx.doi.org/10.1021/acs.nanolett.6b04339] [PMID: 28026960]

[111] Lin, H.; Wang, Y.; Gao, S.; Chen, Y.; Shi, J. Theranostic 2D tantalum carbide (MXene). *Adv. Mater.,* **2018**, *30*(4), 1703284.
[http://dx.doi.org/10.1002/adma.201703284] [PMID: 29226386]

[112] Lin, H.; Gao, S.; Dai, C.; Chen, Y.; Shi, J. A two-dimensional biodegradable niobium carbide (MXene) for photothermal tumor eradication in NIR-I and NIR-II biowindows. *J. Am. Chem. Soc.,* **2017**, *139*(45), 16235-16247.
[http://dx.doi.org/10.1021/jacs.7b07818] [PMID: 29063760]

[113] Feng, W.; Wang, R.; Zhou, Y.; Ding, L.; Gao, X.; Zhou, B.; Hu, P.; Chen, Y. Ultrathin molybdenum carbide MXene with fast biodegradability for highly efficient theory-oriented photonic tumor hyperthermia. *Adv. Funct. Mater.,* **2019**, *29*(22), 1901942.
[http://dx.doi.org/10.1002/adfm.201901942]

[114] Rasool, K.; Mahmoud, K.A.; Johnson, D.J.; Helal, M.; Berdiyorov, G.R.; Gogotsi, Y. Efficient Antibacterial Membrane based on Two-Dimensional $Ti_3C_2T_x$ (MXene) Nanosheets. *Sci. Rep.,* **2017**, *7*(1), 1598.
[http://dx.doi.org/10.1038/s41598-017-01714-3] [PMID: 28487521]

[115] Rasool, K.; Helal, M.; Ali, A.; Ren, C.E.; Gogotsi, Y.; Mahmoud, K.A. Antibacterial Activity of $Ti_3C_2T_x$ MXene. *ACS Nano,* **2016**, *10*(3), 3674-3684.
[http://dx.doi.org/10.1021/acsnano.6b00181] [PMID: 26909865]

[116] He, Q.; Hu, H.; Han, J.; Zhao, Z. Double transition-metal TiVCTX MXene with dual-functional antibacterial capability. *Mater. Lett.,* **2022**, *308*, 131100.
[http://dx.doi.org/10.1016/j.matlet.2021.131100]

[117] Arabi Shamsabadi, A.; Sharifian Gh, M.; Anasori, B.; Soroush, M. Antimicrobial Mode-of-Action of Colloidal $Ti_3C_2T_x$ MXene Nanosheets. *ACS Sustain. Chem.& Eng.,* **2018**, *6*(12), 16586-16596.
[http://dx.doi.org/10.1021/acssuschemeng.8b03823]

[118] Szuplewska, A.; Rozmysłowska-Wojciechowska, A.; Poźniak, S.; Wojciechowski, T.; Birowska, M.; Popielski, M.; Chudy, M.; Ziemkowska, W.; Chlubny, L.; Moszczyńska, D.; Olszyna, A.; Majewski, J.A.; Jastrzębska, A.M. Multilayered stable 2D nano-sheets of Ti_2NT_x MXene: Synthesis, characterization, and anticancer activity. *J. Nanobiotechnology,* **2019**, *17*(1), 114.
[http://dx.doi.org/10.1186/s12951-019-0545-4] [PMID: 31711491]

[119] Jastrzębska, A.M.; Szuplewska, A.; Wojciechowski, T.; Chudy, M.; Ziemkowska, W.; Chlubny, L.; Rozmysłowska, A.; Olszyna, A. In vitro studies on cytotoxicity of delaminated Ti_3C_2 MXene. *J. Hazard. Mater.,* **2017**, *339*, 1-8.
[http://dx.doi.org/10.1016/j.jhazmat.2017.06.004] [PMID: 28601597]

[120] Lim, G.P.; Soon, C.F.; Jastrzębska, A.M.; Ma, N.L.; Wojciechowska, A.R.; Szuplewska, A.; Wan Omar, W.I.; Morsin, M.; Nayan, N.; Tee, K.S. Synthesis, characterization and biophysical evaluation of the 2D Ti_2CT_x MXene using 3D spheroid-type cultures. *Ceram. Int.,* **2021**, *47*(16), 22567-22577.
[http://dx.doi.org/10.1016/j.ceramint.2021.04.268]

[121] Rajavel, K.; Shen, S.; Ke, T.; Lin, D. Achieving high bactericidal and antibiofouling activities of 2D titanium carbide ($Ti_3C_2T_x$) by delamination and intercalation. *2D Materials,* **2019**, *6*(3), 035040.

[122] You, Y.; Yang, C.; Zhang, X.; Lin, H.; Shi, J. Emerging two-dimensional silicene nanosheets for biomedical applications. *Materials Today Nano,* **2021**, *16*, 100132.
[http://dx.doi.org/10.1016/j.mtnano.2021.100132]

[123] Lin, H.; Qiu, W.; Liu, J.; Yu, L.; Gao, S.; Yao, H.; Chen, Y.; Shi, J. Silicene: Wet-chemical exfoliation synthesis and biodegradable tumor nanomedicine. *Adv. Mater.,* **2019**, *31*(37), 1903013.
[http://dx.doi.org/10.1002/adma.201903013] [PMID: 31347215]

[124] Zeng, J.; Goldfeld, D.; Xia, Y. A plasmon-assisted optofluidic (PAOF) system for measuring the photothermal conversion efficiencies of gold nanostructures and controlling an electrical switch. *Angew. Chem. Int. Ed.,* **2013**, *52*(15), 4169-4173.

[http://dx.doi.org/10.1002/anie.201210359] [PMID: 23494970]

[125] Bashkatov, A.N.; Genina, E.A.; Kochubey, V.I.; Tuchin, V.V. Optical properties of human skin, subcutaneous and mucous tissues in the wavelength range from 400 to 2000 nm. *J. Phys. D Appl. Phys.,* **2005**, *38*(15), 2543-2555.
[http://dx.doi.org/10.1088/0022-3727/38/15/004]

[126] Luo, Y.; Ge, M.; Lin, H.; He, R.; Yuan, X.; Yang, C.; Wang, W.; Zhang, X. Anti-Infective Application of Graphene-Like Silicon Nanosheets *via* Membrane Destruction. *Adv. Healthc. Mater.,* **2020**, *9*(3), 1901375.
[http://dx.doi.org/10.1002/adhm.201901375] [PMID: 31894648]

[127] Ares, P.; Aguilar-Galindo, F.; Rodríguez-San-Miguel, D.; Aldave, D.A.; Díaz-Tendero, S.; Alcamí, M.; Martín, F.; Gómez-Herrero, J.; Zamora, F. Mechanical Isolation of Highly Stable Antimonene under Ambient Conditions. *Adv. Mater.,* **2016**, *28*(30), 6332-6336.
[http://dx.doi.org/10.1002/adma.201602128] [PMID: 27272099]

[128] Gibaja, C.; Rodriguez-San-Miguel, D.; Ares, P.; Gómez-Herrero, J.; Varela, M.; Gillen, R.; Maultzsch, J.; Hauke, F.; Hirsch, A.; Abellán, G.; Zamora, F. Few-Layer Antimonene by Liquid-Phase Exfoliation. *Angew. Chem. Int. Ed.,* **2016**, *55*(46), 14345-14349.
[http://dx.doi.org/10.1002/anie.201605298] [PMID: 27529687]

[129] Srivastava, S.; Singh, S.; Mishra, S.; Pandey, M.; Khan, M.Y. Nanopoxia: Antimonene-Based Nanoplatform Targeting Cancer Hypoxia for Precision Cancer Therapy.*Smart Nanomaterials Targeting Pathological Hypoxia*; Springer, **2023**, pp. 103-113.
[http://dx.doi.org/10.1007/978-981-99-1718-1_6]

[130] Wang, Y.; Ding, Y. Electronic structure and carrier mobilities of arsenene and antimonene nanoribbons: a first-principle study. *Nanoscale Res. Lett.,* **2015**, *10*(1), 254.
[http://dx.doi.org/10.1186/s11671-015-0955-7] [PMID: 26058516]

[131] Xie, Z.; Chen, S.; Duo, Y.; Zhu, Y.; Fan, T.; Zou, Q.; Qu, M.; Lin, Z.; Zhao, J.; Li, Y.; Liu, L.; Bao, S.; Chen, H.; Fan, D.; Zhang, H. Biocompatible Two-Dimensional Titanium Nanosheets for Multimodal Imaging-Guided Cancer Theranostics. *ACS Appl. Mater. Interfaces,* **2019**, *11*(25), 22129-22140.
[http://dx.doi.org/10.1021/acsami.9b04628] [PMID: 31144494]

[132] Tao, W.; Ji, X.; Xu, X.; Islam, M.A.; Li, Z.; Chen, S.; Saw, P.E.; Zhang, H.; Bharwani, Z.; Guo, Z.; Shi, J.; Farokhzad, O.C. Antimonene Quantum Dots: Synthesis and Application as Near□Infrared Photothermal Agents for Effective Cancer Therapy. *Angew. Chem. Int. Ed.,* **2017**, *56*(39), 11896-11900.
[http://dx.doi.org/10.1002/anie.201703657] [PMID: 28640986]

[133] Lu, G.; Lv, C.; Bao, W.; Li, F.; Zhang, F.; Zhang, L.; Wang, S.; Gao, X.; Zhao, D.; Wei, W.; Xie, H. Antimonene with two-orders-of-magnitude improved stability for high-performance cancer theranostics. *Chem. Sci.,* **2019**, *10*(18), 4847-4853.
[http://dx.doi.org/10.1039/C9SC00324J] [PMID: 31183034]

[134] Bertrand, N.; Wu, J.; Xu, X.; Kamaly, N.; Farokhzad, O.C. Cancer nanotechnology: The impact of passive and active targeting in the era of modern cancer biology. *Adv. Drug Deliv. Rev.,* **2014**, *66*, 2-25.
[http://dx.doi.org/10.1016/j.addr.2013.11.009] [PMID: 24270007]

CHAPTER 4

Nanotechnology for Drug Design and Drug Delivery

Abstract: The development of ideal, secure, efficient, non-invasive drug delivery systems is now a top priority in this field of drug delivery. Nanoparticles are being employed more frequently for effective medication delivery, exerting the desired therapeutic effect at the expected site of action with the least amount of activity or volume loss. Size, surface chemistry, biological destiny, toxicity, *in vivo* dispersion, and targeting capabilities all play a role in these systems. The stability and interactions of nanoparticles with cells are regulated by their surface chemistry, and they can access a greater variety of targets. The development of nano-drug delivery systems has opened up new avenues for the treatment and prevention of disease, as well as for enhancing pharmacological properties, enhancing targeting, overcoming drug resistance, and lowering immunogenicity and toxicity. This chapter will first discuss the desirable characteristics of an effective drug delivery system and will cover recent developments in nano drug delivery systems used in clinical research, including dendrimers, solid lipid nanoparticles, nanogels, nanoemulsions, polymeric micelles, and polymer nanofibers.

Keywords: Dendrimers, Nano-drug delivery, Nanogels, Nanoemulsions, Polymeric micelles, Polymer nanofibers, Solid-lipid nanoparticles, Solid lipid nanoemulsions.

1. INTRODUCTION

Nanotechnology is being used in drug development at every level, from formulation to effective dosage to administration using the best possible delivery methods. Poor solubility, large molecular size, and inadequate bioavailability for clinical candidates are the primary issues that drug delivery experts face.

Nano-drug delivery systems (NDDS) are crucial in addressing the challenges of conventional drug delivery. The focus is increasingly shifting towards nanoparticles for precise and targeted drug delivery. The effectiveness of nanoparticle targeting relies on factors such as size, surface charge, hydrophobicity, and surface modification. NDDS enhances drug solubility by downsizing drugs to the nanoscale, ensuring sustained and controlled release for improved patient compliance. Furthermore, nano-drug delivery formulations offer

Laksiri Weerasinghe, Imalka Munaweera and Senuri Kumarage

a viable alternative for unstable formulations with shorter shelf lives, reduce the required dosage, thereby increasing safety by mitigating side effects. These systems enhance therapeutic outcomes by prolonging drug action, enhancing efficacy and specificity, combating drug resistance, and decreasing immunogenicity and toxicity.

This chapter will first discuss the desirable characteristics of an effective drug delivery system and will cover recent developments in NDDS used in clinical research, including liposomes, dendrimers, solid-lipid nanoparticles, nanogels, nanoemulsions, polymeric micelles, inorganic NPs, and polymer nanofibers.

2. ATTRIBUTES OF AN EFFECTIVE DELIVERY SYSTEM

Nanoparticles designed as drug delivery systems work by trapping pharmaceuticals or biomolecules inside their internal structures, adhering them to the surfaces of the particles. Currently, drugs, proteins, genes, vaccines, polypeptides, nucleic acids, and other substances are delivered using nanoparticles (NPs). Different uses of the NP-based drug delivery system have seen tremendous growth in recent years in industries including pharmaceutical, medical, biological, and others. Considering the impact of NPs in drug delivery systems, this section will brief on how NP delivery systems circumvent the limitations of conventional delivery methods, the characteristics of NPs that affect on being an efficient delivery system, different targeting methods, and then the existing nano drug delivery systems will be discussed.

While it might be challenging to deliver free drugs in traditional dosage forms to the target place at the recommended doses, during the right time period or after it, drug targeting to specific organs and tissues has emerged as one of the key research efforts. Thus, one of the breakthrough research fields is the hunt for novel drug delivery systems and therapeutic mechanisms [1]. Poor solubility, large molecular size, and inadequate bioavailability for clinical candidates are the major constraints experienced by drug delivery experts. Drug administration for children and the elderly, drug delivery for proteins and peptides, and other issues are concerns in this discipline. The development of ideal, secure, efficient, non-invasive drug delivery systems is now a top priority in this field of drug delivery.

To treat chronic human illnesses, regulated drug release and tailored drug delivery have greatly benefited from nanotechnology. Given that they are composed of substances that have been created at the atomic or molecular level, nanoparticles are frequently very small nanospheres [2]. They might therefore move through the body with more suppleness than larger materials. Nanoparticles have different structural, chemical, mechanical, magnetic, electrical, and biological properties. *In vivo* instability, poor body absorption, issues with target-specific distribution, low bioavailability and solubility, issues with therapeutic effectiveness, and perhaps even negative pharmacological effects are major obstacles when employing large-scale materials for drug administration [1, 3]. Additionally, investigations claim that nanostructures enhance the delivery of medications that are only weakly water-soluble to their target locations and prevent pharmaceuticals from being contaminated in the gastrointestinal tract. Because they are often absorbed by absorptive endocytosis, nanopharmaceuticals have a higher oral bioavailability.

Due to their long-term persistence in the blood circulation system, nanostructures enable the release of integrated medicines at the specified dose. As a consequence, they have fewer adverse effects and less variability in plasma [4]. Due to their nanoscale size, these structures may easily enter the tissue system, allow more efficient drug delivery and administration to cells and ensure that the drug acts where it is targeted. Compared to larger particles between 1 µm and 10 µm in size, cells absorb nanostructures at substantially faster rates [5, 6].

There are a number of things to take into account while developing a nanoparticulate drug delivery system. One of the most crucial characteristics of NPs is their particle size, which affects their biological destiny, toxicity, *in vivo* dispersion, and targeting potential. Additionally, drug loading, drug stability, and drug release are all impacted by NPs. Being smaller yet more mobile than microparticles, nanoparticles can reach a wider array of cellular and intracellular targets [7]. The release of drugs depends on particle size. Accelerated drug release is caused by the large surface area-to-volume ratio of small particles. Instead, bigger particles' massive cores enable the extra drug to be confined per particle, resulting in a delayed drug release [8]. The shape of NPs, in addition to particle size, influences biological processes such as endocytosis [9], transportation through the vasculature [10], consequent intracellular transport [11], circulation half-life [12], targeting efficiency [13], and phagocytosis [14], related to the therapeutic administration of a drug [15 - 17]. When compared to particles shaped like cubes or squat cylinders, it was discovered that rod-shaped nanoparticles, which resemble the form of bacteria that are adept at infecting cells, were faster in accessing the cells [18].

The surface chemistry of nanoparticles plays a significant role in the nanoparticulate drug delivery system in addition to size and shape. Particle stability and interactions with cells [19, 20] as well as opsonization, biodistribution, blood circulation, and phagocytosis [21] are affected by the surface charge and hydrophobicity of the particles. Highly positively or negatively charged NPs showed very high liver absorption in *in vivo* biodistribution studies, which is most likely because of the macrophages (Kupffer cells) in the liver, which actively engage in phagocytosis. In contrast, when the surface charge of the NPs was slightly negative, liver absorption was extremely low but tumour uptake was extremely high. This leads to the conclusion that slightly negatively charged nanoparticles have the potential to reduce undesired reticuloendothelial system (RES) clearance (such as liver and spleen), improve blood compatibility, and assure targeted anti-cancer drug delivery to the cancer or tumour locations [22 - 24]. The hydrophobicity of foreign particle surfaces shows a significant impact during opsonization. Plasma proteins and immunoglobulin complement proteins will coat these hydrophobic particles, and will then be removed by RES. The surface hydrophobicity of NPs rises as a result of the increased protein adsorption at the surface. In order to improve the circulation half-life and to promote the accumulation of NPs in tumour tissue, NPs are coated with polyethylene glycol (PEG) and its analogues [25]. The hydrophilic steric barrier that the PEG coating surrounding nanoparticles create inhibits them from interacting with macrophage or plasma proteins, lowering RES absorption and extending blood circulation time. By preventing the build-up of nanoparticles in the liver, this coating further guarantees that they are mostly eliminated *via* the spleen [26].

A profound range of drug-loading capacity is a need for a suitable nano delivery system. Two approaches can be used to achieve drug loading. The incorporation approach is used when the drug is integrated during the nanoparticle formulation. In contrast, the drug is absorbed by the adsorption/absorption approach following nanoparticle creation, which is accomplished by incubating the nanocarrier with the concentrated drug solution. The effectiveness of medication loading depends on the drug's solubility in the matrix material of the NP. To avoid contamination and little to no effects on drug loading, a suitable polymer, such as PEG, should be chosen for nanoparticle formation [27]. Drugs exhibit the highest loading efficiency when loaded close to or at their isoelectric point [28].

When creating a nanoparticulate delivery system, the release of drugs and polymer biodegradation in polymer nanocomposites should be taken into account. The solubility of the drugs, the rate of desorption of the adsorbed drug, the diffusion of the drug using nanoparticle matrixes, the degradation or erosion of the nanoparticle matrixes, and the combination of the diffusion and erosion processes all determine the efficiency of drugs releasing into the body [29]. The mechanism of release is controlled by the biodegradation, diffusion, and solubility of the particle-matrix. The drug is evenly dispersed in nanospheres and delivered by diffusion or matrix erosion. The release of dimly bound drugs on the surfaces of the NP delivery system can be attributed to the quick 'burst' of the drugs in the initial stages. A sustained release of the drugs with minor burst properties can be accomplished by employing the incorporation method for drug loading. Drug release of polymer-coated NPs occurs by diffusion *via* the polymeric membrane [30].

In order for a drug delivery system to be effective, NPs must be able to reach the expected site of action with the least loss of activity or volume. Second, once within the target, they must be able to perform the intended therapeutic effect. Both of these prerequisites are met by nanoparticles [31]. NPs must always appropriately reach the target site, recognize it, and attach to it before delivering the drug materials to the desired tissues and minimizing the harm that the drugs induce to healthy tissues. The most popular method for directing NPs to the targeted location is to keep coating-specific ligands on the NPs' surface. Nanoparticles can either stick to specific biological structures in the targeted tissue by molecular recognition of surface-bound ligands, or they can collect passively or actively in the intended tissue *via* transit through leaky vessels and particular intra-organ pressures (Fig. **1**). Small molecules, antibodies, protein molecules, nucleic acid aptamer, *etc.* are utilized in creating these ligands [32, 33].

There are now a number of medications based on nanocarriers that rely on passive targeting *via* "enhanced permeability and retention." Nanoparticles may circulate in circulation for a long time and have a greater chance of reaching the tumour site or targeted tissues because of their shape, size, and surface characteristics. They can also escape through blood vessel walls and enter tissues [35]. Additionally, nanoparticles tend to aggregate in tumours due to leaky blood vessels and poor lymphatic drainage, which concentrate the associated cytotoxic drug where it is required, preserving healthy tissue, and dramatically reduce negative side effects. The use of myeloid cells like macrophages, which absorb nanoparticles and concentrate them like a Trojan horse in the area to be treated, is another method of passive targeting.

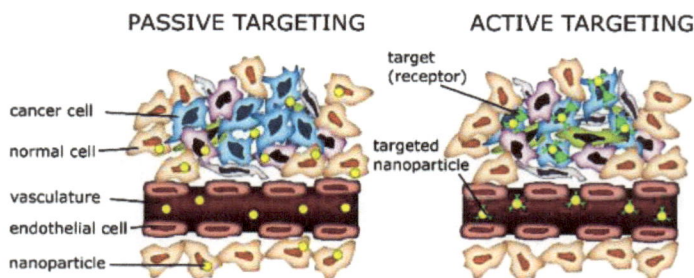

Fig. (1). Comparison of passive targeting, active targeting. Adapted from [34] Copyright (2021) of Hafeez, M. N. *et al.*, published by MDPI and distributed under the terms and conditions of the Creative Commons Attribution (CC BY) license (https://creativecommons.org/licenses/by/4.0/).

In addition to being able to attach to target tissues and interact with or be picked up by targeted cells, nanoparticles should also be stealthy to evade immune clearance and avoid non-specific cell uptake. Scientists have created smarter NPs with switchable sticky and stealthy modes for biodistribution and targeting of NPs to diseased tissues inspired by nature by exploiting the concepts of viruses, transport proteins, and their interactions with cell membranes. Different envelope-type [36] or shell-sheddable nanocarriers [37] have been investigated to improve the dispersion of NPs in target tissue by mimicking envelope-type viruses. PEG or zwitterionic polymers, which have excellent antifouling capabilities, were connected to NPs by cleavable anchor groups that are sensitive to a variety of stimuli, including pH, redox, and proteolytic enzymes. Due to the EPR effect, or passive targeting, the NPs with the stealthy shell exhibited longer circulation durations and increased accumulation in solid tumours. The specific triggers in the targeted tissue provide the NP the ability to release its shell, changing its stealthy state to sticky [38]. In addition, Neoglycoconjugates, or sugar-like functional groups, and other functions like thiol groups can be used to coat nanoparticles in order to change them from stealthy to sticky. Such glycan-based ligands offer extraordinarily high stability in biofluids while limiting nonspecific cell internalization, while being normally uncharged [39, 40]. Optimizing NP sizes is also crucial for tumour accumulation, penetration, and ultimately therapeutic effectiveness in addition to modifying the surface features of NPs, especially when focusing on stroma-rich tumours [41, 42].

In addition to passive targeting NPs, the actively targeted drugs to malignant cells, depending on the chemicals those cells display on their surfaces, has also been demonstrated. A nanoparticle can be modified to carry molecules that bind to certain biological receptors, allowing it to target cells that express that receptor alone [43]. By inducing the diseased cell to absorb the nanocarrier, active targeting can even be utilized to deliver medications within the cancerous cell. Another example of using active targeting is the magnetic focussing of drug carriers on the tumour cites. Iron oxide NPs in the tumour area can be enriched by magnetic focusing. Metal or metal oxide NPs, such as SPIONs, are present in the materials most frequently utilized for magnetic drug delivery. In order to promote colloidal stability and prevent separation into NPs and carrier media, superparamagnetic iron oxide NPs typically have an organic coating made of fatty acids, polysaccharides, or polymers on top of their iron oxide core [44]. To further decrease the interaction of transported drugs with healthy tissue, active targeting can be used in conjunction with passive targeting. Active and passive targeting made possible by nanotechnology can also boost the effectiveness of a chemotherapeutic, resulting in a more profound tumour decrease with reduced drug dosages [45]. Table 01 summarizes the comparison between active and passive target drug designs.

Table 1. Comparison between active and passive target drug designs.

Active Targeting	Passive Targeting
Specific targeting with the NPs modified with affinity ligands modified with affinity ligands, ligand receptor, antibody-antigen or another form of molecular recognition/reactions specific to the targeting site.	Targeting is determined by the size, shape, and surface charge of nanoparticles, as well as the physiological condition or anatomic barriers. Delivery by EPR due to leaky blood vessels and poor lymphatic drainage in tumour/inflammation sites.
Higher efficacy due to more concentrated and focused delivery.	Modest efficacy due to limited focus.
Less toxicity and potential side effects.	More toxicity and potential side effects.
A smaller amount of drug needs to be administered due to specific targeting.	Generally, high amounts of drugs need to be administered due to non-specificity in targeting.
Synthesizing ligands attached to NPs and simultaneously maintaining their desired targeting activity are challenging.	Less challenging to engineer the NPs.

The advent of nano-drug delivery systems (NDDSs) opens up new avenues for disease prevention and therapy. Liposomes, polymeric micelles, nanogels, nanoemulsions, solid lipid nanoparticles, dendrimers, inorganic nanoparticles, and polymer nanofibers have all been employed as NDDS in pre-clinical and clinical research in recent years [46]. These systems have the potential to enhance the pharmacological and pharmaceutical features of therapeutics by prolonging the period of action, enhancing efficacy and targeting, conquering drug resistance, and minimizing immunogenicity and toxicity [47, 48].

3. UP-TO-DATE DRUG DELIVERY SYSTEMS

3.1. Liposomes

Liposomes are potential drug delivery vehicles composed of lipid vesicles with one or more concentric lipid bilayers surrounding an aqueous space (Fig **2**). By modifying the technique of preparation, liposomes can change their chemical content, colloidal size, and shape [49]. Liposomes of various sizes, ranging from a few nanometres to micrometres, allow for the inclusion of different bilayer components during liposome formulation, permitting them to be impermeable or permeable, rigid and less stable [50]. Liposomes have the unique capacity to load and distribute compounds with various solubilities attributed to their well-organized structure. Amphiphilic molecules can be loaded at the water/lipid bilayer interface, hydrophobic molecules can be incorporated into the lipid bilayer, and hydrophilic molecules can be located in the interior aqueous core [51]. It has been discovered that by properly charging charges on the surface of liposomes, cationic liposomes, anionic liposomes, and neutral liposomes may be produced. Endocytosis and fusion being the two basic ways that liposomes and cells interact could be readily linked with additional targeting macromolecules (such as antibodies, proteins, or enzymes) to transport drugs to the infection site efficiently [52]. With multiple formulations authorized by the U.S. Food and Drug Administration, liposomes are among the most technologically sophisticated delivery systems in terms of clinical translation [53]. Some cancer treatments currently employ drug delivery methods based on liposomes (*e.g.*, Myocet, Doxil, and Daunoxome). However, liposomes have some notable disadvantages, including a limited ability to sterilize due to physical and chemical degradation of liposomes [54], the use of organic solvents in their manufacturing methods, a tendency to leak often, and instability in biological fluids and aqueous solutions [55].

Glioblastoma multiforme (GBM), which often develops from brain astrocytes, continues to be one of the most prevalent and aggressive tumours globally, accounting for 60–70% of malignant gliomas [56]. For targeted administration across the BBB, Shi *et al.* [57] created the drug (doxorubicin)-encapsulated dual-functionalized thermosensitive liposomal system by conjugating anti-GBM antibody (TN-C) and a cell-penetrating peptide (P1NS) specific for GBM to the liposome surface. The liposomes were further co-loaded with superparamagnetic iron oxide nanoparticles (SPIONs) to produce thermo triggered drug release while using an alternating magnetic field (AMF). The results demonstrated that the developed liposomal system readily transported across an *in vitro* BBB model and displayed a thermo-responsive and GBM-specific cellular uptake while suppressing the tumour cell proliferation without causing any significant impact on healthy brain cell function. $ATB^{0,+}$ which is an amino acid transporter coupled with Na^+/Cl^-, is overexpressed in many cancer cells and has been considered as a target for improved liposomal drug delivery for liver cancer treatment. As such, the ability of a lysine amino acid conjugated liposome to penetrate $ATB^{0,+}$-positive tumour cells has been evaluated, as well as the therapeutic value of these liposomes for the treatment of pancreatic cancer [56]. The internalization of liposomes and their payload entails endocytosis, with the eventual release of the cargo inside the cells, just after lysine-functionalized liposomes attach to the transporter on the cell surface. During the endocytotic process, although the transporter protein is itself partially destroyed, the protein levels eventually recover. This frequent overexpression of the amino acid transporter in cancer cells would present an intriguing delivery route for amino acid functionalized liposomes for the targeted administration of chemotherapeutics for cancer treatment. Recently, Valle *et al.* created a mucoadhesive vehicle based on lyophilized liposomes for drug delivery *via* the sublingual mucosa [58]. Egg phosphatidylcholine and cholesterol at a ratio of 7:3 were used for the liposome fabrication, and lyophilisation was carried out in the presence of mixtures of sodium alginate and carboxymethylcellulose for mucoadhesive properties and lactose and mannitol for taste-masking properties. Round and capsule-shaped tablets made from compressed lyophilized products were tested on healthy participants. The observations demonstrated that lyophilized liposomes in unidirectional round tablets had appropriate buccal retention, palatability, small size and comfort for sublingual administration.

3.2. Polymeric Micelles

Self-assembled amphiphilic block copolymers create polymer micelles in aqueous liquids, which are solid, spherical aggregates with diameters between 10 and 100 nm that are made of hydrophobic and hydrophilic units [59]. Amphiphilic polymer molecules in aqueous solutions exist as single molecules at low concentrations, similar to small-molecule surfactants. Pursuant to hydrophobic, electrostatic, hydrogen bonding, and other molecular interactions, the hydrophobic areas of the polymer interact with one another to form micelles when the concentration surpasses the critical micelle concentration (CMC) (Fig **3**). The interior of the micelles acts as a hydrophobic container when in water, while their exteriors act as a hydrophilic interface. They have displayed significant potential in NDDS because of their biophysical and chemical characteristics [60]. Additionally, polymeric micelles containing drugs might lessen negative side effects and accelerate circulation [61]. For instance, adding cisplatin to polymeric micelles considerably lowers nephrotoxicity [62]. By lowering acute renal build-up of polymeric micelles, shielding the cisplatin-loaded core with PEG prolongs blood circulation. Polymeric micelles, in comparison to other nanocarriers, have a smaller size, easy preparation and sterilizing methods, and strong solubilization capabilities; yet, they have poorer stability in biological fluids and a more difficult characterisation [63].

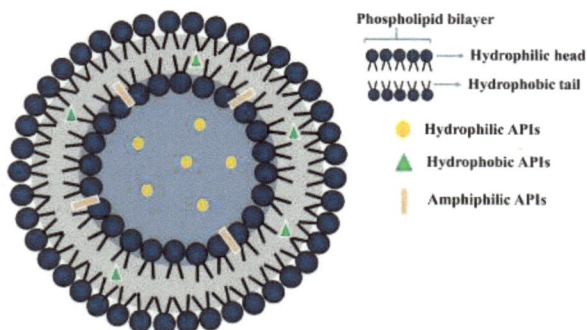

Fig. (2). General structure of liposomes.

The most researched method of administering micelles is intravenous injection/infusion [64, 65], yet oral and topical (ocular, buccal, and nasal) [66 - 69] delivery has also shown some very intriguing outcomes in terms of enhanced drug bioavailability. Surface features, which govern the stability of micelles after administration, have a significant influence on their *in vivo* behaviour. A hydrophilic and neutral surface decreases protein corona formation and increases circulation time after intravenous administration [70]. The non-specific protein binding and enhanced aggregation *in vivo*, on the other hand, make micelles with positive zeta potential exhibit very low stability in biological fluids [71, 72]. In addition, it has been demonstrated that micelles with sizes ranging from 30 to 100 nm may easily collect in highly permeable tumours, but less permeable tumours are only penetrated by micelles with dimensions of 30 nm, highlighting the significance of size [73]. The shape of these nanocarriers is a major factor in regulating circulation time, biodistribution, and cellular absorption [74]. Filomicelles, for example, have been shown to have a slower clearing process and a longer circulation time compared to spherical micelles due to their elongated form, flexibility, and fragmentation capability [75, 76]. In specific, compared to spherical micelles (40 nm) and long filo micelles (2.5 μm), shorter filo micelles (180 nm) have demonstrated the deepest tumour penetration and the most effective cellular uptake [77]. A similar study evaluating the role of micelle morphology on the drug pharmacological performance has demonstrated that the morphology of polymeric micelles is dependent on the polymer type, molecular mass and the drug loading ratio [78]. Overall, the spherical micelles have shown a rapid accumulation and even distribution in the tumour sites while retaining a large amount of the loaded drug. In contrast, the worm-like micelles have shown prolonged circulation in the plasma and a slow accumulation at the tumour sites, which happens only after they have released a significant amount of the loaded drugs. Hence more effective antitumor activity has been exhibited by spherical micelles. Core cross-linked polymeric micelles have been recently proposed to impede the limitation of instability of polymeric micelles in biological fluids and at tumour sites. A zinc coordination-induced core-crosslinked polymeric micelle prepared using a block copolymer bearing imidazole pendants has been synthesized [79]. The core-crosslinking of the polymeric micelles significantly lowered the critical micelle concentration compared to that of the non-crosslinked polymeric micelles. The fragile DOX loaded core-crosslinked polymeric micelles are easily affected by the slightly acidic tumour milieu which transforms the polymeric micelles back into hydrophilic polymers disassembling the micelles, thereby unloading the cargoes. An adequate toxicity was exhibited by those micelles with a low IC_{50} value of 3.713 ± 0.166 μg/mL.

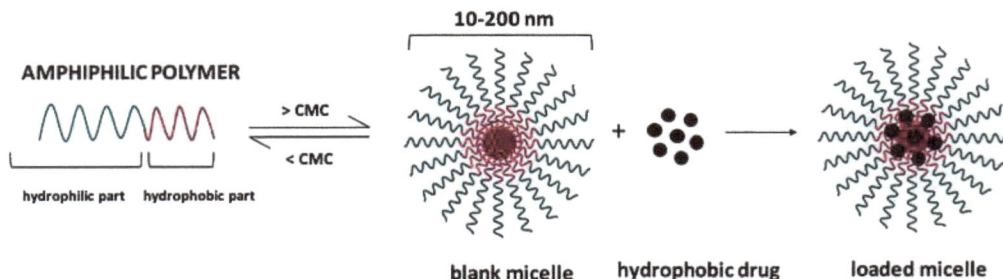

AMPHIPHILIC POLYMER

10-200 nm

> CMC

< CMC

hydrophilic part   hydrophobic part

blank micelle   hydrophobic drug   loaded micelle

Fig. (3). Schematic representation of polymeric micelles. Reprinted from [63] Copyright (2021) of Ghezzi *et al.*, published by Elsevier and distributed under the terms of the Creative Commons Attribution 4.0 International http://creativecommons.org/licenses/by/4.0/.

3.3. Nanogels

The nanoscale three-dimensional hydrogels known as nanogels have a network of hydrophilic polymers that are sustained by physical or chemical interactions, in which drugs can be entrapped [80]. Nanogels are advantageous NDDSs because of their facile dispersion in water, hydrophilicity, flexible and soft appearance, high permeability, high water content, capacity to encapsulate a large number of physiologically active molecules, and good compatibility with the body [80, 81]. Additionally, by adjusting the chemical makeup of the nanogels, properties, including size, charge, porosity, amphiphilicity, softness, and degradability, may be fine-tuned [82]. Basic nanogel formulations typically have diameters of 5 to 500 nm. This effective size range is crucial in preventing fast renal separation, which is enough to prevent reticuloendothelial system uptake. Nanogels can readily pass the blood-brain barrier (BBB) and exhibit potential permeability because of their nanosize properties [83]. The hydrophilic surface of nanogels hampers its ability to be opsonized in blood and can inhibit macrophage phagocytosis [84]. Different types of drugs, including hydrophilic drugs, hydrophobic drugs, peptide and protein drugs, and nucleic acid drugs, can be enclosed in nanogels with various structures and chemical compositions, which is a scarce property found in other nanoparticulate systems [85, 86]. Nanogels are a highly promising approach because they have a high degree of encapsulation efficiency, strong stability, and environmental sensitivity (such as ionic strength, pH, and temperature). Due to their distinctive characteristics, including stimuli-responsive behaviour, softness, and swelling, nanogels not only shield the cargo from deterioration and removal but also actively engage in the delivery process to help produce a regulated, triggered response at the target region [87, 88]. Nanogels also have strong biocompatibility, biodegradability, and other qualities that increase the effectiveness of drug-loaded chemotherapeutics on drug-sensitive and drug-resistant cancer cells and make antibiotic-resistant bacteria more susceptible to treatment [89].

A major advantage of the nanogels is their rapid response to environmental condition variations. A series of events that are triggered by an external signal, such as a change in pH, enzyme concentration, redox conditions, or temperature, or by a stimulus that may be produced externally, such as light or a magnetic field, brings out the stimulus-responsive behaviour of nanogels [90]. This stimulation will result in conformational or structural alterations in the nanogel, (Fig **4**) which is often spurred by the ionization of functional groups on the polymer chains or a shift in temperature below or above its lower critical solution temperature. These alterations will, in turn, modify the hydrophobicity or hydrophilicity of the nanogel, which will change the extent to which the system interacts with water molecules [91, 92]. This will consequently lead to swelling or shrinking of the nanogel network, which will bring out responses such as the release of the entrapped cargo [93, 94]. Controlling the structure of the materials used to fabricate the nanogels allows for precise regulation of the responsiveness of the nanogels to external physical or chemical signals [88, 95].

PEGylation of the nanogels has often been used to impart stealth properties to prolong its circulation time by avoiding opsonization and clearance *via* the spleen and the liver. Although this mechanism is highly reliant on the structural characteristics such as the size and shape of the nanogel and molecular weight and surface density of the PEG used, PEGylation will induce more hydrophilicity to the nanogel surface and will shield the charges of the payload within the core of the nanogel thus producing steric hindrance for serum protein interaction [96, 97].

The softness and deformability of nanogels, which resemble erythrocytes, aids the nanogels to evade the splenic filtration process [98]. The passive targeting of inflamed tissues of nanogels is achieved through EPR, as a result of their ability to accumulate at inflamed sites with unique structural features such as leaky blood vessels and impaired lymphatic drainage and typically, nanogels are too large to pass past the tight connections of the regular endothelium, thus avoiding the healthy cells [99, 100].

It has been shown that nanoparticles with a surface charge that is almost neutral have longer circulation durations. However, the charged groups inserted into the network of nanogels are generally responsible for the most significant characteristic of their stimuli-responsive activity. Nevertheless, it is frequently preferred that such groups exist in order to aid in the binding of pharmacological cargo. Because of this, attaining a precise balance between charge-related responsive behaviour and avoiding interactions between the nanogels and other *in vivo* components is particularly challenging [90]. In spite of the many advances in the field of nanogel design, only a few nanogels have been studied in clinical trials. The intricate and complicated structural features necessitate careful engineering of the nanogel to produce the desired result [90].

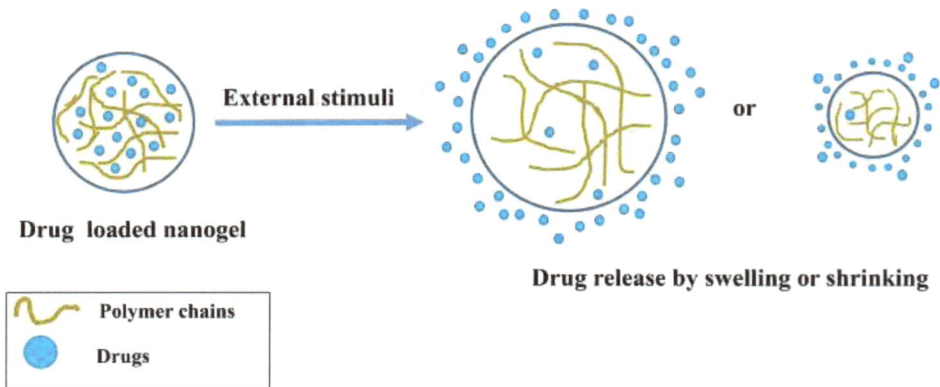

Fig. (4). Diagrammatic representation mechanism of drug release from nanogels.

3.4. Nanoemulsions

A colloidal particulate nanosystem called a nanoemulsion (NE), often referred to as a microemulsion, is made up of a combination of water, oil, and an appropriate stabilizing surfactant [101 - 104]. Emulsions are majorly two types; oil-in-water, where oil is dispersed through water and water-in-oil, where water is dispersed through oil (Fig 5). Due to the smaller particle sizes and increased surface area when compared to traditional emulsions, nanoemulsions (NE) are often more stable and permeable. They are made up of nanometre-sized droplets stabilized by emulsifiers. The NE's stability and solubility in aqueous environments enabled them with efficient drug delivery [105]. However, nanoemulsions are thermodynamically unstable entities that gradually separate into two distinct phases with time. When surfactants are used to stabilize emulsions, this time period is extended, effectively turning emulsions kinetically stable, allowing a well-designed emulsion to have a longer shelf life while preserving its original qualities for months or years. Hence, to guarantee that nanoemulsions are appropriately synthesized and stored, it is critical to understand the mechanisms of emulsion instability and stabilization in nanomedicine applications [106].

Recent advances in immunotherapy, vaccines, and photo/thermal therapies, among other innovative medicines for cancer, autoimmune, and chronic diseases, may be enhanced by making use of the special characteristics of nanoemulsions as a delivery vector. As they have been used often in the clinical context and have favourable pharmacokinetic profiles and safety, nanoemulsions are an appealing adjuvant to augment the immunogenic response. Kim *et al.* demonstrated a multifunctional nanoemulsion by encapsulating Toll-like receptor 7/8 agonists within a nanoemulsion that successfully reprogramme immunosuppression at the tumour site, inducing the recruitment and activation of innate immune cells, infiltration of lymphocytes, and polarization of tumour-associated M2 macrophages, which resulted in the inhibition of tumour growth [107]. Without the use of additional adjuvants, Zeng *et al.* described a PEGylated antigen-Clec9A nanoemulsion that promoted dendritic cell uptake, enhanced immunogenic responses in tumour-specific $CD4^+$ and $CD8^+$ T-cells, and subsequently inhibited tumour development [108]. Furthermore, Pellosi *et al.* also reported the development of a low-density nanoemulsion system incorporating magnetic-maghemite nanoparticles and chlorin e6, for dual magnetic hyperthermia and phototherapy treatment [109].

Due to their inherent antimicrobial properties, the capacity to increase drug solubility, stability, and bioavailability, the potential for organ and cellular targeting, the ability to target biofilms, and the potential to overcome antimicrobial resistance, NE have been recognized as a possible method of antimicrobial delivery. NE can be delivered *via* a variety of different means, including oral, parenteral, dermal, transdermal, ocular, pulmonary, nasal, and rectal [110]. In a study, it was discovered that using nanoemulsions of essential oils rather than pure essential oil improves the antibacterial activity [111]. They contend that bringing the essential oil in close contact with the cell membrane is the key to the antibacterial nanoemulsion's ability to combat E. coli. Due to this, hydrophobic compounds in essential oils have the ability to damage cell membranes, either by affecting the structure of the phospholipid bilayer or by interfering with active transporters that are encapsulated inside the phospholipid bilayer. Nucleic acids, proteins, and potassium escape from inside the damaged cell membrane as a result of changes in its permeability, causing cell death within five minutes. Nanoemulsions may therefore be particularly efficient delivery mechanisms for essential oils.

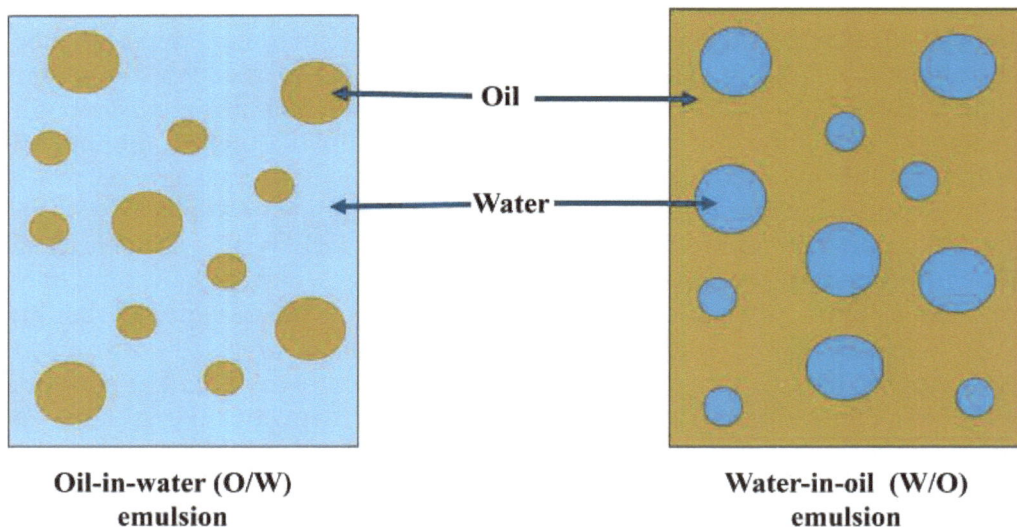

Oil-in-water (O/W)
emulsion

Water-in-oil (W/O)
emulsion

Fig. (5). Schematic representation of emulsions.

3.5. Solid Lipid Nanoparticles

Solid lipid nanoparticles (SLNs) are a type of aqueous dispersion of solid lipids that have been stabilized by an emulsifying layer and are commonly spherical in shape with diameters ranging from 50 nm- 1000 nm [112]. They are similar to nanoemulsions but have an inner solid lipid rather than an inner liquid lipid (Fig. 6) [113]. These are a particular class of lipid-based vesicular structures that have gained recognition for their ability to distribute drugs in a regulated and site-specific manner [114]. Surfactants are also used in the emulsification process to increase SLN stability. They are biopolymers with either synthetic or natural origins that are appropriate for encasing lipophilic drugs [115]. It is stated that the SLNs, by fusing all the beneficial traits of polymeric nanoparticles, liposomes, and microemulsions, have revolutionized the field of drug delivery [116]. The lipid content, surfactant concentration, and temperature adjustment during production are primarily responsible for the stability of SLNs [112]. Furthermore, compared to other nanoparticulate formulations, the stability pattern of solid lipid nanoparticles (SLNs) is more appealing. Aqueous SLNs may be kept in storage for up to three years or more, and the propensity to gel, brought on by prolonged storage and exposure to light, can be sustained by preventing transitions by lipid modification [117].

Nanostructured lipid carriers, lipid drug conjugates, polymeric lipid hybrid nanoparticles, and long-circulating SLNs are new generations of SLNs that increase their role as adaptable drug carriers for many forms of chemotherapy, parasite infections, and tuberculosis treatment [118, 119]. The cell line studies have demonstrated efficient cell uptake and substitution capability of SLNs as a colloidal drug carrier when administering chemotherapeutic agents, particularly for the treatment of malignant melanoma and colorectal cancer [120]. Furthermore, SLNs can prevent the adhesion of malignant cells, including those deriving from breast, prostate, and melanoma malignancies, to the cells found on human umbilical vein endothelium [121]. Doxorubicin concentrations were also shown to be greater in the lungs, spleen, and brain of rats, according to a pharmacokinetic investigation, when SLNs were used instead of normal commercial drug solutions [122].

In addition, due to their non-toxic and non-irritating compositional materials, they have found their application in topical formulations as well [123]. Owing to the higher surface area as a result of the smaller size of SLNs, they adhere strongly. Thus, they have been used to treat several skin diseases by incorporating lipids such as glyceryl palmitostearate and glyceryl behenate [124, 125]. When compared to the cell penetration of coenzyme Q10 with liquid paraffin and isopropanol, the enzyme demonstrated an effective penetration of stratum corneum as SLNs [126]. In addition, when compared to conventional drug carriers, SLNs exhibit an efficient drug release. For instance, the release kinetics of Compritol® (Retinol-loaded) SLNs has shown a controlled release during the first 6 hrs and after 12-24 hrs, an increased release rate that exceeded that of comparable nanoemulsions has been observed [127].

DNA may be successfully delivered to binding sites using cationically modified SLNs, where cytotoxicity and transfection efficiency are equally very low [128]. Additionally, it has been proposed that solid lipid nanoparticles and nanostructured lipid carriers are efficient and secure substitutes that may be used to treat both genetic and non-genetic disorders. The primary biological challenges to cell transfection, such as nuclease breakdown, cell uptake, and intracellular trafficking, are easily surmounted by lipid nanoparticles. Hence, SLNs have been established to be efficient in treating ocular diseases, infectious diseases, and lysosomal storage disorders and can be used in gene therapy as well.

Numerous studies have demonstrated that SLNs can also be envisaged as new possible vehicles for the pulmonary delivery of antitubercular medications like rifabutin due to a number of qualities, including stability, full release, and minimal toxicity [129]. In comparison to pure antitubercular pharmaceuticals, antitubercular drugs incorporated in SLN prepared with a microemulsion technique demonstrated a two-fold suppression of *Mycobacterium marinum* [130]. According to Jalal *et al.*, SLNs loaded with rifampicin (Rif) performed better against *B. abortus* than unbound rifampicin by a factor of two [131].

Vancomycin's performance, entrapment, release profile, and antibacterial activity against sensitive and resistant strains are all improved by co-encapsulating multiple lipids and polymers in lipid polymer hybrid nanoparticles, according to research by Seedat *et al.* This prevents side effects like renal failure and neutropenia [132 - 135].

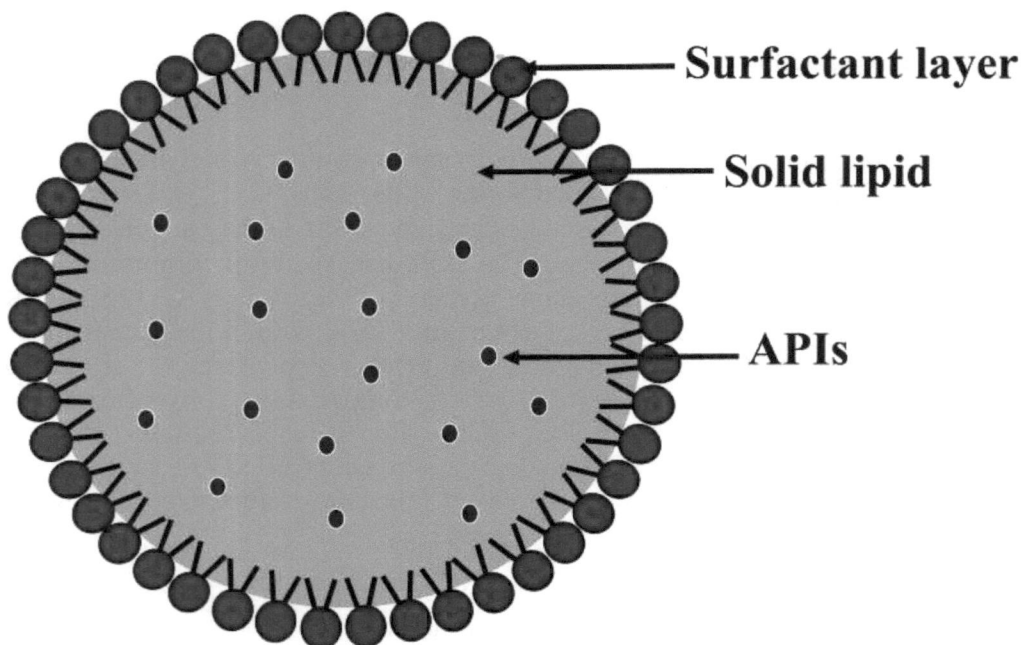

Fig. (6). Schematic representation of solid lipid nanoparticles.

3.6. Dendrimers

Another type of polymeric NPs are dendrimers, (Fig 7) which have the benefit of being almost monodisperse in comparison to other polymerization products and having a known structure and content [136, 137]. In addition dendrimers are highly symmetrical and possess surface polyvalency [138]. Surprisingly, unlike liposomes and polymer micelles, dendrimers with sufficient hydrophilicity lack the crucial micelle concentration [139]. Dendrimers should therefore "in theory" not fragment upon dilution [140]. Additionally, as the number of generations rises, the number of functional groupings increases exponentially. Hence dendrimers are a potent delivery system for drugs. Different methods, such as covalent binding or encapsulation, can be used to load drugs into dendrimers, while unimolecular micelles or supramolecular complexes can be used to encapsulate drugs [141].

The most commonly used chemotherapy drugs, such as DOX, methotrexate, paclitaxel, and camptothecin, can be encapsulated using this method [137]. Covalent drug binding has been employed to solve the encapsulation issues. The pharmaceuticals are attached to the dendrimer surface utilizing groups that will break after cellular absorption (*e.g.*, cis-aconityl or acyl hydrazine groups, ester groups or disulfide groups) [137]. All of these qualities make these materials a possible therapeutic drug carrier [142].

Over 100 dendritic structures have been described thus far, including polypropyleneimine (PPI) dendrimers, polyamide-, polyamidoamine (PAMAM) dendrimers, polyester-, polyether-, and phosphorus-based dendrimers among the most widely known dendritic families [137, 143 - 146]. One major challenge in dendrimers as a drug delivery carrier is their size limitation. While PAMAM dendrimers of generation 6 and above require a greater reliance on the hepatic clearance pathway for clearance, dendrimers of generation 5 or below can be effectively removed by glomerular filtration *via* the renal excretion pathway [147, 148]. Dendrimers that range in size from 4 to 10 nm can interact with nanometric cellular components and overcome the cellular endocytosis barrier [149, 150]. The higher generation of PAMAM dendrimers that are 6 and above, are rarely utilized since they are expensive and extremely hazardous [147]. The internalization of cells is facilitated by the strong binding ability of cationic dendrimers with nuclei or anion compounds [151]. However, non-specific plasma protein adsorptions and reticuloendothelial system-accelerated elimination are frequent problems for cationic dendrimers [149]. In addition, there's minimal intracellular dissociation of dendrimers with nucleic acids [152]. Particularly at high doses, the toxicity of cationic dendrimers is frequently greater than that of neutral or anionic dendrimers because their interaction with negatively charged cell membranes may cause the membrane to become unstable and so cause cell lysis [153 - 155]. These facts were proven in a study of the toxicity of PAMAM in embryonic zebrafish models, where, at the same dose, cationic PAMAM generation 6 was statistically more hazardous than neutral PAMAM generation 6 and anionic PAMAM generation 6 [156].

To overcome these constraints, size and charge adaptive electrostatically bound azithromycin (AZM) conjugated PAMAM dendrimer (PAMAM-AZM) and 2, 3-dimethyl maleic anhydride modified poly (ethylene glycol)-block-polylysine (PEG-b-PLys) clustered nanoparticle that can be readily disintegrated in an acidic biofilm microenvironment (pH 6.0), releasing the PAMAM-AZM while simultaneously decreasing its size from 112.0 to 6.5 nm and reversing its charge from 2.2 to 23.8 mV, have been synthesized [157]. Small and positively-charged PAMAM-AZM nanoparticles demonstrated outstanding penetration and retention capabilities inside biofilms both *in vitro* and *in vivo*. Bacterial membranes bound by the cationic PAMAM-AZM NPs, will experience increased permeabilization of both the inner and outer membranes, which will lead to enhanced internalization of AZM. As a result, AZM-DA NPs outperformed free AZM in terms of antibacterial activity during the treatment of a persistent lung infection brought on by *P. aeruginosa*. Another size-switchable nanotherapy platform with self-destruction and tumour penetration characteristics for site-specific phototherapy of cancer has been developed by binding photothermal agent indocyanine green conjugated poly(amidoamine) dendrimer (PAMAM-ICG) with the amphiphilic polymer poly(ethylene glycol)-b-poly(ε-caprolactone) (PEG--PCL) through a singlet oxygen-responsive thioketal linker and then loading with photosensitizer chlorin e6 (Ce6) [158]. The nanoparticulate system aggregated at the perivascular sites of the tumour after intravenous injection. In the hypoxic milieu, the singlet oxygen generated by Ce6 can release tiny PAMAM-ICGs with increased tumour penetration by killing tumour cells in the normoxic microenvironment while simultaneously cleaving the thioketal linker.

PEGylation, which is widely used to preserve the cationic surface of dendrimers to minimize their toxicity and prolong their circulation length, hinders dendrimer penetration into tissues and consequent cell internalization [159, 160]. Although PEGylated dendrimers can also improve DNA transfection, increase the flexibility for dendrimer conjugation, increase the solubilization of hydrophobic medicines, and facilitate tumour targeting [159, 161], alternate methods have to be used. The acetylation of amine groups is one technique that can be used to lessen the toxicity of PAMAM dendrimers by lowering their positive surface charges. According to Waite *et al.*, PAMAM may be modestly acetylated (about 20% of the amine was acetylated) to retain the efficiency of siRNA delivery while lowering toxicity [162]. Recently, it has been claimed that zwitterionic-modified nanomaterials have greater antifouling properties than their PEGylated counterparts [163]. According to Wang *et al.*, a zwitterionic nanocarrier was self-assembled from a Janus dendrimer with two different dendrons, one of which was modified with positively charged arginine groups and hydrophobic moieties and the other with hydrophilic and zwitterionic end-group functionalization [164]. Using zwitterionic moieties as the outer layer, this Janus dendrimer may self-assemble into a larger nanoparticle. In comparison to PEGylated nanocarriers, it was demonstrated that they could resist against proteins and have extended blood circulation time.

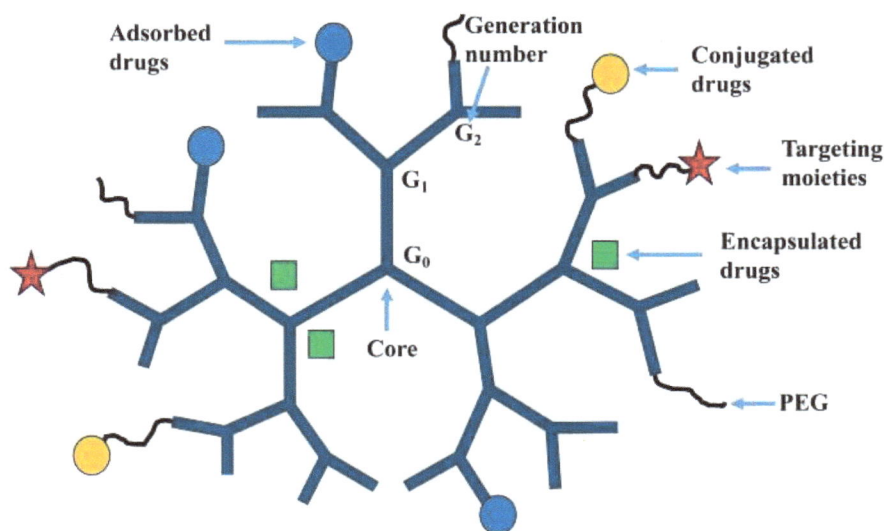

Fig. (7). Schematic structure of dendrimers.

3.7. Inorganic Nanoparticles

Similar to organic NPs, inorganic NPs are commonly utilized as delivery systems. Metal and metal oxides, such as iron (Fe), gold (Au), silver (Ag), platinum (Pt), titanium (TiO_2), copper oxide (CuO), and zinc oxide (ZnO), are examples of inorganic NPs [165, 166]. Inorganic NPs have long been investigated for a range of therapeutic uses, including the treatment of cancer and pathogens. Inorganic pharmaceuticals can also be beneficial as NDDSs in a manner similar to that of organic medications by enhancing their pharmacokinetic characteristics, such as improved targeting, drug loading, and immune system resistance [167]. Metal nanoparticles' antibacterial properties rely on their shape and size. They inhibit the growth of bacteria in a variety of ways, including by binding to and altering the properties of polymers and by releasing free radicals through reactive oxygen species (ROS) [168, 169]. By targeting many cell components, including the cell wall, membrane, DNA, and protein, metal NPs are seen as promising possibilities for antibacterial drugs [170].

One of the noble metals noted for distinctive optical characteristics brought about by the well-known phenomena of localized surface plasmon resonance is AuNPs (LSPR). The primary cause of AuNP's capacity to penetrate biological tissues is this phenomenon, which is significantly impacted by the form of the particle [171]. An oral administration of Resveratrol-coated gold nanoparticles with a median size of 20 nm to streptozotocin (STZ)-induced diabetic rats demonstrated a protective effect against diabetic retinopathy and contributed to the restoration of the balance of the stimulators and inhibitors of the angiogenesis [172]. Exner *et al.* have recently studied the effect of grafting drug-binding peptides (DBP) onto gold nanoparticles as a delivery vehicle for transporting Doxorubicin [173]. The increase of DBP:DOX ratio from 1:1 to 1:2 in order to check the feasibility of increasing drug loading capacity resulted in the second DOX molecule being adhered to the nanoparticles for 195 ns and then dissociating into surrounding solution. The chain length of the DBP has been considered as the limiting factor for the drug-loading capacity. A mucin1 aptamer and PEG-modified, targeted, photothermal therapeutic(PTT) gold nanoparticle for paclitaxel delivery have displayed a dual near-infrared/pH-dependent sustained release [174]. The system has shown the desired selectivity towards mucin1-positive breast cancer cells. Furthermore, combining PTT with targeted drug delivery resulted in a synergistic effect that boosted cell death compared to either PTT or chemotherapy independently.

The class of nanotechnology-based materials known as magnetic nanoparticles includes those made of magnetic elements, including iron, cobalt, chromium, and manganese. As their reactive surface may be functionalized with biocompatible coatings or bioactive chemicals, increasing their selectivity toward biological targets and preventing contact with healthy cells, it creates a potent drug delivery method, particularly due to targeting ability by an external magnetic force [175]. A nanoconjugate of anti-folate receptor modified-methotrexate loaded-magnetic nanoparticles has shown efficient eradication of tumour exhibiting a cell cytotoxicity of 80% in 24 hrs against HeLa cells, and the cell internalization of these nanosystems from their uptake by folate receptors on tumour cells' surface in antibody-mediated endocytosis [176]. In order to produce superparamagnetic Fe_3O_4 nanoparticles, chia seed water extract was employed, which was subsequently chitosan-coated and used for the delivery of oxaliplatin and irinotecan to colorectal cancer cells [177]. The two nanodrugs showed IC_{50} values of 79.6 and 61.1 ppm, respectively.

ZnO Nps are among the most used nanoparticles in the medicinal field due to their affordability, less toxicity and good absorbance by the body. ZnO Nps have been used in antimicrobial, anti-aging, anti-inflammatory, anti-diabetic, and also in wound healing [178, 179]. Furthermore, because ZnO NPs dissolve easily at low pH, they have been used as a pH-sensitive nanocarrier for tumour-targeted medicine delivery and intracellular drug release [180, 181]. Targeted drug delivery systems have utilised porous ZnO structures, such as porous nanobelts, porous nanotubes, porous cages and porous nanorods, with success [182, 183]. A pH-responsive drug releasing phenylboronic acid modified- quercetin loaded-ZnO Np has been used for targeting sialic acid over-expressing cancer cells. It caused apoptosis in human breast cancer cells (MCF-7) by increasing oxidative stress and mitochondrial damage and has been found to diminish tumour-associated toxicity in the liver, kidney and spleen [184]. Polyethylamine-coated $ZnO-SiO_2$ core-shell Nps functionalized with cholic acid have shown efficient delivery of Ruthenium pro-drugs that exhibit anticancer effects by directly binding with DNA for cervical cancer cells [185].

Mesoporous silica nanoparticles (MSNPs) have distinguished themselves among the inorganic nanocarriers as a multifaceted platform that permits the design of specially tailored therapeutic approaches for disease-specific applications. The use of MSNPs to address problems unique to cancer, such as the dysplastic stroma of pancreatic ductal adenocarcinoma, is one example [186, 187].

Theranostic fluorescence type- MSNps for pH-responsive delivery of Doxorubicin have been synthesized by doping with gold and quantum dots nanoparticles [188]. By incorporating gold and quantum dot nanoparticles into MSNPs, their optical properties have been transferred to the mesoporous matrix. Doxorubicin has been conjugated to the MSNPs *via* Schiff-base linkage with the amine groups functionalized on the MSNPs. To circumvent the limitation of using brimonidine, an eye drop due to rapid clearance from the preocular space, amino-functionalized MSNps have been employed [189]. The amino-functionalized MSNps adhered to the mucous layer and allowed a prolonged preocular time. The presence of mesopores to encapsulate the brimonidine facilitated the sustained release of the drug for 8 hrs.

The utilization of NPs as multifunctional and tailored drug delivery systems with revolutionary benefits in the medical industry is demonstrated by these recent discoveries. However, further research should be done to evaluate any potential toxicity on the human body and negative impacts on the environment.

3.8. Electrospun Polymeric Nanofiber

To achieve the intended therapeutic effects, specific drug release based on target location and timing is extensively applicable in nanofiber-based drug delivery systems. Electrospinning, which may be utilized for the continuous production of nanofibers on an industrial scale, is the process that is most often employed for creating drug-loaded nanofibers [190]. Typically, a drug-specific nanofiber formulation is developed, and using a different medication might dramatically change the release kinetics from the same delivery device [191]. Recent investigations explore nanofiber-based local delivery systems for combination of chemotherapy, photodynamic therapy, gene therapy, and thermal therapy, following electrospun nanofibers' use in chemotherapeutic agents' delivery [192, 193].

Due to their special and desirable properties for use as localized drug delivery devices, electrospun nanofibers have drawn a lot of attention over the past two decades. These characteristics include microscale or nanoscale diameters with a structure similar to extracellular matrix (ECM), extremely high surface area, controllable surface morphology, high drug-loading capacity and entrapment efficiency, high porosity with interconnectivity, and simultaneous delivery of multiple drugs. Nanofibers can also prevent a drug from breaking down in the body before it reaches the desired target [194]. Electrospun nanofibers are researched for local, sustained anticancer drug-loaded implants, offering reduced side effects and easy access to effective dosages [195]. Electrospun nanofibrous mats used for local chemotherapy following surgical resection have been infused with a variety of chemotherapy drugs, including cisplatin, docetaxel, doxorubicin (DOX), paclitaxel (PTX), dichloroacetate (DCA), 5-fluorouracil, platinum complexes, and curcumin [196]. Preclinical and clinical research on electrospun nanofiber-mediated drug delivery systems for cancer treatment is still ongoing [197]. In addition to anticancer drugs, anti-inflammatory drugs, antimicrobial drugs, cardiovascular drugs, antihistamine drugs, gastrointestinal drugs, palliative drugs, and contraceptive drugs have also been incorporated in electrospun fibers and tested for their efficacy [198]. They can be administered in many different ways, including oral, topical, transdermal, and transmucosal [199 - 202]. Furthermore, their release kinetics may be varied by the preparation ingredients, constituent proportions, and preparation techniques, allowing them to be used in a variety of medicinal disciplines [203].

Recently a dual drug delivery system has been constructed *via* coaxial electrospinning technique to be used as a wound dressing. In order to create a core-shell electrospun nanofibrous membrane that simultaneously exhibits cell proliferation and antibacterial activity, polycaprolactone (PCL) was loaded with phenytoin (Ph), a well-known proliferative agent, as the shell membrane and silver-chitosan nanoparticles (Ag-CS NPs), as prepared biocidal agents, was embedded in polyvinyl alcohol (PVA), as the core layer [204]. In comparison to PVA/PCL-Ph NFs, the coaxial PVA-Ag CS NPs/PCL-Ph nanofibers (NFs) demonstrated better regulated Ph release. A notable enhancement of morphology, mechanical, thermal, antibacterial properties and cytobiocompatibility of the fibers has been observed with the incorporation of Ph and Ag-CS Nps.

A preliminary study on fast-dissolving oral film fabrication by electrospinning chitosan/pullulan composite has been carried out by Qin *et al.* and they have reported that the ratio of chitosan and pullulan had an influence on the solution property of the composite [205]. A composite exhibiting a complete dissolution within 60s in water has been achieved. This composite, with excellent thermal stability and fast solubility, has been successfully loaded with aspirin as a model drug. Although antibacterial electrospun nanofibers are widespread, the inability to incorporate a high loading has restricted its usage. In order to impede this drawback, nanofibers based on natural excipients such as cyclodextrin have created a novel platform in electrospinning drug delivery nanofibers without the use of a polymer carrier since the hydrogen bonds of cyclodextrin will drive the nanofiber formation [206]. These nanofibers have a high loading capacity and have achieved better stability *via* inclusion complexes between the drugs and the excipient. Hence, electrospun nanofibers have been fabricated using cyclodextrin as the excipient to carry antibiotics, including Kanamycin, chloramphenicol, gentamicin and ampicillin with a good antibiotic encapsulation (45–90%). The research demonstrates that polymer-free cyclodextrin-antibiotic nanofibers can dissolve in water and synthetic saliva in a matter of seconds, delivering CD-antibiotic complexes with significant antibacterial activity against Gram-negative *Escherichia coli.* This study suggests polymer-free cyclodextrin-antibiotic nanofibers as fast-dissolving oral drug delivery devices.

CONCLUSION

Pharmaceuticals or biomolecules are efficiently delivered and administered to cells by using nanoparticles (NPs) as drug-delivery devices. Numerous sectors, including the pharmaceutical, medical, and biological industries, have witnessed tremendous growth for these systems. Nanostructures enable greater oral bioavailability, avoid gastrointestinal contamination, and enhance the absorption of water-soluble drugs. Nanoparticles can infiltrate the tissue system and act where they are intended, enabling more effective drug administration and delivery.

Drug delivery techniques heavily depend on the size, surface chemistry, biological fate, toxicity, *in vivo* dispersion, and targeting capabilities of nanoparticles. Nanoparticles can access a greater variety of cellular and intracellular targets because they are more mobile and smaller than microparticles. Particle stability and interactions with cells are also impacted by surface charge and hydrophobicity. Drug solubility, rate of desorption, diffusion, degradation, and erosion processes, as well as drug solubility, all affect how well a drug delivery system works. Nanoparticles must exert the desired therapeutic effect at the expected site of action with the least amount of activity or volume loss.

New opportunities for disease prevention and treatment have emerged with the development of nano-drug delivery systems (NDDS). These systems can improve the pharmacological and pharmaceutical characteristics of therapies by lengthening the duration of action, improving efficacy and targeting, overcoming drug resistance, and reducing immunogenicity and toxicity. In recent years, preclinical and clinical research has used NDDS, such as liposomes, polymeric micelles, nanogels, nanoemulsions, solid lipid nanoparticles, dendrimers, inorganic nanoparticles, and polymer nanofibers.

PRACTICE QUESTIONS

1. Define controlled drug delivery systems with examples.
2. Differentiate active and passive targeting.
3. Describe the various strategies and modifications of the drug delivery systems to achieve targeted drug delivery.
4. Describe the various criteria and physicochemical and pharmaceutical factors to be considered for drug candidates that must be satisfied before being formulated into a controlled drug delivery system.
5. Describe the strategies for the formulations of controlled release based on diffusion, dissolution, and ion exchange methods.
6. Compare and contrast the different drug delivery systems available up-to-date.
7. Explain the mechanism of drug release in controlled and sustained release dosage form.
8. Explain biodegradable and non-biodegradable polymers used for controlled drug delivery systems with examples.

REFERENCES

[1]   Martinho, N.; Damgé, C.; Reis, C.P. Recent advances in drug delivery systems. *J. Biomater. Nanobiotechnol.,* **2011,** *2*(5), 510-526.
        [http://dx.doi.org/10.4236/jbnb.2011.225062]

[2]   Rudramurthy, G.; Swamy, M.; Sinniah, U.; Ghasemzadeh, A. Nanoparticles: Alternatives against drug-resistant pathogenic microbes. *Molecules,* **2016,** *21*(7), 836.
        [http://dx.doi.org/10.3390/molecules21070836] [PMID: 27355939]

[3]   Jahangirian, H.; Ghasemian lemraski, E.; Webster, T.J.; Rafiee-Moghaddam, R.; Abdollahi, Y. A review of drug delivery systems based on nanotechnology and green chemistry: green nanomedicine. *Int. J. Nanomedicine,* **2017,** *12*, 2957-2978.
        [http://dx.doi.org/10.2147/IJN.S127683] [PMID: 28442906]

[4]   De Villiers, M.M.; Aramwit, P.; Kwon, G.S. *Nanotechnology in drug delivery*; Springer Science & Business Media, **2008.**

[5]   Mirza, A.Z.; Siddiqui, F.A. Nanomedicine and drug delivery: a mini review. *Int. Nano Lett.,* **2014,** *4*(1), 94.
        [http://dx.doi.org/10.1007/s40089-014-0094-7]

[6]   Kabanov, A.V.; Lemieux, P.; Vinogradov, S.; Alakhov, V. Pluronic® block copolymers: Novel functional molecules for gene therapy. *Adv. Drug Deliv. Rev.,* **2002,** *54*(2), 223-233.
        [http://dx.doi.org/10.1016/S0169-409X(02)00018-2] [PMID: 11897147]

[7]   Panyam, J.; Labhasetwar, V. Biodegradable nanoparticles for drug and gene delivery to cells and tissue. *Adv. Drug Deliv. Rev.,* **2003,** *55*(3), 329-347.
        [http://dx.doi.org/10.1016/S0169-409X(02)00228-4] [PMID: 12628320]

[8]   Redhead, H.M.; Davis, S.S.; Illum, L. Drug delivery in poly(lactide-co-glycolide) nanoparticles surface modified with poloxamer 407 and poloxamine 908: *in vitro* characterisation and *in vivo*

evaluation. *J. Control. Release,* **2001**, *70*(3), 353-363.
[http://dx.doi.org/10.1016/S0168-3659(00)00367-9] [PMID: 11182205]

[9]   Hutter, E.; Boridy, S.; Labrecque, S.; Lalancette-Hébert, M.; Kriz, J.; Winnik, F.M.; Maysinger, D. Microglial response to gold nanoparticles. *ACS Nano,* **2010**, *4*(5), 2595-2606.
[http://dx.doi.org/10.1021/nn901869f] [PMID: 20329742]

[10]   Decuzzi, P.; Godin, B.; Tanaka, T.; Lee, S.Y.; Chiappini, C.; Liu, X.; Ferrari, M. Size and shape effects in the biodistribution of intravascularly injected particles. *J. Control. Release,* **2010**, *141*(3), 320-327.
[http://dx.doi.org/10.1016/j.jconrel.2009.10.014] [PMID: 19874859]

[11]   Yoo, J.W.; Doshi, N.; Mitragotri, S. Endocytosis and intracellular distribution of plga particles in endothelial cells: Effect of particle geometry. *Macromol. Rapid Commun.,* **2010**, *31*(2), 142-148.
[http://dx.doi.org/10.1002/marc.200900592] [PMID: 21590886]

[12]   Geng, Y.; Dalhaimer, P.; Cai, S.; Tsai, R.; Tewari, M.; Minko, T.; Discher, D.E. Shape effects of filaments versus spherical particles in flow and drug delivery. *Nat. Nanotechnol.,* **2007**, *2*(4), 249-255.
[http://dx.doi.org/10.1038/nnano.2007.70] [PMID: 18654271]

[13]   Park, J.H.; von Maltzahn, G.; Zhang, L.; Schwartz, M.P.; Ruoslahti, E.; Bhatia, S.N.; Sailor, M.J. Magnetic Iron Oxide Nanoworms for Tumor Targeting and Imaging. *Adv. Mater.,* **2008**, *20*(9), 1630-1635.
[http://dx.doi.org/10.1002/adma.200800004] [PMID: 21687830]

[14]   Champion, J.A.; Mitragotri, S. Role of target geometry in phagocytosis. *Proc. Natl. Acad. Sci. USA,* **2006**, *103*(13), 4930-4934.
[http://dx.doi.org/10.1073/pnas.0600997103] [PMID: 16549762]

[15]   Canelas, D.A.; Herlihy, K.P.; DeSimone, J.M. Top-down particle fabrication: Control of size and shape for diagnostic imaging and drug delivery. *Wiley Interdiscip. Rev. Nanomed. Nanobiotechnol.,* **2009**, *1*(4), 391-404.
[http://dx.doi.org/10.1002/wnan.40] [PMID: 20049805]

[16]   Doshi, N.; Zahr, A.S.; Bhaskar, S.; Lahann, J.; Mitragotri, S. Red blood cell-mimicking synthetic biomaterial particles. *Proc. Natl. Acad. Sci. USA,* **2009**, *106*(51), 21495-21499.
[http://dx.doi.org/10.1073/pnas.0907127106] [PMID: 20018694]

[17]   Petros, R.A.; DeSimone, J.M. Strategies in the design of nanoparticles for therapeutic applications. *Nat. Rev. Drug Discov.,* **2010**, *9*(8), 615-627.
[http://dx.doi.org/10.1038/nrd2591] [PMID: 20616808]

[18]   Gratton, S.E.A.; Ropp, P.A.; Pohlhaus, P.D.; Luft, J.C.; Madden, V.J.; Napier, M.E.; DeSimone, J.M. The effect of particle design on cellular internalization pathways. *Proc. Natl. Acad. Sci. USA,* **2008**, *105*(33), 11613-11618.
[http://dx.doi.org/10.1073/pnas.0801763105] [PMID: 18697944]

[19]   Hillaireau, H.; Couvreur, P. Nanocarriers' entry into the cell: relevance to drug delivery. *Cell. Mol. Life Sci.,* **2009**, *66*(17), 2873-2896.
[http://dx.doi.org/10.1007/s00018-009-0053-z] [PMID: 19499185]

[20]   Verma, A.; Stellacci, F. Effect of surface properties on nanoparticle-cell interactions. *Small,* **2010**, *6*(1), 12-21.
[http://dx.doi.org/10.1002/smll.200901158] [PMID: 19844908]

[21]   Schipper, M.L.; Iyer, G.; Koh, A.L.; Cheng, Z.; Ebenstein, Y.; Aharoni, A.; Keren, S.; Bentolila, L.A.; Li, J.; Rao, J.; Chen, X.; Banin, U.; Wu, A.M.; Sinclair, R.; Weiss, S.; Gambhir, S.S. Particle size, surface coating, and PEGylation influence the biodistribution of quantum dots in living mice. *Small,* **2009**, *5*(1), 126-134.
[http://dx.doi.org/10.1002/smll.200800003] [PMID: 19051182]

[22]   Xiao, K.; Li, Y.; Luo, J.; Lee, J.S.; Xiao, W.; Gonik, A.M.; Agarwal, R.G.; Lam, K.S. The effect of

surface charge on *in vivo* biodistribution of PEG-oligocholic acid based micellar nanoparticles. *Biomaterials,* **2011**, *32*(13), 3435-3446.
[http://dx.doi.org/10.1016/j.biomaterials.2011.01.021] [PMID: 21295849]

[23]   Yamamoto, Y.; Nagasaki, Y.; Kato, Y.; Sugiyama, Y.; Kataoka, K. Long-circulating poly(ethylene glycol)–poly(d,l-lactide) block copolymer micelles with modulated surface charge. *J. Control. Release,* **2001**, *77*(1-2), 27-38.
[http://dx.doi.org/10.1016/S0168-3659(01)00451-5] [PMID: 11689257]

[24]   Blau, S.; Jubeh, T. T.; Haupt, S. M.; Rubinstein, A. Drug targeting by surface cationization. *Critical Reviews™ in Therapeutic Drug Carrier Systems,* **2000**, *17*(5)

[25]   Esmaeili, F.; Ghahremani, M.H.; Esmaeili, B.; Khoshayand, M.R.; Atyabi, F.; Dinarvand, R. PLGA nanoparticles of different surface properties: Preparation and evaluation of their body distribution. *Int. J. Pharm.,* **2008**, *349*(1-2), 249-255.
[http://dx.doi.org/10.1016/j.ijpharm.2007.07.038] [PMID: 17875373]

[26]   Duan, X.; Li, Y. Physicochemical characteristics of nanoparticles affect circulation, biodistribution, cellular internalization, and trafficking. *Small,* **2013**, *9*(9-10), 1521-1532.
[http://dx.doi.org/10.1002/smll.201201390] [PMID: 23019091]

[27]   Singh, R.; Lillard, J.W., Jr Nanoparticle-based targeted drug delivery. *Exp. Mol. Pathol.,* **2009**, *86*(3), 215-223.
[http://dx.doi.org/10.1016/j.yexmp.2008.12.004] [PMID: 19186176]

[28]   Calvo, P.; Remuñan-López, C.; Vila-Jato, J.L.; Alonso, M.J. Chitosan and chitosan/ethylene oxide-propylene oxide block copolymer nanoparticles as novel carriers for proteins and vaccines. *Pharm. Res.,* **1997**, *14*(10), 1431-1436.
[http://dx.doi.org/10.1023/A:1012128907225] [PMID: 9358557]

[29]   Uddin, M.D.S. Nanoparticles as Nanopharmaceuticals: Smart Drug Delivery Systems.*Nanoparticulate Drug Delivery Systems*; Apple Academic Press, **2019**, pp. 85-120.
[http://dx.doi.org/10.1201/9781351137263-3]

[30]   Zahin, N.; Anwar, R.; Tewari, D.; Kabir, M.T.; Sajid, A.; Mathew, B.; Uddin, M.S.; Aleya, L.; Abdel-Daim, M.M. Nanoparticles and its biomedical applications in health and diseases: special focus on drug delivery. *Environ. Sci. Pollut. Res. Int.,* **2020**, *27*(16), 19151-19168.
[http://dx.doi.org/10.1007/s11356-019-05211-0] [PMID: 31079299]

[31]   Cho, K.; Wang, X.; Nie, S.; Chen, Z.G.; Shin, D.M. Therapeutic nanoparticles for drug delivery in cancer. *Clin. Cancer Res.,* **2008**, *14*(5), 1310-1316.
[http://dx.doi.org/10.1158/1078-0432.CCR-07-1441] [PMID: 18316549]

[32]   Rizvi, S.A.A.; Saleh, A.M. Applications of nanoparticle systems in drug delivery technology. *Saudi Pharm. J.,* **2018**, *26*(1), 64-70.
[http://dx.doi.org/10.1016/j.jsps.2017.10.012] [PMID: 29379334]

[33]   Attia, M.F.; Anton, N.; Wallyn, J.; Omran, Z.; Vandamme, T.F. An overview of active and passive targeting strategies to improve the nanocarriers efficiency to tumour sites. *J. Pharm. Pharmacol.,* **2019**, *71*(8), 1185-1198.
[http://dx.doi.org/10.1111/jphp.13098] [PMID: 31049986]

[34]   Hafeez, M.N.; Celia, C.; Petrikaite, V. Challenges towards targeted drug delivery in cancer nanomedicines. *Processes (Basel),* **2021**, *9*(9), 1527.
[http://dx.doi.org/10.3390/pr9091527]

[35]   Matsumura, Y.; Maeda, H. A new concept for macromolecular therapeutics in cancer chemotherapy: mechanism of tumoritropic accumulation of proteins and the antitumor agent smancs. *Cancer Res.,* **1986**, *46*(12 Pt 1), 6387-6392.
[PMID: 2946403]

[36]   Zhang, J.; Yuan, Z.F.; Wang, Y.; Chen, W.H.; Luo, G.F.; Cheng, S.X.; Zhuo, R.X.; Zhang, X.Z.

Multifunctional envelope-type mesoporous silica nanoparticles for tumor-triggered targeting drug delivery. *J. Am. Chem. Soc.,* **2013**, *135*(13), 5068-5073.
[http://dx.doi.org/10.1021/ja312004m] [PMID: 23464924]

[37]   Chen, W.; Zou, Y.; Meng, F.; Cheng, R.; Deng, C.; Feijen, J.; Zhong, Z. Glyco-nanoparticles with sheddable saccharide shells: a unique and potent platform for hepatoma-targeting delivery of anticancer drugs. *Biomacromolecules,* **2014**, *15*(3), 900-907.
[http://dx.doi.org/10.1021/bm401749t] [PMID: 24460130]

[38]   Yuan, Y.Y.; Mao, C.Q.; Du, X.J.; Du, J.Z.; Wang, F.; Wang, J. Surface charge switchable nanoparticles based on zwitterionic polymer for enhanced drug delivery to tumor. *Adv. Mater.,* **2012**, *24*(40), 5476-5480.
[http://dx.doi.org/10.1002/adma.201202296] [PMID: 22886872]

[39]   Marradi, M.; Chiodo, F.; García, I.; Penadés, S. Glyconanoparticles as multifunctional and multimodal carbohydrate systems. *Chem. Soc. Rev.,* **2013**, *42*(11), 4728-4745.
[http://dx.doi.org/10.1039/c2cs35420a] [PMID: 23288339]

[40]   García, I.; Sánchez-Iglesias, A.; Henriksen-Lacey, M.; Grzelczak, M.; Penadés, S.; Liz-Marzán, L.M. Glycans as biofunctional ligands for gold nanorods: Stability and targeting in protein-rich media. *J. Am. Chem. Soc.,* **2015**, *137*(10), 3686-3692.
[http://dx.doi.org/10.1021/jacs.5b01001] [PMID: 25706836]

[41]   Wang, J.; Mao, W.; Lock, L.L.; Tang, J.; Sui, M.; Sun, W.; Cui, H.; Xu, D.; Shen, Y. The role of micelle size in tumor accumulation, penetration, and treatment. *ACS Nano,* **2015**, *9*(7), 7195-7206.
[http://dx.doi.org/10.1021/acsnano.5b02017] [PMID: 26149286]

[42]   Huo, S.; Ma, H.; Huang, K.; Liu, J.; Wei, T.; Jin, S.; Zhang, J.; He, S.; Liang, X.J. Superior penetration and retention behavior of 50 nm gold nanoparticles in tumors. *Cancer Res.,* **2013**, *73*(1), 319-330.
[http://dx.doi.org/10.1158/0008-5472.CAN-12-2071] [PMID: 23074284]

[43]   Peer, D.; Karp, J.M.; Hong, S.; Farokhzad, O.C.; Margalit, R.; Langer, R. *Nanocarriers as an emerging platform for cancer therapy*; Nano-Enabled Medical Applications, **2020**, pp. 61-91.
[http://dx.doi.org/10.1201/9780429399039-2]

[44]   Saadat, M.; Manshadi, M.K.D.; Mohammadi, M.; Zare, M.J.; Zarei, M.; Kamali, R.; Sanati-Nezhad, A. Magnetic particle targeting for diagnosis and therapy of lung cancers. *J. Control. Release,* **2020**, *328*, 776-791.
[http://dx.doi.org/10.1016/j.jconrel.2020.09.017] [PMID: 32920079]

[45]   Boisseau, P.; Loubaton, B. Nanomedicine, nanotechnology in medicine. *C. R. Phys.,* **2011**, *12*(7), 620-636.
[http://dx.doi.org/10.1016/j.crhy.2011.06.001]

[46]   Chen, X.; Gambhir, S.S.; Cheon, J. Theranostic Nanomedicine. *Acc. Chem. Res.,* **2011**, *44*(10), 841-841.
[http://dx.doi.org/10.1021/ar200231d] [PMID: 22004477]

[47]   Chen, D.; Lian, S.; Sun, J.; Liu, Z.; Zhao, F.; Jiang, Y.; Gao, M.; Sun, K.; Liu, W.; Fu, F. Design of novel multifunctional targeting nano-carrier drug delivery system based on CD44 receptor and tumor microenvironment pH condition. *Drug Deliv.,* **2016**, *23*(3), 798-803.
[http://dx.doi.org/10.3109/10717544.2014.917130] [PMID: 24892632]

[48]   Karthik, V.; Poornima, S.; Vigneshwaran, A.; Raj, D.P.R.D.D.; Subbaiya, R.; Manikandan, S.; Saravanan, M. Nanoarchitectonics is an emerging drug/gene delivery and targeting strategy -a critical review. *J. Mol. Struct.,* **2021**, *1243*, 130844.
[http://dx.doi.org/10.1016/j.molstruc.2021.130844]

[49]   El Bayoumi, T. A.; Torchilin, V. P., Current Trends in *Liposome Research. In Liposomes: Methods and Protocols, Volume 1: Pharmaceutical Nanocarriers*, Weissig, V., Ed. Humana Press: Totowa, NJ, *2010*; pp 1-27.

[50]   Lamichhane, N.; Udayakumar, T.; D'Souza, W.; Simone, C., II; Raghavan, S.; Polf, J.; Mahmood, J. Liposomes: Clinical applications and potential for image-guided drug delivery. *Molecules,* **2018**, *23*(2), 288.
[http://dx.doi.org/10.3390/molecules23020288] [PMID: 29385755]

[51]   Laouini, A.; Jaafar-Maalej, C.; Limayem-Blouza, I.; Sfar, S.; Charcosset, C.; Fessi, H. Preparation, characterization and applications of liposomes: State of the art. *Journal of colloid Science and Biotechnology,* **2012**, *1*(2), 147-168.

[52]   Ferreira, M.; Aguiar, S.; Bettencourt, A.; Gaspar, M.M. Lipid-based nanosystems for targeting bone implant-associated infections: current approaches and future endeavors. *Drug Deliv. Transl. Res.,* **2021**, *11*(1), 72-85.
[http://dx.doi.org/10.1007/s13346-020-00791-8] [PMID: 32514703]

[53]   Fan, Y.; Zhang, Q. Development of liposomal formulations: From concept to clinical investigations. *Asian Journal of Pharmaceutical Sciences,* **2013**, *8*(2), 81-87.
[http://dx.doi.org/10.1016/j.ajps.2013.07.010]

[54]   Guimarães, D.; Cavaco-Paulo, A.; Nogueira, E. Design of liposomes as drug delivery system for therapeutic applications. *Int. J. Pharm.,* **2021**, *601*, 120571.
[http://dx.doi.org/10.1016/j.ijpharm.2021.120571] [PMID: 33812967]

[55]   Huynh, N.T.; Passirani, C.; Saulnier, P.; Benoît, J.P. Lipid nanocapsules: A new platform for nanomedicine. *Int. J. Pharm.,* **2009**, *379*(2), 201-209.
[http://dx.doi.org/10.1016/j.ijpharm.2009.04.026] [PMID: 19409468]

[56]   Brown, C.E.; Alizadeh, D.; Starr, R.; Weng, L.; Wagner, J.R.; Naranjo, A.; Ostberg, J.R.; Blanchard, M.S.; Kilpatrick, J.; Simpson, J.; Kurien, A.; Priceman, S.J.; Wang, X.; Harshbarger, T.L.; D'Apuzzo, M.; Ressler, J.A.; Jensen, M.C.; Barish, M.E.; Chen, M.; Portnow, J.; Forman, S.J.; Badie, B. Regression of glioblastoma after chimeric antigen receptor T-cell therapy. *N. Engl. J. Med.,* **2016**, *375*(26), 2561-2569.
[http://dx.doi.org/10.1056/NEJMoa1610497] [PMID: 28029927]

[57]   Shi, D.; Mi, G.; Shen, Y.; Webster, T.J. Glioma-targeted dual functionalized thermosensitive Ferri-liposomes for drug delivery through an *in vitro* blood–brain barrier. *Nanoscale,* **2019**, *11*(32), 15057-15071.
[http://dx.doi.org/10.1039/C9NR03931G] [PMID: 31369016]

[58]   De Jesús Valle, M.J.; Zarzuelo Castañeda, A.; Maderuelo, C.; Cencerrado Treviño, A.; Loureiro, J.; Coutinho, P.; Sánchez Navarro, A. Development of a mucoadhesive vehicle based on lyophilized liposomes for drug delivery through the sublingual mucosa. *Pharmaceutics,* **2022**, *14*(7), 1497.
[http://dx.doi.org/10.3390/pharmaceutics14071497] [PMID: 35890395]

[59]   He, B.; Hu, H.; Tan, T.; Wang, H.; Sun, K.; Li, Y.; Zhang, Z. IR-780-loaded polymeric micelles enhance the efficacy of photothermal therapy in treating breast cancer lymphatic metastasis in mice. *Acta Pharmacol. Sin.,* **2018**, *39*(1), 132-139.
[http://dx.doi.org/10.1038/aps.2017.109] [PMID: 28795690]

[60]   Torchilin, V.P. Micellar nanocarriers: Pharmaceutical perspectives. *Pharm. Res.,* **2006**, *24*(1), 1-16.
[http://dx.doi.org/10.1007/s11095-006-9132-0] [PMID: 17109211]

[61]   Jones, M.C.; Leroux, J.C. Polymeric micelles : A new generation of colloidal drug carriers. *Eur. J. Pharm. Biopharm.,* **1999**, *48*(2), 101-111.
[http://dx.doi.org/10.1016/S0939-6411(99)00039-9] [PMID: 10469928]

[62]   Nishiyama, N.; Okazaki, S.; Cabral, H.; Miyamoto, M.; Kato, Y.; Sugiyama, Y.; Nishio, K.; Matsumura, Y.; Kataoka, K. Novel cisplatin-incorporated polymeric micelles can eradicate solid tumors in mice. *Cancer Res.,* **2003**, *63*(24), 8977-8983.
[PMID: 14695216]

[63]   Ghezzi, M.; Pescina, S.; Padula, C.; Santi, P.; Del Favero, E.; Cantù, L.; Nicoli, S. Polymeric micelles

in drug delivery: An insight of the techniques for their characterization and assessment in biorelevant conditions. *J. Control. Release,* **2021**, *332*, 312-336.
[http://dx.doi.org/10.1016/j.jconrel.2021.02.031] [PMID: 33652113]

[64] Cho, H.; Lai, T.C.; Tomoda, K.; Kwon, G.S. Polymeric micelles for multi-drug delivery in cancer. *AAPS PharmSciTech,* **2015**, *16*(1), 10-20.
[http://dx.doi.org/10.1208/s12249-014-0251-3] [PMID: 25501872]

[65] Zhang, Y.; Huang, Y.; Li, S. Polymeric micelles: nanocarriers for cancer-targeted drug delivery. *AAPS PharmSciTech,* **2014**, *15*(4), 862-871.
[http://dx.doi.org/10.1208/s12249-014-0113-z] [PMID: 24700296]

[66] Sosnik, A.; Menaker Raskin, M. Polymeric micelles in mucosal drug delivery: Challenges towards clinical translation. *Biotechnol. Adv.,* **2015**, *33*(6), 1380-1392.
[http://dx.doi.org/10.1016/j.biotechadv.2015.01.003] [PMID: 25597531]

[67] Mandal, A.; Bisht, R.; Rupenthal, I.D.; Mitra, A.K. Polymeric micelles for ocular drug delivery: From structural frameworks to recent preclinical studies. *J. Control. Release,* **2017**, *248*, 96-116.
[http://dx.doi.org/10.1016/j.jconrel.2017.01.012] [PMID: 28087407]

[68] Khan, A.R.; Liu, M.; Khan, M.W.; Zhai, G. Progress in brain targeting drug delivery system by nasal route. *J. Control. Release,* **2017**, *268*, 364-389.
[http://dx.doi.org/10.1016/j.jconrel.2017.09.001] [PMID: 28887135]

[69] Grimaudo, M.A.; Pescina, S.; Padula, C.; Santi, P.; Concheiro, A.; Alvarez-Lorenzo, C.; Nicoli, S. Topical application of polymeric nanomicelles in ophthalmology: A review on research efforts for the noninvasive delivery of ocular therapeutics. *Expert Opin. Drug Deliv.,* **2019**, *16*(4), 397-413.
[http://dx.doi.org/10.1080/17425247.2019.1597848] [PMID: 30889977]

[70] Logie, J.; Owen, S.C.; McLaughlin, C.K.; Shoichet, M.S. PEG-graft density controls polymeric nanoparticle micelle stability. *Chem. Mater.,* **2014**, *26*(9), 2847-2855.
[http://dx.doi.org/10.1021/cm500448x]

[71] Zhu, Y.; Meng, T.; Tan, Y.; Yang, X.; Liu, Y.; Liu, X.; Yu, F.; Wen, L.; Dai, S.; Yuan, H.; Hu, F. Negative surface shielded polymeric micelles with colloidal stability for intracellular endosomal/lysosomal escape. *Mol. Pharm.,* **2018**, *15*(11), 5374-5386.
[http://dx.doi.org/10.1021/acs.molpharmaceut.8b00842] [PMID: 30204446]

[72] Honary, S.; Zahir, F. Effect of zeta potential on the properties of nano-drug delivery systems-a review (Part 2). *Trop. J. Pharm. Res.,* **2013**, *12*(2), 265-273.

[73] Cabral, H.; Matsumoto, Y.; Mizuno, K.; Chen, Q.; Murakami, M.; Kimura, M.; Terada, Y.; Kano, M.R.; Miyazono, K.; Uesaka, M.; Nishiyama, N.; Kataoka, K. Accumulation of sub-100 nm polymeric micelles in poorly permeable tumours depends on size. *Nat. Nanotechnol.,* **2011**, *6*(12), 815-823.
[http://dx.doi.org/10.1038/nnano.2011.166] [PMID: 22020122]

[74] Truong, N.P.; Whittaker, M.R.; Mak, C.W.; Davis, T.P. The importance of nanoparticle shape in cancer drug delivery. *Expert Opin. Drug Deliv.,* **2015**, *12*(1), 129-142.
[http://dx.doi.org/10.1517/17425247.2014.950564] [PMID: 25138827]

[75] Christian, D.A.; Cai, S.; Garbuzenko, O.B.; Harada, T.; Zajac, A.L.; Minko, T.; Discher, D.E. Flexible filaments for *in vivo* imaging and delivery: persistent circulation of filomicelles opens the dosage window for sustained tumor shrinkage. *Mol. Pharm.,* **2009**, *6*(5), 1343-1352.
[http://dx.doi.org/10.1021/mp900022m] [PMID: 19249859]

[76] Oltra, N.S.; Swift, J.; Mahmud, A.; Rajagopal, K.; Loverde, S.M.; Discher, D.E. Filomicelles in nanomedicine – from flexible, fragmentable, and ligand-targetable drug carrier designs to combination therapy for brain tumors. *J. Mater. Chem. B Mater. Biol. Med.,* **2013**, *1*(39), 5177-5185.
[http://dx.doi.org/10.1039/c3tb20431f] [PMID: 32263324]

[77] Ke, W.; Lu, N.; Japir, A.A.W.M.M.; Zhou, Q.; Xi, L.; Wang, Y.; Dutta, D.; Zhou, M.; Pan, Y.; Ge, Z. Length effect of stimuli-responsive block copolymer prodrug filomicelles on drug delivery efficiency.

J. Control. Release, **2020,** *318,* 67-77.
[http://dx.doi.org/10.1016/j.jconrel.2019.12.012] [PMID: 31837355]

[78]   Lim, C.; Ramsey, J.D.; Hwang, D.; Teixeira, S.C.M.; Poon, C.D.; Strauss, J.D.; Rosen, E.P.; Sokolsky-Papkov, M.; Kabanov, A.V. Drug-Dependent Morphological Transitions in Spherical and Worm-Like Polymeric Micelles Define Stability and Pharmacological Performance of Micellar Drugs. *Small,* **2022,** *18*(4), 2103552.
[http://dx.doi.org/10.1002/smll.202103552] [PMID: 34841670]

[79]   Bai, J.; Wang, J.; Feng, Y.; Yao, Y.; Zhao, X. Stability-tunable core-crosslinked polymeric micelles based on an imidazole-bearing block polymer for pH-responsive drug delivery. *Colloids Surf. A Physicochem. Eng. Asp.,* **2022,** *639,* 128353.
[http://dx.doi.org/10.1016/j.colsurfa.2022.128353]

[80]   Pashirova, T.N.; Fernandes, A.R.; Sanchez-Lopez, E.; Garcia, M.L.; Silva, A.M.; Zakharova, L.Y.; Souto, E.B. Polymer nanogels: Fabrication, structural behavior, and biological applications.*Theory and Applications of Nonparenteral Nanomedicines*; Kesharwani, P.; Taurin, S.; Greish, K., Eds.; Academic Press, **2021,** pp. 97-111.
[http://dx.doi.org/10.1016/B978-0-12-820466-5.00005-3]

[81]   Suhail, M.; Rosenholm, J.M.; Minhas, M.U.; Badshah, S.F.; Naeem, A.; Khan, K.U.; Fahad, M. Nanogels as drug-delivery systems: a comprehensive overview. *Ther. Deliv.,* **2019,** *10*(11), 697-717.
[http://dx.doi.org/10.4155/tde-2019-0010] [PMID: 31789106]

[82]   Soni, K. S.; Desale, S. S.; Bronich, T. K. Nanogels: An overview of properties, biomedical applications and obstacles to clinical translation. *Journal of controlled release : official journal of the Controlled Release Society,* **2016,** *240,* 109-126.

[83]   Cheng, J.; Teply, B.; Sherifi, I.; Sung, J.; Luther, G.; Gu, F.; Levynissenbaum, E.; Radovicmoreno, A.; Langer, R.; Farokhzad, O. Formulation of functionalized PLGA–PEG nanoparticles for *in vivo* targeted drug delivery. *Biomaterials,* **2007,** *28*(5), 869-876.
[http://dx.doi.org/10.1016/j.biomaterials.2006.09.047] [PMID: 17055572]

[84]   Gao, D.; Xu, H.; Philbert, M.A.; Kopelman, R. Bioeliminable nanohydrogels for drug delivery. *Nano Lett.,* **2008,** *8*(10), 3320-3324.
[http://dx.doi.org/10.1021/nl8017274] [PMID: 18788823]

[85]   Malmsten, M. Soft drug delivery systems. *Soft Matter,* **2006,** *2*(9), 760-769.
[http://dx.doi.org/10.1039/b608348j] [PMID: 32680216]

[86]   Napier, M.E.; DeSimone, J.M. Nanoparticle drug delivery platform. *J. Macromol. Sci. Part C Polym. Rev.,* **2007,** *47*(3), 321-327.

[87]   Zha, L.; Banik, B.; Alexis, F. Stimulus responsive nanogels for drug delivery. *Soft Matter,* **2011,** *7*(13), 5908-5916.
[http://dx.doi.org/10.1039/c0sm01307b]

[88]   Motornov, M.; Roiter, Y.; Tokarev, I.; Minko, S. Stimuli-responsive nanoparticles, nanogels and capsules for integrated multifunctional intelligent systems. *Prog. Polym. Sci.,* **2010,** *35*(1-2), 174-211.
[http://dx.doi.org/10.1016/j.progpolymsci.2009.10.004]

[89]   Simonson, A.W.; Lawanprasert, A.; Goralski, T.D.P.; Keiler, K.C.; Medina, S.H. Bioresponsive peptide-polysaccharide nanogels : A versatile delivery system to augment the utility of bioactive cargo. *Nanomedicine,* **2019,** *17,* 391-400.
[http://dx.doi.org/10.1016/j.nano.2018.10.008] [PMID: 30399437]

[90]   Soni, K.S.; Desale, S.S.; Bronich, T.K. Nanogels: An overview of properties, biomedical applications and obstacles to clinical translation. *J. Control. Release,* **2016,** *240,* 109-126.
[http://dx.doi.org/10.1016/j.jconrel.2015.11.009] [PMID: 26571000]

[91]   Jochum, F.D.; Theato, P. Temperature- and light-responsive smart polymer materials. *Chem. Soc. Rev.,* **2013,** *42*(17), 7468-7483.

[http://dx.doi.org/10.1039/C2CS35191A] [PMID: 22868906]

[92]   Mok, H.; Jeong, H.; Kim, S.J.; Chung, B.H. Indocyanine green encapsulated nanogels for hyaluronidase activatable and selective near infrared imaging of tumors and lymph nodes. *Chem. Commun.,* **2012**, *48*(69), 8628-8630.
[http://dx.doi.org/10.1039/c2cc33555g] [PMID: 22745939]

[93]   Canal, T.; Peppas, N.A. Correlation between mesh size and equilibrium degree of swelling of polymeric networks. *J. Biomed. Mater. Res.,* **1989**, *23*(10), 1183-1193.
[http://dx.doi.org/10.1002/jbm.820231007] [PMID: 2808463]

[94]   Lustig, S.R.; Peppas, N.A. Solute diffusion in swollen membranes. IX. Scaling laws for solute diffusion in gels. *J. Appl. Polym. Sci.,* **1988**, *36*(4), 735-747.
[http://dx.doi.org/10.1002/app.1988.070360401]

[95]   Kabanov, A.V.; Vinogradov, S.V. Nanogels as pharmaceutical carriers: finite networks of infinite capabilities. *Angew. Chem. Int. Ed.,* **2009**, *48*(30), 5418-5429.
[http://dx.doi.org/10.1002/anie.200900441] [PMID: 19562807]

[96]   Mitragotri, S.; Lahann, J. Physical approaches to biomaterial design. *Nat. Mater.,* **2009**, *8*(1), 15-23.
[http://dx.doi.org/10.1038/nmat2344] [PMID: 19096389]

[97]   Jeon, S.I.; Lee, J.H.; Andrade, J.D.; De Gennes, P.G. Protein—surface interactions in the presence of polyethylene oxide. *J. Colloid Interface Sci.,* **1991**, *142*(1), 149-158.
[http://dx.doi.org/10.1016/0021-9797(91)90043-8]

[98]   Moghimi, S.M.; Hunter, A.C.; Murray, J.C. Long-circulating and target-specific nanoparticles: Theory to practice. *Pharmacol. Rev.,* **2001**, *53*(2), 283-318.
[PMID: 11356986]

[99]   Maeda, H.; Bharate, G.Y.; Daruwalla, J. Polymeric drugs for efficient tumor-targeted drug delivery based on EPR-effect. *Eur. J. Pharm. Biopharm.,* **2009**, *71*(3), 409-419.
[http://dx.doi.org/10.1016/j.ejpb.2008.11.010] [PMID: 19070661]

[100] Maeda, H. The enhanced permeability and retention (EPR) effect in tumor vasculature: the key role of tumor-selective macromolecular drug targeting. *Adv. Enzyme Regul.,* **2001**, *41*(1), 189-207.
[http://dx.doi.org/10.1016/S0065-2571(00)00013-3] [PMID: 11384745]

[101] Ahmed-Farid, O.A.H.; Nasr, M.; Ahmed, R.F.; Bakeer, R.M. Beneficial effects of curcumin nano-emulsion on spermatogenesis and reproductive performance in male rats under protein deficient diet model: enhancement of sperm motility, conservancy of testicular tissue integrity, cell energy and seminal plasma amino acids content. *J. Biomed. Sci.,* **2017**, *24*(1), 66.
[http://dx.doi.org/10.1186/s12929-017-0373-5] [PMID: 28865467]

[102] Ismail, A.; Nasr, M.; Sammour, O. Nanoemulsion as a feasible and biocompatible carrier for ocular delivery of travoprost: Improved pharmacokinetic/pharmacodynamic properties. *Int. J. Pharm.,* **2020**, *583*, 119402.
[http://dx.doi.org/10.1016/j.ijpharm.2020.119402] [PMID: 32387308]

[103] Nasr, M. Development of an optimized hyaluronic acid-based lipidic nanoemulsion co-encapsulating two polyphenols for nose to brain delivery. *Drug Deliv.,* **2016**, *23*(4), 1444-1452.
[http://dx.doi.org/10.3109/10717544.2015.1092619] [PMID: 26401600]

[104] Ramez, S. A.; Soliman, M. M.; Fadel, M.; Nour El-Deen, F.; Nasr, M.; Youness, E. R.; Aboel-Fadl, D. M. Novel methotrexate soft nanocarrier/fractional erbium YAG laser combination for clinical treatment of plaque psoriasis. *Artificial Cells, Nanomedicine, and Biotechnology,* **2018**, *46* 1, 996-1002.

[105] Silva, R.C.S.; de Souza Arruda, I.R.; Malafaia, C.B.; de Moraes, M.M.; Beck, T.S.; Gomes da Camara, C.A.; Henrique da Silva, N.; Vanusa da Silva, M.; dos Santos Correia, M.T.; Frizzo, C.P.; Machado, G. Synthesis, characterization and antibiofilm/antimicrobial activity of nanoemulsions containing Tetragastris catuaba (Burseraceae) essential oil against disease-causing pathogens. *J. Drug Deliv. Sci.*

Technol., **2022**, *67*, 102795.
[http://dx.doi.org/10.1016/j.jddst.2021.102795]

[106] Wilson, R.J.; Li, Y.; Yang, G.; Zhao, C.X. Nanoemulsions for drug delivery. *Particuology,* **2022**, *64*, 85-97.
[http://dx.doi.org/10.1016/j.partic.2021.05.009]

[107] Kim, S.Y.; Kim, S.; Kim, J.E.; Lee, S.N.; Shin, I.W.; Shin, H.S.; Jin, S.M.; Noh, Y.W.; Kang, Y.J.; Kim, Y.S.; Kang, T.H.; Park, Y.M.; Lim, Y.T. Lyophilizable and Multifaceted Toll-like Receptor 7/8 Agonist-Loaded Nanoemulsion for the Reprogramming of Tumor Microenvironments and Enhanced Cancer Immunotherapy. *ACS Nano,* **2019**, *13*(11), 12671-12686.
[http://dx.doi.org/10.1021/acsnano.9b04207] [PMID: 31589013]

[108] Zeng, B.; Middelberg, A.P.J.; Gemiarto, A.; MacDonald, K.; Baxter, A.G.; Talekar, M.; Moi, D.; Tullett, K.M.; Caminschi, I.; Lahoud, M.H.; Mazzieri, R.; Dolcetti, R.; Thomas, R. Self-adjuvanting nanoemulsion targeting dendritic cell receptor Clec9A enables antigen-specific immunotherapy. *J. Clin. Invest.,* **2018**, *128*(5), 1971-1984.
[http://dx.doi.org/10.1172/JCI96791] [PMID: 29485973]

[109] Pellosi, D.S.; Macaroff, P.P.; Morais, P.C.; Tedesco, A.C. Magneto low-density nanoemulsion (MLDE): A potential vehicle for combined hyperthermia and photodynamic therapy to treat cancer selectively. *Mater. Sci. Eng. C,* **2018**, *92*, 103-111.
[http://dx.doi.org/10.1016/j.msec.2018.06.033] [PMID: 30184726]

[110] Garcia, C.R.; Malik, M.H.; Biswas, S.; Tam, V.H.; Rumbaugh, K.P.; Li, W.; Liu, X. Nanoemulsion delivery systems for enhanced efficacy of antimicrobials and essential oils. *Biomater. Sci.,* **2022**, *10*(3), 633-653.
[http://dx.doi.org/10.1039/D1BM01537K] [PMID: 34994371]

[111] Moghimi, R.; Ghaderi, L.; Rafati, H.; Aliahmadi, A.; McClements, D.J. Superior antibacterial activity of nanoemulsion of Thymus daenensis essential oil against E. coli. *Food Chem.,* **2016**, *194*, 410-415.
[http://dx.doi.org/10.1016/j.foodchem.2015.07.139] [PMID: 26471573]

[112] Duan, Y.; Dhar, A.; Patel, C.; Khimani, M.; Neogi, S.; Sharma, P.; Siva Kumar, N.; Vekariya, R.L. A brief review on solid lipid nanoparticles: part and parcel of contemporary drug delivery systems. *RSC Advances,* **2020**, *10*(45), 26777-26791.
[http://dx.doi.org/10.1039/D0RA03491F] [PMID: 35515778]

[113] Hallan, S.S.; Kaur, P.; Kaur, V.; Mishra, N.; Vaidya, B. Lipid polymer hybrid as emerging tool in nanocarriers for oral drug delivery. *Artif. Cells Nanomed. Biotechnol.,* **2016**, *44*(1), 334-349.
[http://dx.doi.org/10.3109/21691401.2014.951721] [PMID: 25237838]

[114] Briones, E.; Colino, C.I.; Lanao, J.M. Delivery systems to increase the selectivity of antibiotics in phagocytic cells. *J. Control. Release,* **2008**, *125*(3), 210-227.
[PMID: 18077047]

[115] Khatak, S.; Mehta, M.; Awasthi, R.; Paudel, K.R.; Singh, S.K.; Gulati, M.; Hansbro, N.G.; Hansbro, P.M.; Dua, K.; Dureja, H. Solid lipid nanoparticles containing anti-tubercular drugs attenuate the Mycobacterium marinum infection. *Tuberculosis (Edinb.),* **2020**, *125*, 102008.
[http://dx.doi.org/10.1016/j.tube.2020.102008] [PMID: 33059322]

[116] Yang, S.C.; Lu, L.F.; Cai, Y.; Zhu, J.B.; Liang, B.W.; Yang, C.Z. Body distribution in mice of intravenously injected camptothecin solid lipid nanoparticles and targeting effect on brain. *J. Control. Release,* **1999**, *59*(3), 299-307.
[http://dx.doi.org/10.1016/S0168-3659(99)00007-3] [PMID: 10332062]

[117] Freitas, C.; Müller, R.H. Correlation between long-term stability of solid lipid nanoparticles (SLN™) and crystallinity of the lipid phase. *Eur. J. Pharm. Biopharm.,* **1999**, *47*(2), 125-132.
[http://dx.doi.org/10.1016/S0939-6411(98)00074-5] [PMID: 10234536]

[118] Dhakad, R.; Tekade, R.; Jain, N. Cancer targeting potential of folate targeted nanocarrier under comparative influence of tretinoin and dexamethasone. *Curr. Drug Deliv.,* **2013**, *10*(4), 477-491.

[http://dx.doi.org/10.2174/1567201811310040012] [PMID: 23062180]

[119] Bocca, C.; Caputo, O.; Cavalli, R.; Gabriel, L.; Miglietta, A.; Gasco, M.R. Phagocytic uptake of fluorescent stealth and non-stealth solid lipid nanoparticles. *Int. J. Pharm.*, **1998**, *175*(2), 185-193.
[http://dx.doi.org/10.1016/S0378-5173(98)00282-8]

[120] Miglietta, A.; Cavalli, R.; Bocca, C.; Gabriel, L.; Rosa Gasco, M. Cellular uptake and cytotoxicity of solid lipid nanospheres (SLN) incorporating doxorubicin or paclitaxel. *Int. J. Pharm.*, **2000**, *210*(1-2), 61-67.
[http://dx.doi.org/10.1016/S0378-5173(00)00562-7] [PMID: 11163988]

[121] Dianzani, C.; Zara, G. P.; Maina, G.; Pettazzoni, P.; Pizzimenti, S.; Rossi, F.; Gigliotti, C. L.; Ciamporcero, E. S.; Daga, M.; Barrera, G. *Drug delivery nanoparticles in skin cancers., BioMed research intern.*, **2014**, *2014*
[http://dx.doi.org/10.1155/2014/895986]

[122] Zara, G.P.; Cavalli, R.; Fundarò, A.; Bargoni, A.; Caputo, O.; Gasco, M.R. Pharmacokinetics of doxorubicin incorporated in solid lipid nanospheres (SLN). *Pharmacol. Res.*, **1999**, *40*(3), 281-286.
[http://dx.doi.org/10.1006/phrs.1999.0509] [PMID: 10479474]

[123] Jenning, V.; Gysler, A.; Schäfer-Korting, M.; Gohla, S.H. Vitamin A loaded solid lipid nanoparticles for topical use: Occlusive properties and drug targeting to the upper skin. *Eur. J. Pharm. Biopharm.*, **2000**, *49*(3), 211-218.
[http://dx.doi.org/10.1016/S0939-6411(99)00075-2] [PMID: 10799811]

[124] Müller-Goymann, C. C. Physicochemical characterization of colloidal drug delivery systems such as reverse micelles, vesicles, liquid crystals and nanoparticles for topical administration. *European journal of pharmaceutics and biopharmaceutics : official journal of Arbeitsgemeinschaft fur Pharmazeutische Verfahrenstechnik e.V,* **2004**, *58*(2), 343-356.

[125] Schäferkorting, M.; Mehnert, W.; Korting, H. Lipid nanoparticles for improved topical application of drugs for skin diseases. *Adv. Drug Deliv. Rev.*, **2007**, *59*(6), 427-443.
[http://dx.doi.org/10.1016/j.addr.2007.04.006] [PMID: 17544165]

[126] Müller, R.H.; Radtke, M.; Wissing, S.A. Solid lipid nanoparticles (SLN) and nanostructured lipid carriers (NLC) in cosmetic and dermatological preparations. *Adv. Drug Deliv. Rev.*, **2002**, *54* 1, S131-S155.
[http://dx.doi.org/10.1016/S0169-409X(02)00118-7] [PMID: 12460720]

[127] Jenning, V.; Schäfer-Korting, M.; Gohla, S. Vitamin A-loaded solid lipid nanoparticles for topical use: drug release properties. *J. Control. Release*, **2000**, *66*(2-3), 115-126.
[http://dx.doi.org/10.1016/S0168-3659(99)00223-0] [PMID: 10742573]

[128] Olbrich, C.; Bakowsky, U.; Lehr, C.M.; Müller, R.H.; Kneuer, C. Cationic solid-lipid nanoparticles can efficiently bind and transfect plasmid DNA. *J. Control. Release,* **2001**, *77*(3), 345-355.
[http://dx.doi.org/10.1016/S0168-3659(01)00506-5] [PMID: 11733101]

[129] Gaspar, D.P.; Faria, V.; Gonçalves, L.M.D.; Taboada, P.; Remuñán-López, C.; Almeida, A.J. Rifabutin-loaded solid lipid nanoparticles for inhaled antitubercular therapy: Physicochemical and *in vitro* studies. *Int. J. Pharm.*, **2016**, *497*(1-2), 199-209.
[http://dx.doi.org/10.1016/j.ijpharm.2015.11.050] [PMID: 26656946]

[130] Ghaderkhani, J.; Yousefimashouf, R.; Arabestani, M.; Roshanaei, G.; Asl, S.S.; Abbasalipourkabir, R. Improved antibacterial function of Rifampicin-loaded solid lipid nanoparticles on *Brucella abortus*. *Artif. Cells Nanomed. Biotechnol.*, **2019**, *47*(1), 1181-1193.
[http://dx.doi.org/10.1080/21691401.2019.1593858] [PMID: 30942627]

[131] Bush, K.; Courvalin, P.; Dantas, G.; Davies, J.; Eisenstein, B.; Huovinen, P.; Jacoby, G.A.; Kishony, R.; Kreiswirth, B.N.; Kutter, E.; Lerner, S.A.; Levy, S.; Lewis, K.; Lomovskaya, O.; Miller, J.H.; Mobashery, S.; Piddock, L.J.V.; Projan, S.; Thomas, C.M.; Tomasz, A.; Tulkens, P.M.; Walsh, T.R.; Watson, J.D.; Witkowski, J.; Witte, W.; Wright, G.; Yeh, P.; Zgurskaya, H.I. Tackling antibiotic resistance. *Nat. Rev. Microbiol.*, **2011**, *9*(12), 894-896.

[http://dx.doi.org/10.1038/nrmicro2693] [PMID: 22048738]

[132]   Zhang, L.; Pornpattananangkul, D.; Hu, C.M.; Huang, C.M. Development of nanoparticles for antimicrobial drug delivery. *Curr. Med. Chem.,* **2010,** *17*(6), 585-594.
[http://dx.doi.org/10.2174/092986710790416290] [PMID: 20015030]

[133]   Baker-Austin, C.; Wright, M.S.; Stepanauskas, R.; McArthur, J.V. Co-selection of antibiotic and metal resistance. *Trends Microbiol.,* **2006,** *14*(4), 176-182.
[http://dx.doi.org/10.1016/j.tim.2006.02.006] [PMID: 16537105]

[134]   Friedman, M. Chemistry and multibeneficial bioactivities of carvacrol (4-isopropyl-2-methylphenol), a component of essential oils produced by aromatic plants and spices. *J. Agric. Food Chem.,* **2014,** *62*(31), 7652-7670.
[http://dx.doi.org/10.1021/jf5023862] [PMID: 25058878]

[135]   Seedat, N.; Kalhapure, R.S.; Mocktar, C.; Vepuri, S.; Jadhav, M.; Soliman, M.; Govender, T. Co-encapsulation of multi-lipids and polymers enhances the performance of vancomycin in lipid–polymer hybrid nanoparticles: *In vitro* and in silico studies. *Mater. Sci. Eng. C,* **2016,** *61,* 616-630.
[http://dx.doi.org/10.1016/j.msec.2015.12.053] [PMID: 26838890]

[136]   Wei, T.; Chen, C.; Liu, J.; Liu, C.; Posocco, P.; Liu, X.; Cheng, Q.; Huo, S.; Liang, Z.; Fermeglia, M.; Pricl, S.; Liang, X.J.; Rocchi, P.; Peng, L. Anticancer drug nanomicelles formed by self-assembling amphiphilic dendrimer to combat cancer drug resistance. *Proc. Natl. Acad. Sci. USA,* **2015,** *112*(10), 2978-2983.
[http://dx.doi.org/10.1073/pnas.1418494112] [PMID: 25713374]

[137]   Mintzer, M.A.; Grinstaff, M.W. Biomedical applications of dendrimers: A tutorial. *Chem. Soc. Rev.,* **2011,** *40*(1), 173-190.
[http://dx.doi.org/10.1039/B901839P] [PMID: 20877875]

[138]   Abbasi, E.; Aval, S.F.; Akbarzadeh, A.; Milani, M.; Nasrabadi, H.T.; Joo, S.W.; Hanifehpour, Y.; Nejati-Koshki, K.; Pashaei-Asl, R. Dendrimers: synthesis, applications, and properties. *Nanoscale Res. Lett.,* **2014,** *9*(1), 247.
[http://dx.doi.org/10.1186/1556-276X-9-247] [PMID: 24994950]

[139]   Rolland, O.; Turrin, C.O.; Caminade, A.M.; Majoral, J.P. Dendrimers and nanomedicine: multivalency in action. *New J. Chem.,* **2009,** *33*(9), 1809-1824.
[http://dx.doi.org/10.1039/b901054h]

[140]   Bussy, C.; Alexiou, C.; Petros, A. Therapeutic applications. In Adverse effects of engineered nanomaterials: exposure, toxicology, and impact on human health, 1 ed.; Fadeel, B.; Pietroiusti, A.; Shvedova, A. A., Eds. Academic Press: 2012; pp 286-313.

[141]   Raghupathi, K.R.; Guo, J.; Munkhbat, O.; Rangadurai, P.; Thayumanavan, S. Supramolecular disassembly of facially amphiphilic dendrimer assemblies in response to physical, chemical, and biological stimuli. *Acc. Chem. Res.,* **2014,** *47*(7), 2200-2211.
[http://dx.doi.org/10.1021/ar500143u] [PMID: 24937682]

[142]   Nyström, A.M.; Wooley, K.L. The importance of chemistry in creating well-defined nanoscopic embedded therapeutics: devices capable of the dual functions of imaging and therapy. *Acc. Chem. Res.,* **2011,** *44*(10), 969-978.
[http://dx.doi.org/10.1021/ar200097k] [PMID: 21675721]

[143]   Liko, F.; Hindré, F.; Fernandez-Megia, E. Dendrimers as Innovative Radiopharmaceuticals in Cancer Radionanotherapy. *Biomacromolecules,* **2016,** *17*(10), 3103-3114.
[http://dx.doi.org/10.1021/acs.biomac.6b00929] [PMID: 27608327]

[144]   Wang, D.; Astruc, D. Dendritic catalysis—Basic concepts and recent trends. *Coord. Chem. Rev.,* **2013,** *257*(15-16), 2317-2334.
[http://dx.doi.org/10.1016/j.ccr.2013.03.032]

[145]   Wang, J.; Li, B.; Qiu, L.; Qiao, X.; Yang, H. Dendrimer-based drug delivery systems: history,

challenges, and latest developments. *J. Biol. Eng.,* **2022,** *16*(1), 18.
[http://dx.doi.org/10.1186/s13036-022-00298-5] [PMID: 35879774]

[146] Idris, A.O.; Mamba, B.; Feleni, U. Poly (propylene imine) dendrimer: A potential nanomaterial for electrochemical application. *Mater. Chem. Phys.,* **2020,** *244*, 122641.
[http://dx.doi.org/10.1016/j.matchemphys.2020.122641]

[147] Surekha, B.; Kommana, N.S.; Dubey, S.K.; Kumar, A.V.P.; Shukla, R.; Kesharwani, P. PAMAM dendrimer as a talented multifunctional biomimetic nanocarrier for cancer diagnosis and therapy. *Colloids Surf. B Biointerfaces,* **2021,** *204*, 111837.
[http://dx.doi.org/10.1016/j.colsurfb.2021.111837] [PMID: 33992888]

[148] Yang, H. Targeted nanosystems: Advances in targeted dendrimers for cancer therapy. *Nanomedicine,* **2016,** *12*(2), 309-316.
[http://dx.doi.org/10.1016/j.nano.2015.11.012] [PMID: 26706410]

[149] Kannan, R.M.; Nance, E.; Kannan, S.; Tomalia, D.A. Emerging concepts in dendrimer-based nanomedicine: from design principles to clinical applications. *J. Intern. Med.,* **2014,** *276*(6), 579-617.
[http://dx.doi.org/10.1111/joim.12280] [PMID: 24995512]

[150] Pandita, D.; Madaan, K.; Kumar, S.; Poonia, N.; Lather, V. Dendrimers in drug delivery and targeting: Drug-dendrimer interactions and toxicity issues. *J. Pharm. Bioallied Sci.,* **2014,** *6*(3), 139-150.
[http://dx.doi.org/10.4103/0975-7406.130965] [PMID: 25035633]

[151] Kesharwani, P.; Banerjee, S.; Gupta, U.; Mohd Amin, M.C.I.; Padhye, S.; Sarkar, F.H.; Iyer, A.K. PAMAM dendrimers as promising nanocarriers for RNAi therapeutics. *Mater. Today,* **2015,** *18*(10), 565-572.
[http://dx.doi.org/10.1016/j.mattod.2015.06.003]

[152] Zhou, L.; Gan, L.; Li, H.; Yang, X. Studies on the interactions between DNA and PAMAM with fluorescent probe [Ru(phen)2dppz]2+. *J. Pharm. Biomed. Anal.,* **2007,** *43*(1), 330-334.
[http://dx.doi.org/10.1016/j.jpba.2006.06.021] [PMID: 16872783]

[153] Thiagarajan, G.; Greish, K.; Ghandehari, H. Charge affects the oral toxicity of poly(amidoamine) dendrimers. *Eur. J. Pharm. Biopharm.,* **2013,** *84*(2), 330-334.
[http://dx.doi.org/10.1016/j.ejpb.2013.01.019] [PMID: 23419816]

[154] Chauhan, A.S.; Jain, N.K.; Diwan, P.V. Pre-clinical and behavioural toxicity profile of PAMAM dendrimers in mice. *Proc.- Royal Soc., Math. Phys. Eng. Sci.,* **2010,** *466*(2117), 1535-1550.
[http://dx.doi.org/10.1098/rspa.2009.0448]

[155] Araújo, R.; Santos, S.; Igne Ferreira, E.; Giarolla, J. New Advances in General Biomedical Applications of PAMAM Dendrimers. *Molecules,* **2018,** *23*(11), 2849.
[http://dx.doi.org/10.3390/molecules23112849] [PMID: 30400134]

[156] Pryor, J.B.; Harper, B.J.; Harper, S.L. Comparative toxicological assessment of PAMAM and thiophosphoryl dendrimers using embryonic zebrafish. *Int. J. Nanomedicine,* **2014,** *9*, 1947-1956.
[PMID: 24790436]

[157] Gao, Y.; Wang, J.; Chai, M.; Li, X.; Deng, Y.; Jin, Q.; Ji, J. Size and charge adaptive clustered nanoparticles targeting the biofilm microenviroment for chronic lung infection management. *ACS Nano,* **2020,** *14*(5), 5686-5699.
[http://dx.doi.org/10.1021/acsnano.0c00269] [PMID: 32320228]

[158] Wang, K.; Tu, Y.; Yao, W.; Zong, Q.; Xiao, X.; Yang, R.M.; Jiang, X.Q.; Yuan, Y. Size-switchable nanoparticles with self-destructive and tumor penetration characteristics for site-specific phototherapy of cancer. *ACS Appl. Mater. Interfaces,* **2020,** *12*(6), 6933-6943.
[http://dx.doi.org/10.1021/acsami.9b21525] [PMID: 31951372]

[159] Luong, D.; Kesharwani, P.; Deshmukh, R.; Mohd Amin, M.C.I.; Gupta, U.; Greish, K.; Iyer, A.K. PEGylated PAMAM dendrimers: Enhancing efficacy and mitigating toxicity for effective anticancer drug and gene delivery. *Acta Biomater.,* **2016,** *43*, 14-29.

[http://dx.doi.org/10.1016/j.actbio.2016.07.015] [PMID: 27422195]

[160] Ho, M.N.; Bach, L.G.; Nguyen, D.H.; Nguyen, C.H.; Nguyen, C.K.; Tran, N.Q.; Nguyen, N.V.; Hoang Thi, T.T. PEGylated PAMAM dendrimers loading oxaliplatin with prolonged release and high payload without burst effect. *Biopolymers,* **2019**, *110*(7), e23272.
[http://dx.doi.org/10.1002/bip.23272] [PMID: 30897210]

[161] Yuan, Q.; Yeudall, W.A.; Yang, H. PEGylated polyamidoamine dendrimers with bis-aryl hydrazone linkages for enhanced gene delivery. *Biomacromolecules,* **2010**, *11*(8), 1940-1947.
[http://dx.doi.org/10.1021/bm100589g] [PMID: 20593893]

[162] Waite, C.L.; Sparks, S.M.; Uhrich, K.E.; Roth, C.M. Acetylation of PAMAM dendrimers for cellular delivery of siRNA. *BMC Biotechnol.,* **2009**, *9*(1), 38.
[http://dx.doi.org/10.1186/1472-6750-9-38] [PMID: 19389227]

[163] Xiong, Z.; Shen, M.; Shi, X. Zwitterionic Modification of Nanomaterials for Improved Diagnosis of Cancer Cells. *Bioconjug. Chem.,* **2019**, *30*(10), 2519-2527.
[http://dx.doi.org/10.1021/acs.bioconjchem.9b00543] [PMID: 31502829]

[164] Wang, L.; Shi, C.; Wang, X.; Guo, D.; Duncan, T.M.; Luo, J. Zwitterionic Janus Dendrimer with distinct functional disparity for enhanced protein delivery. *Biomaterials,* **2019**, *215*, 119233.
[http://dx.doi.org/10.1016/j.biomaterials.2019.119233] [PMID: 31176068]

[165] Wang, T.; Zhang, D.; Sun, D.; Gu, J. Current status of *in vivo* bioanalysis of nano drug delivery systems. *J. Pharm. Anal.,* **2020**, *10*(3), 221-232.
[http://dx.doi.org/10.1016/j.jpha.2020.05.002] [PMID: 32612868]

[166] Bayda, S.; Hadla, M.; Palazzolo, S.; Riello, P.; Corona, G.; Toffoli, G.; Rizzolio, F. Inorganic nanoparticles for cancer therapy: A transition from lab to clinic. *Curr. Med. Chem.,* **2018**, *25*(34), 4269-4303.
[http://dx.doi.org/10.2174/0929867325666171229141156] [PMID: 29284391]

[167] Nisar, P.; Ali, N.; Rahman, L.; Ali, M.; Shinwari, Z.K. Antimicrobial activities of biologically synthesized metal nanoparticles: an insight into the mechanism of action. *J. Biol. Inorg. Chem.,* **2019**, *24*(7), 929-941.
[http://dx.doi.org/10.1007/s00775-019-01717-7] [PMID: 31515623]

[168] Gallo, G.; Schillaci, D. Bacterial metal nanoparticles to develop new weapons against bacterial biofilms and infections. *Appl. Microbiol. Biotechnol.,* **2021**, *105*(13), 5357-5366.
[http://dx.doi.org/10.1007/s00253-021-11418-4] [PMID: 34184105]

[169] Ren, E.; Zhang, C.; Li, D.; Pang, X.; Liu, G. Leveraging metal oxide nanoparticles for bacteria tracing and eradicating. *VIEW,* **2020**, *1*(3), 20200052.
[http://dx.doi.org/10.1002/VIW.20200052]

[170] Ghaffar, N.; Javad, S.; Farrukh, M.A.; Shah, A.A.; Gatasheh, M.K.; AL-Munqedhi, B.M.A.; Chaudhry, O. Metal nanoparticles assisted revival of Streptomycin against MDRS Staphylococcus aureus. *PLoS One,* **2022**, *17*(3), e0264588.
[http://dx.doi.org/10.1371/journal.pone.0264588] [PMID: 35324924]

[171] Boken, J.; Khurana, P.; Thatai, S.; Kumar, D.; Prasad, S. Plasmonic nanoparticles and their analytical applications: A review. *Appl. Spectrosc. Rev.,* **2017**, *52*(9), 774-820.
[http://dx.doi.org/10.1080/05704928.2017.1312427]

[172] Dong, Y.; Wan, G.; Yan, P.; Qian, C.; Li, F.; Peng, G. Fabrication of resveratrol coated gold nanoparticles and investigation of their effect on diabetic retinopathy in streptozotocin induced diabetic rats. *J. Photochem. Photobiol. B,* **2019**, *195*, 51-57.
[http://dx.doi.org/10.1016/j.jphotobiol.2019.04.012] [PMID: 31082734]

[173] Exner, K.S.; Ivanova, A. A doxorubicin–peptide–gold nanoparticle conjugate as a functionalized drug delivery system: exploring the limits. *Phys. Chem. Chem. Phys.,* **2022**, *24*(24), 14985-14992.
[http://dx.doi.org/10.1039/D2CP00707J] [PMID: 35687051]

[174] Kadkhoda, J.; Aghanejad, A.; Safari, B.; Barar, J.; Rasta, S.H.; Davaran, S. Aptamer-conjugated gold nanoparticles for targeted paclitaxel delivery and photothermal therapy in breast cancer. *J. Drug Deliv. Sci. Technol.,* **2022**, *67*, 102954.
[http://dx.doi.org/10.1016/j.jddst.2021.102954]

[175] Giannaccini, M.; Giannini, M.; Calatayud, M.; Goya, G.; Cuschieri, A.; Dente, L.; Raffa, V. Magnetic nanoparticles as intraocular drug delivery system to target retinal pigmented epithelium (RPE). *Int. J. Mol. Sci.,* **2014**, *15*(1), 1590-1605.
[http://dx.doi.org/10.3390/ijms15011590] [PMID: 24451140]

[176] Lodhi, M.S.; Khalid, F.; Khan, M.T.; Samra, Z.Q.; Muhammad, S.; Zhang, Y.J.; Mou, K. A Novel Method of Magnetic Nanoparticles Functionalized with Anti-Folate Receptor Antibody and Methotrexate for Antibody Mediated Targeted Drug Delivery. *Molecules,* **2022**, *27*(1), 261.
[http://dx.doi.org/10.3390/molecules27010261] [PMID: 35011493]

[177] Farmanbar, N.; Mohseni, S.; Darroudi, M. Green synthesis of chitosan-coated magnetic nanoparticles for drug delivery of oxaliplatin and irinotecan against colorectal cancer cells. *Polym. Bull.,* **2022**, *79*(12), 10595-10613.
[http://dx.doi.org/10.1007/s00289-021-04066-1]

[178] Mishra, P.K.; Mishra, H.; Ekielski, A.; Talegaonkar, S.; Vaidya, B. Zinc oxide nanoparticles: A promising nanomaterial for biomedical applications. *Drug Discov. Today,* **2017**, *22*(12), 1825-1834.
[http://dx.doi.org/10.1016/j.drudis.2017.08.006] [PMID: 28847758]

[179] Anjum, S.; Hashim, M.; Malik, S.A.; Khan, M.; Lorenzo, J.M.; Abbasi, B.H.; Hano, C. Recent Advances in Zinc Oxide Nanoparticles (ZnO NPs) for Cancer Diagnosis, Target Drug Delivery, and Treatment. *Cancers (Basel),* **2021**, *13*(18), 4570.
[http://dx.doi.org/10.3390/cancers13184570] [PMID: 34572797]

[180] Wang, Y.; Song, S.; Liu, J.; Liu, D.; Zhang, H. ZnO-functionalized upconverting nanotheranostic agent: multi-modality imaging-guided chemotherapy with on-demand drug release triggered by pH. *Angew. Chem. Int. Ed.,* **2015**, *54*(2), 536-540.
[http://dx.doi.org/10.1002/anie.201409519] [PMID: 25366670]

[181] Muhammad, F.; Guo, M.; Qi, W.; Sun, F.; Wang, A.; Guo, Y.; Zhu, G. pH-Triggered controlled drug release from mesoporous silica nanoparticles *via* intracelluar dissolution of ZnO nanolids. *J. Am. Chem. Soc.,* **2011**, *133*(23), 8778-8781.
[http://dx.doi.org/10.1021/ja200328s] [PMID: 21574653]

[182] Zheng, J.; Jiang, Z.Y.; Kuang, Q.; Xie, Z.X.; Huang, R.B.; Zheng, L.S. Shape-controlled fabrication of porous ZnO architectures and their photocatalytic properties. *J. Solid State Chem.,* **2009**, *182*(1), 115-121.
[http://dx.doi.org/10.1016/j.jssc.2008.10.009]

[183] Vimala, K.; Sundarraj, S.; Paulpandi, M.; Vengatesan, S.; Kannan, S. Green synthesized doxorubicin loaded zinc oxide nanoparticles regulates the Bax and Bcl-2 expression in breast and colon carcinoma. *Process Biochem.,* **2014**, *49*(1), 160-172.
[http://dx.doi.org/10.1016/j.procbio.2013.10.007]

[184] Sadhukhan, P.; Kundu, M.; Chatterjee, S.; Ghosh, N.; Manna, P.; Das, J.; Sil, P.C. Targeted delivery of quercetin *via* pH-responsive zinc oxide nanoparticles for breast cancer therapy. *Mater. Sci. Eng. C,* **2019**, *100*, 129-140.
[http://dx.doi.org/10.1016/j.msec.2019.02.096] [PMID: 30948047]

[185] Zhou, W. Cholic acid-functionalized mesoporous silica nanoparticles loaded with ruthenium pro-drug delivery to cervical cancer therapy. *J. Inorg. Organomet. Polym. Mater.,* **2021**, *31*(1), 311-318.
[http://dx.doi.org/10.1007/s10904-020-01710-7]

[186] Meng, H.; Zhao, Y.; Dong, J.; Xue, M.; Lin, Y.S.; Ji, Z.; Mai, W.X.; Zhang, H.; Chang, C.H.; Brinker, C.J.; Zink, J.I.; Nel, A.E. Two-wave nanotherapy to target the stroma and optimize gemcitabine delivery to a human pancreatic cancer model in mice. *ACS Nano,* **2013**, *7*(11), 10048-10065.

[http://dx.doi.org/10.1021/nn404083m] [PMID: 24143858]

[187] Meng, H.; Wang, M.; Liu, H.; Liu, X.; Situ, A.; Wu, B.; Ji, Z.; Chang, C.H.; Nel, A.E. Use of a lipid-coated mesoporous silica nanoparticle platform for synergistic gemcitabine and paclitaxel delivery to human pancreatic cancer in mice. *ACS Nano,* **2015**, *9*(4), 3540-3557.
[http://dx.doi.org/10.1021/acsnano.5b00510] [PMID: 25776964]

[188] Akbarian, M.; Gholinejad, M.; Mohammadi-Samani, S.; Farjadian, F. Theranostic mesoporous silica nanoparticles made of multi-nuclear gold or carbon quantum dots particles serving as pH responsive drug delivery system. *Microporous Mesoporous Mater.,* **2022**, *329*, 111512.
[http://dx.doi.org/10.1016/j.micromeso.2021.111512]

[189] Kim, S.N.; Ko, S.A.; Park, C.G.; Lee, S.H.; Huh, B.K.; Park, Y.H.; Kim, Y.K.; Ha, A.; Park, K.H.; Choy, Y.B. Amino-Functionalized Mesoporous Silica Particles for Ocular Delivery of Brimonidine. *Mol. Pharm.,* **2018**, *15*(8), 3143-3152.
[http://dx.doi.org/10.1021/acs.molpharmaceut.8b00215] [PMID: 30020792]

[190] Persano, L.; Camposeo, A.; Tekmen, C.; Pisignano, D. Industrial Upscaling of Electrospinning and Applications of Polymer Nanofibers: A Review. *Macromol. Mater. Eng.,* **2013**, *298*(5), 504-520.
[http://dx.doi.org/10.1002/mame.201200290]

[191] Kajdič, S.; Planinšek, O.; Gašperlin, M.; Kocbek, P. Electrospun nanofibers for customized drug-delivery systems. *J. Drug Deliv. Sci. Technol.,* **2019**, *51*, 672-681.
[http://dx.doi.org/10.1016/j.jddst.2019.03.038]

[192] Deldar, Y.; Pilehvar-Soltanahmadi, Y.; Dadashpour, M.; Montazer Saheb, S.; Rahmati-Yamchi, M.; Zarghami, N. An *in vitro* examination of the antioxidant, cytoprotective and anti-inflammatory properties of chrysin-loaded nanofibrous mats for potential wound healing applications. *Artif. Cells Nanomed. Biotechnol.,* **2018**, *46*(4), 706-716.
[http://dx.doi.org/10.1080/21691401.2017.1337022] [PMID: 28595461]

[193] Deldar, Y.; Zarghami, F.; Pilehvar-Soltanahmadi, Y.; Dadashpour, M.; Zarghami, N. Antioxidant effects of chrysin-loaded electrospun nanofibrous mats on proliferation and stemness preservation of human adipose-derived stem cells. *Cell Tissue Bank.,* **2017**, *18*(4), 475-487.
[http://dx.doi.org/10.1007/s10561-017-9654-1] [PMID: 28808812]

[194] Patel, G.C.; Yadav, B.K. Polymeric nanofibers for controlled drug delivery applications.*Organic materials as smart nanocarriers for drug delivery*; Elsevier, **2018**, pp. 147-175.
[http://dx.doi.org/10.1016/B978-0-12-813663-8.00004-X]

[195] Wang, S.; Zhao, Y.; Shen, M.; Shi, X. Electrospun hybrid nanofibers doped with nanoparticles or nanotubes for biomedical applications. *Ther. Deliv.,* **2012**, *3*(10), 1155-1169.
[http://dx.doi.org/10.4155/tde.12.103] [PMID: 23116009]

[196] Norouzi, M.; Nazari, B.; Miller, D.W. Electrospun-based systems in cancer therapy.*Electrospun materials for tissue engineering and biomedical applications*; Elsevier, **2017**, pp. 337-356.
[http://dx.doi.org/10.1016/B978-0-08-101022-8.00013-2]

[197] Khodadadi, M.; Alijani, S.; Montazeri, M.; Esmaeilizadeh, N.; Sadeghi-Soureh, S.; Pilehvar-Soltanahmadi, Y. Recent advances in electrospun nanofiber- mediated drug delivery strategies for localized cancer chemotherapy. *J. Biomed. Mater. Res. A,* **2020**, *108*(7), 1444-1458.
[http://dx.doi.org/10.1002/jbm.a.36912] [PMID: 32246745]

[198] Torres-Martínez, E.J.; Cornejo Bravo, J.M.; Serrano Medina, A.; Pérez González, G.L.; Villarreal Gómez, L.J. A summary of electrospun nanofibers as drug delivery system: Drugs loaded and biopolymers used as matrices. *Curr. Drug Deliv.,* **2018**, *15*(10), 1360-1374.
[http://dx.doi.org/10.2174/1567201815666180723114326] [PMID: 30033869]

[199] Samprasit, W.; Akkaramongkolporn, P.; Ngawhirunpat, T.; Rojanarata, T.; Kaomongkolgit, R.; Opanasopit, P. Fast releasing oral electrospun PVP/CD nanofiber mats of taste-masked meloxicam. *Int. J. Pharm.,* **2015**, *487*(1-2), 213-222.
[http://dx.doi.org/10.1016/j.ijpharm.2015.04.044] [PMID: 25899284]

[200] Liu, Y.; Zhou, S.; Gao, Y.; Zhai, Y. Electrospun nanofibers as a wound dressing for treating diabetic foot ulcer. *Asian Journal of Pharmaceutical Sciences,* **2019**, *14*(2), 130-143.
[http://dx.doi.org/10.1016/j.ajps.2018.04.004] [PMID: 32104445]

[201] Mendes, A.C.; Gorzelanny, C.; Halter, N.; Schneider, S.W.; Chronakis, I.S. Hybrid electrospun chitosan-phospholipids nanofibers for transdermal drug delivery. *Int. J. Pharm.,* **2016**, *510*(1), 48-56.
[http://dx.doi.org/10.1016/j.ijpharm.2016.06.016] [PMID: 27286632]

[202] Brako, F.; Thorogate, R.; Mahalingam, S.; Raimi-Abraham, B.; Craig, D.Q.M.; Edirisinghe, M. Mucoadhesion of Progesterone-Loaded Drug Delivery Nanofiber Constructs. *ACS Appl. Mater. Interfaces,* **2018**, *10*(16), 13381-13389.
[http://dx.doi.org/10.1021/acsami.8b03329] [PMID: 29595052]

[203] Duan, X.; Chen, H.; Guo, C. Polymeric Nanofibers for Drug Delivery Applications: A Recent Review. *J. Mater. Sci. Mater. Med.,* **2022**, *33*(12), 78.
[http://dx.doi.org/10.1007/s10856-022-06700-4] [PMID: 36462118]

[204] Mohamady Hussein, M.A.; Guler, E.; Rayaman, E.; Cam, M.E.; Sahin, A.; Grinholc, M.; Sezgin Mansuroglu, D.; Sahin, Y.M.; Gunduz, O.; Muhammed, M.; El-Sherbiny, I.M.; Megahed, M. Dual-drug delivery of Ag-chitosan nanoparticles and phenytoin *via* core-shell PVA/PCL electrospun nanofibers. *Carbohydr. Polym.,* **2021**, *270*, 118373.
[http://dx.doi.org/10.1016/j.carbpol.2021.118373] [PMID: 34364617]

[205] Qin, Z.; Jia, X.W.; Liu, Q.; Kong, B.; Wang, H. Fast dissolving oral films for drug delivery prepared from chitosan/pullulan electrospinning nanofibers. *Int. J. Biol. Macromol.,* **2019**, *137*, 224-231.
[http://dx.doi.org/10.1016/j.ijbiomac.2019.06.224] [PMID: 31260763]

[206] Manasco, J.L.; Saquing, C.D.; Tang, C.; Khan, S.A. Cyclodextrin fibers *via* polymer-free electrospinning. *RSC Advances,* **2012**, *2*(9), 3778-3784.
[http://dx.doi.org/10.1039/c2ra00004k]

CHAPTER 5

Fate of Nanoparticles

Abstract: Gaining insight into the process that ingested nanoparticles/nanodrugs is crucial to maximize therapeutic advantages and avoid side effects. In the process of drug development, it is critical to consider how nanodrugs are ingested, how they interact with body fluids, how particles are absorbed by cells, and how they are eliminated to achieve effective treatments. In addition, consideration of the toxicity of the ingested nanoparticles is of utmost significance.

Hence the fate of ingested nanoparticles within the body will be covered in this chapter, including ingestion, endocytosis, exocytosis, and lastly the toxicity of the ingested NPs *in vivo* and *in vitro*. Initially, the chapter will brief about how the ingested nanoparticles undergo interactions with proteins in body fluids to form a protein corona and then will discuss comprehensively the different endocytic routes. Then the nanoparticle's excretion from cells which is essential for preserving homeostasis and receptor function will be discussed. Finally, the toxicity such as DNA damage, protein damage, cell membrane damage, oxidative stress, inflammation, impaired protein synthesis, deregulated cellular functions, and neurotoxicity of some commonly used nanoparticles will be outlined.

Keywords: Cellular damages, Endocytosis, Exocytosis, *In-vivo* toxicology, *In-vitro* toxicity, Nanoparticles, Neurotoxicity, Oxidative stress.

1. INTRODUCTION

Understanding the destiny of NPs in the human body is a crucial step in evaluating their safety and effectiveness in various consumer or medicinal applications. To better understand real-time behaviour, enhance targeted region absorption, and improve diagnostic techniques and treatment outcomes, it is imperative to study NP absorption, distribution, metabolism, and excretion in vivo systematically. For the purpose of industrializing nanoparticle formulations and creating novel nanodrug formulations, it is crucial to comprehend the absorption processes and toxicity of nanoparticle formulations. Hence the fate of ingested nanoparticles within the body will be covered in this chapter, including ingestion, endocytosis, exocytosis, and lastly the toxicity of the ingested NPs *in vivo* and *in vitro*.

Laksiri Weerasinghe, Imalka Munaweera and Senuri Kumarage

2. CELL UPTAKE AND METABOLISM

The nanodrugs can be administered to the body *via* four major routes; orally, transdermally, intravenously, and by inhalation [1]. Serum proteins attach non-specifically onto the nanoparticle surface when they come into contact with blood, forming a protein corona. The protein corona affects the physicochemical characteristics of nanoparticles by giving them an unintentional biological identity; subsequently, affecting how it interacts with biological systems such as organs, tissues, cells, and subcellular organelles. As a result, rather than the intentionally created synthetic nanoparticle features, this biological identity predominantly regulates nanoparticle *in vivo* circulation and biodistribution. Engineering of nanomedicines faces substantial difficulties since a nanoparticle's physicochemical characteristics may alter considerably after being exposed to the biological environment [2]. In order to optimize the therapeutic advantages of nanomedicines while avoiding adverse effects, it is crucial to investigate what happens to nanoparticles after they are introduced to the body.

Nanoparticles' absorption in cells requires regulated systems and biomolecular interactions to penetrate the cell plasma membrane, which acts as a barrier. The membrane's negative charge with few cationic areas and selective permeability to ions, biomolecules, and nanoparticles make it crucial to understand their fundamental absorption processes, as they impact their function, intracellular fate, and biological response [3, 4].

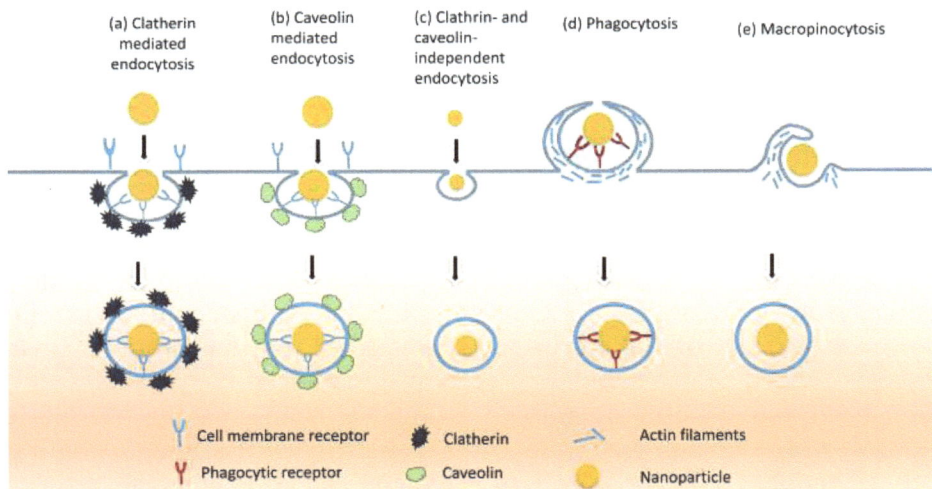

Fig. (1). Schematic diagram of endocytosis mechanisms (a) (a) clathrin-mediated; (b) caveolin-mediated; (c) clathrin- and caveolin-independent; (d) phagocytosis; and (e) macropinocytosis pathways.

The internalization mechanism significantly affects the rate of nanoparticle uptake, whereas the physical characteristics of the nanoparticles, such as size, shape, surface chemistry, including surface electrical charge, hydrophobicity, hydrophilicity, and ligand binding, influence the cell uptake process [5]. Furthermore, each cell has its own mode of internalization. Identifying the techniques of internalization can therefore assist scientists in determining which cells are more likely to ingest nanoparticles designed to target certain routes. When studying nanoparticles with different cell lines or shifting nanoparticles from *in vitro* to *in vivo* studies, a lack of understanding of internalization routes may result in poorly built nanoparticles with inadequate therapeutic efficacy. Additionally, diverse cell types may absorb a single nanoparticle in different ways [6, 7]. Direct fusion with the plasma membrane and endocytosis are the two primary routes into the cell.

2.1. Endocytosis

Nanoparticles may enter cells by a variety of different techniques and routes, which are referred to together as endocytosis. These processes are classified into five mechanistically distinct groups: (a) clathrin-dependent endocytosis, (b) caveolin-dependent endocytosis, (c) clathrin- and caveolin-independent endocytosis, (d) phagocytosis, and (e) macro-pinocytosis (Fig 1). Several lipids and transport proteins, including lipid rafts clathrin, dynamin, caveolin, and pattern recognition receptors, regulate and govern various absorption pathways at the biomolecular level [8, 9].

Nanoparticle cell absorption mechanisms are controlled by biomolecules, affecting intracellular transport and influencing biological responses and therapeutic outcomes.

2.1.1. Clathrin-mediated Endocytosis

Clathrin-dependent endocytosis is characterized by the clustering and binding of nanoparticle surface ligands to cell membrane receptors such as transferrin receptors, β2 adrenergic receptors, low density lipoprotein receptors, and epidermal growth factor, resulting in complicated multistep processes [10]. It entails the formation of a clathrin-coated pit from the nucleation of cytosolic endocytosis-related proteins, bending and invagination of the plasma membrane, scission from the plasma membrane, which is then usually transported to endosomes with the aid of intracellular actin filaments, and uncoating and recovery of endocytic proteins from intracellular vesicles [11]. Nanoparticles with diameters between 100 and 500 nm are entrapped in intracellular vesicles through the clathrin-dependent endocytosis mechanism [12]. In intracellular vesicles, which are detached from the membrane with the aid of conformational changes from the GTPase enzyme dynamin, nanoparticles are trapped [13]. The consumed vesicular contents and payloads are broken down enzymatically as a result of endosome recycling or fusion with lysosomes.

2.1.2. Caveolin-dependent Endocytosis

A receptor-specific mechanism for nanoparticle internalization called a caveolin-dependent endocytosis relies on invaginations of the plasma membrane known as caveolae that are coated with caveolin. Vesicles covered with caveolin are carried by the cytoplasm to intracellular locations like the Golgi apparatus and the endoplasmic reticulum. Using nanoparticle surface ligands including albumin, cholesterol, and folic acid, nanoparticle surface engineering techniques have been demonstrated to encourage cellular internalization *via* caveolin-dependent endocytosis [14 - 16]. There is evidence that caveolae are transported across cells through caveolin-dependent endocytosis. Exploring caveolin-mediated transcytosis in endothelial cells, which could allow nanoparticles to enter and traverse the endothelium, has been the subject of recent investigations. This shuttle mechanism may aid in the effective transport of therapeutic nanoparticles and their payloads to the body's sick regions [17, 18].

2.1.3. Clathrin and Caveolin-independent Endocytosis

Nanoparticles can pass across the cell plasma membrane without the aid of clathrin and caveolin-dependent pathways, including virus-like particles and other nanoparticles. One example of clathrin- and caveolin-independent endocytosis is lipid rafts, which are cholesterol- and sphingolipid-rich regions of the plasma membrane that undergo endocytosis when stimulated [19]. In immunological situations, a common mechanism where lymphocytes ingest and process interleukins is lipid raft-mediated endocytosis. The route is controlled by the actin regulatory complex Arp2/3, the small GTPase Cdc42, specific BAR domain protein, IRSp53, and GRAF1 [20].

2.1.4. Phagocytosis

Immune cells including neutrophils, macrophages, dendritic cells, and B lymphocytes use an uptake mechanism called phagocytosis to remove infections, diseased cells, and synthetic or biological elements that are alien to the bod [21]. In most cases, physical binding to phagocyte cell surface receptors, such as mannose receptors, Fc receptors, complement receptors, and scavenger receptors, triggers the phagocytosis of nanoparticles [22, 23]. Following cellular absorption, nanoparticles become caught in phagosome vesicles, which eventually unite with lysosomes to create a structure known as a phagolysosome. Phagolysosomes use enzymes and biochemical reactions to digest foreign "non-self" materials, including nanoparticles [6, 24]. Nanoparticle surface alterations have been created to lessen nanoparticle opsonization in order to decrease nanoparticle MPS sequestration. For instance, PEGylation of NPs may impact blood circulation rates and nanoparticle opsonization [25].

2.1.5. Macropinocytosis

Macropinocytosis involves extracellular fluids and solutes being engulfed by actin-stabilized plasma membrane extensions. In this mechanism, actin signalling causes membrane ruffling, which traps nanoparticles and other ingested components inside macropinosome vesicle forms [26, 27]. These vesicles can be anywhere from 0.5 and 1.5 μm in size [28]. It has been proposed that macropinosomes are porous intracellular vesicles that might let nanoparticles escape before being destroyed by lysosomes. As part of their sentinel role, immature dendritic cells regularly perform macropinocytosis of extracellular components for antigen presentation, which makes them desirable targets for vaccines. Macropinocytosis is a crucial process required for the immune system's appropriate defensive mechanisms. Recent studies have shown that Nab-paclitaxel is absorbed by macrophages by a process called macropinocytosis, which has been shown to polarize tumour-associated macrophages (TAMs) towards the M1 immuno-stimulatory phenotype. These nanoparticle systems may be effective in decreasing cancer's capacity to evade immune surveillance through intratumoral immunomodulation [29, 30].

2.2. Direct Fusion with the Plasma Membrane

Nanoparticles have the ability to physically or biochemically pass through the cell plasma membrane and into the cytoplasm. With the ability to target and interact with intracellular structures and subcellular organelles, nanoparticles that are freely diffused throughout the cytoplasm can perform specific biological and therapeutic roles. Some encapsulated viruses utilize direct fusion to the plasma membrane, and fascinating nanoparticle systems have been created to take advantage of this mechanism.

2.2.1. Cytoplasmic Entry by Direct Translocation

By interacting with the lipid bilayer molecules through direct translocation pathways, nanoparticles may rupture the cell plasma membrane and enter the cytoplasm [31]. In order to enter the cytoplasm of the cell, this approach bypasses endosomal trapping and energy-dependent transport systems. The size, shape, charge, and surface ligands of the nanoparticles as well as their attachment to their surface all affect how effectively they may enter the cytoplasm *via* direct translocation. For example, it has been found that worm- and rod-shaped nanoparticles diffuse across cell plasma membranes more effectively than spherical micelles [32]. Direct translocation of semiconductor quantum dot nanoparticles with an average size of 8 nm and zwitterionic surface chemistry was also seen, with the lipid softening layer by layer leading to flexible membrane conformation in red blood cells [33]. Another group discovered that zwitterionic gold NPs of 2-4 nm are directly translocated into HeLa cells, but slightly larger NPs of roughly 6 nm are internalized *via* caveolin/lipid-raft endocytosis, demonstrating a nanoparticle size dependent influence on cellular internalization [34]. Another method for direct translocation uses NPs surfaces functionalized with cell penetrating peptides (CPPs), which are short amino acid sequences (usually less than 40 amino acids) capable of crossing cell membranes [35].

2.2.2. Cytoplasmic Entry by Lipid Fusion

The process by which some varieties of lipid bilayer coatings merge with a cell's plasma membrane is known as lipid fusion. The enclosed contents of the nanoparticle, including proteins, nucleotides, and small molecule payloads, are transferred straight to the cytoplasm after membrane fusion [36, 37].

2.2.3. Electroporation

When electrical pulses are used, electroporation approaches physically damage a cell's plasma membrane. As a result, temporary voids are created in the membrane, allowing nanoparticles to pass from the extracellular area into the cytoplasm. By carefully adjusting the electrical pulse (such as pulse length and voltage), membrane void development caused by electroporation may be managed such that the newly produced pores have no negative effects on cell survival [38].

Internalization is merely the first stage in the delivery of therapeutic nanoparticles. The effectiveness of the distribution mechanism is significantly impacted by the ensuing trafficking. Nanoparticle intracellular trafficking is similar to nanoparticle cellular uptake in that it depends on the type of cell as well as the physicochemical characteristics of the nanoparticles, such as size, shape, and surface chemistry.

Numerous variables connected to the internalization mechanism may influence the destiny of nanoparticles. The rate of internalization, the amount of material internalized, and signalling on the cytosolic end of the internalized receptor are a few of these. Certain internalization routes may impact subsequent cellular trafficking, however it is unclear whether this trafficking is primarily regulated by the internalization pathway or by signalling from the receptor. For instance liposomes with high surface densities of octa-arginine have been demonstrated to improve macropinocytosis and had greater transfection efficiencies than lower-density octa-arginine liposomes, which were absorbed *via* alternative pathways [39].

Although small drug molecules can diffuse through the plasma membrane passively, macromolecular drugs owing to their size and polarity will be internalized *via* endocytosis [40]. When nanoparticles enter the cell by endocytic pathways, they are trapped within a membrane-lined vesicle, such as an endosome, which moves them throughout the cell in intricate trafficking patterns. Endosomes can age, defined by early- to late-stage vesicle metamorphosis associated with changes in intra-vesicle pH, and can merge with lysosomal compartments for enzymatic digestion and disposal of vesicle contents. Endosomal entrapment is frequently a substantial hindrance to nanomedicine attempts. Nanoparticles having therapeutic properties must get through the endosomal barrier before lysosomal degradation. Endosomal escape can be facilitated more efficiently by engineering physicochemical nanoparticle features such as surface charge and surface ligand display.

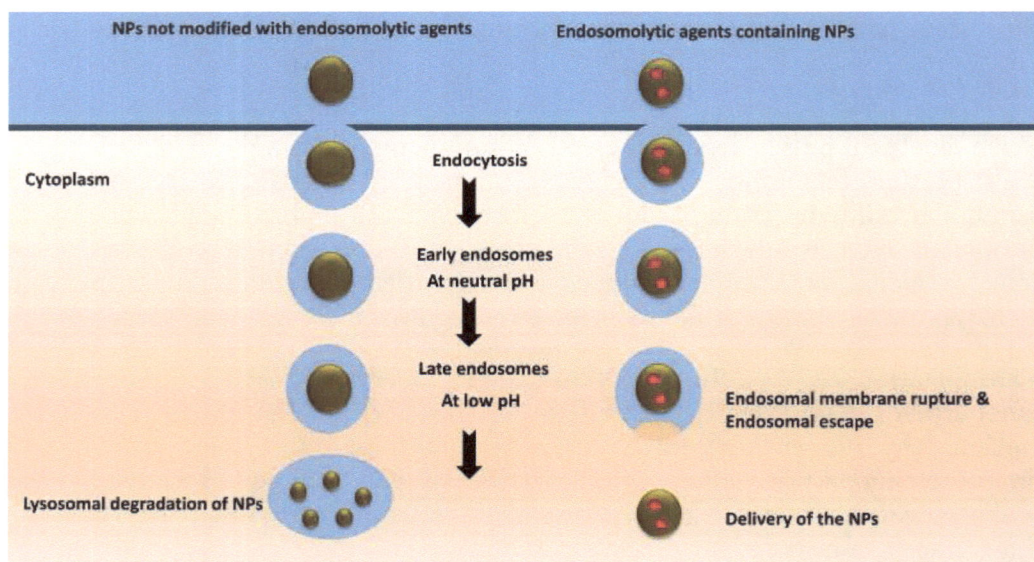

Fig (2). Fate of NPs with and without endosomolytic agents, within a cell.

Lysosomes degrade nanoparticles without endosomal escape agents through hydrolytic enzymes (Fig **2**).

Nanoparticle endosomal escape strategies include the utilization of endosomolytic agents that facilitate the endosomal escape. Several cationic peptides, anionic peptides, polymers synthetic biomimetic peptides, chemicals, and dendrimers have recently been found as having extraordinary efficacy in aiding endosomal escape [41]. Three significant alterations for nanoparticles to breach and evade endosomal barriers have been documented by Donahue *et al.*; Modifications with membrane disrupting polymers and peptides, pH-responsive materials and enzyme-cleavable materials [2].

Cell penetrating peptides (CPPs) and other membrane disruptive nanoparticle surface modifications will result in the endosomal rupture or pore formation leading to the escape of entrapped therapeutic nanodrugs. Gene transfer frequently involves CPPs including R9, R8, TAT, transportan, M918, penetratin, and VP22, among others [2, 42]. The proton-sponge mechanism allows a number of polymers, such as dendrimers made of polyethylenimine (PEI) and polyamidoamine (PAMAM), as well as histidine-rich peptides, to escape from the endosome and enter the cytosol. During endosomal acidification, these amine-rich components can provide significant amounts of buffering action. The vesicle's protons build up, which causes a surge of chloride counter ions and raises the osmotic pressure. When water enters the endosomal vesicle due to the elevated ion concentration, the endosomal compartment swells and the endosome membrane ruptures, releasing the nanoparticles into the cytosol [43]. Exploiting the intracellular acidic pH of endosomes and lysosomes is the other modification pathway for endosomal escape. To transfer cargo into cells, a variety of pH-sensitive natural and man-made polymers, including as carboxymethylcellulose, hyaluronic acid, alginate, polyacids, and polybases, are utilized as nanocarriers. Acid-labile linkers, such as acetal, ketal, hydrazone, imine, boronate ester, orthoester, and oximes, have been introduced to several polymers. These linkers cleave in reaction to low pH and improve drug administration [42]. Enzyme-cleavable nanoparticle modifications, such as linkers and shells, are a third strategy for endosomal escape. Research have been conducted by attaching drug molecules to nanodrug vehicle with endosome-specific enzyme-cleavable linkers [44].

Effective intracellular transport of nanoparticles is frequently crucial to the therapeutic and diagnostic efficacy of nanomedicines. Even though organelle targeting is an effective strategy for boosting the effectiveness of nanomedicines, to improve endosomal escape and transport of nanoparticles and their payloads to intracellular destinations, more study is needed. The difficulty of successfully targeting organelles *in vivo* is evident. Before they can reach their intended cell populations in the body, nanoparticles must first get past several biological and physical obstacles. Second, before nanoparticles may interact with intracellular proteins and organelles after they have entered the targeted cells, they must pass through a number of cellular obstacles. The accumulation of nanoparticles and/or their payloads at sufficiently high concentrations in the targeted cellular structures is another obstacle that must be overcome in order to achieve the intended biological effects.

Organelles with particular biological roles in the energy generation, replication, cell division, intracellular transport, and lipid and protein synthesis include the mitochondria, cell nucleus, Golgi apparatus, and endoplasmic reticulum. Organelle malfunction, change, and deregulation of intracellular systems constitute common markers of illness, whereas these functions are firmly controlled, maintained, and coordinated in healthy cells. In order to diagnose and treat diseases it is crucial to target intracellular organelles and compartments using nanoparticles. While targeting molecules can help with organelle localization, effective nanoparticle distribution depends on a number of other crucial elements. For instance, multiple studies have demonstrated a link between size, charge, and surface chemistry for the transport of nanoparticles into the cell compartments for therapeutic interventions [42, 45 - 48].

The excretion of nanoparticles from cells is less well studied, despite the fact that nanoparticle internalization has been the subject of substantial research. Nanoparticle exocytosis also appears to be cell-dependent, size-dependent, shape-dependent, and surface chemistry (charge and functionality) dependent, similar to nanoparticle endocytosis [49, 50]. Cells must go through exocytosis in order to preserve cellular homeostasis. Membrane-wrapped vesicles and their contents are expelled to the extracellular space during exocytosis. Exocytosis is crucial for optimal receptor operation because endosomes often recycle and transport endocytosed receptors back to the cell periphery. One of the most common ways that cells excrete nanoparticles is by lysosomal-mediated exocytosis. It is interesting to note that vesicle-mediated exocytosis is far more preferred over direct translocation of nanoparticles from the cytoplasm through the cell plasma membrane and into the extracellular environment [51 - 53].

3. *IN-VIVO* AND *IN-VITRO* TOXICITY

With the rising usage of nanomaterials in medicine, it is critical to investigate their toxicity before they reach the clinical stage. Nanotoxicology studies the toxicity of nanomaterials in medicine, focusing on exposure route, concentration, dose, frequency and/or time. Factors like material composition, surface chemistry, shape, size, surface charge, and administered dose and gender are crucial in evaluating their toxicity on human health. Potential negative consequences include neurotoxicity, genotoxicity, vascular dysfunction, pulmonary toxicity, and immunotoxicity [54].

Upon administration into the body, nanoparticles will interact with the tissues or organs that they encounter initially and consequently will translocate and enter the bloodstream to reach other organs/ tissues *via* the systemic transport. Nanoparticles can cause toxicity at cellular and subcellular levels by interacting with cells, intracellular organelles, and various biomolecules, including carbohydrates, nucleic acids, proteins, and lipids. This causes a protein corona to form around the nanoparticle surface, changing its surface characteristics and potentially causing nanotoxicity or impairing the effectiveness of nanodrugs [54].

One of the main mechanisms of toxicity is the generation of reactive oxygen species (ROS), which can lead to oxidative stress, inflammation, and subsequent damage to proteins, cell membranes, and DNA. A general definition of oxidative stress is an imbalance between the production of oxidants and the activity of antioxidants [55]. Peroxynitrite (ONOO), nitric oxide (NO), hydroxyl radical (OH), hydrogen peroxide (H_2O_2), and superoxide radical (O^-) are examples of ROS that are frequently produced as by-products of biochemical reactions, such as mitochondrial respiration, enzymatic metabolism of cytochrome P450, and neutrophil-mediated phagocytosis. The most important biomolecules such as lipids, proteins, and nucleic acids are attacked by ROS, which can activate the NADPH-like system, hamper the electron transport chain, depolarize the mitochondrial membrane, and harm the mitochondrial structure [56, 57]. ROS produced by NPs may adversely impact genetic materials by causing DNA-cros--linking, DNA-strand breakage, and genetic alterations. By stimulating inflammatory cells such as neutrophils, NPs can also boost ROS generation [58].

In addition, the NPs can interfere with the various physicochemical, biochemical, and molecular mechanisms of the cells. TiO_2 nanoparticles, for example, were discovered to interact with tubule heterodimers, microtubules, and tau proteins, causing microtubule instability and thereby contributing to neurotoxicity [59]. It was observed that the TiO_2 NPs interaction resulted in the reduced rate of microtubule development, increased pace at which they shorten, and reduced the span of the new microtubules remained. The NP cytotoxicity can additionally impede protein synthesis, cell differentiation, and the activation of pro-inflammatory genes and production of inflammatory mediators.

Moreover polymer NPs are also used extensively in pharmaceutical industry and have also shown physicochemical properties dependent *in vivo* toxicity [60, 61]. Anionic PAMAM dendrimers did not demonstrate any discernible harmful effects, whereas cationic polypropylenimine dendrimers dramatically reduced zebrafish embryo survival rates and cardiovascular functions [62]. Upon exposing zebrafish embryos to chitosan NPs and Tween 80-modified chitosan NPs (TmCS-NPs) in different concentrations, neurobehavioral abnormalities were observed. In addition, the NPs promoted the ROS generation and impaired the development of muscle and motor neurons revealing their developmental neurotoxicity [63].

Hence polymeric NPs have the potential to occasionally cause autonomic imbalance disruption and can have an impact on cardiac and vascular functioning [64].

According to Sukhanova *et al.* [65], the most common mechanisms of NP cytotoxicity are listed as follows.

1. Through the production of ROS and other free radicals, NPs may lead to oxidation.
2. Cell membrane perforation by NPs might cause damage.
3. NPs disrupt cell division and intracellular trafficking by damaging cytoskeleton components.
4. DNA damage and transcription disruption caused by NPs speed up the process of mutagenesis.
5. NPs disrupt mitochondrial metabolism and damage them, which results in an unbalanced supply of energy within the cell.
6. NPs prevent the development of lysosomes, which prevents autophagy from degrading macromolecules and causes apoptosis.
7. NPs alter the structure of membrane proteins and interfere with intracellular and intercellular transit of chemicals.
8. By interfering with normal cell metabolism, tissue metabolism, and organ metabolism, NPs promote the synthesis of inflammatory mediators.

There have been extensive studies on various nanoparticles for their *in vivo* and *in vitro* toxicity. We have summarized the *in vitro* and *in vivo* toxic effects of the most commonly employed nanoparticles in nano medicines (Table **1**).

There are no serious demerits of polymeric NPs. However, the limited targeting abilities and the problem of discontinuation of the therapy may be considered the major drawbacks.

Table 1. *In vitro* **and** *in vivo* **toxicity of NPs.**

NPs	*In vitro* Toxicity	*In vivo* Toxicity
Ag NPs	Alveolar epithelial cells have undergone morphological alterations such as cell shrinkage, limited cellular extensions, a constrained spreading pattern, cell death, DNA damage, and an overexpression of metallothioneins [66, 67]. PVP-AgNPs and citrate-AgNPs significantly increased ROS production, increased intracellular calcium uptake, and decreased mitochondrial membrane potential in macrophages and bronchial epithelial cells [68]. Increased LDH levels, oxidative stress, increased inflammatory protein release (including interleukin (IL) 8 and tumor necrosis factor (TNF-α)), and decreased albumin production in hepatocytes [69]. Reduced cell viability, cell cycle arrest in the gap/mitotic phase, considerably higher rates of apoptosis, and increased production of ROS in HepG2 cells [70]. Release of cytokines and increased genotoxicity in intestinal cells [71]. Increase in inflammatory cytokines and a decrease in cell viability in HEKs cells [72]. In mice cardiac papillary muscle cells, depolarization of the resting membrane potential and a reduced action potential eventually resulted in a loss of excitability [73]. Human mesenchymal stem cells displayed elevated LDH release, increased ROS generation, and decreased cell viability and mitochondrial membrane potential [74].	Inhalation causes a dose-dependent increase in bile duct hyperplasia in AgNP-exposed liver [75]. Acute pulmonary neutrophilic inflammation with proinflammatory and pro-neutrophil cytokines production [76]. Reduced oestrogen plasma levels are connected with an increase in the number of resorbed foetuses [77]. Exacerbation of myocardial ischemic-reperfusion damage after pulmonary exposure [78]. Cell apoptosis in the heart caused by oxidative stress and DNA damage. Prothrombotic states were induced, and coagulation markers were altered [79]. When exposed orally, it causes oxidative stress in the liver and the heart, as well as a minor inflammatory reaction in the liver [80]. High dose increased sperm morphological defects [81]. Regardless of the route and the type of silver, enters and traverses placenta [82]. Hepatocellular damage caused by increased ROS generation, increased autophagy, and a reduced insulin signalling pathway [83]. In male CD1 mice, intravenous injection changed Leydig cell activity and elevated testosterone levels [84]. Reduced thymus weight, increased spleen weight and spleen cell count, significantly decreased NK cell activity, and decreased IFN- production [85]. Mild thymus and spleen irritation, considerably elevated chromosomal breakage and polyploidy cell rates [86].

(Table 1) cont.....

NPs	*In vitro* Toxicity	*In vivo* Toxicity
Gold Nps	Elevated lipid peroxidase, DNA damage, and cytotoxicity in airway epithelial cells [87]. High lipid peroxidation, antioxidant upregulation, protein and gene expression of stress response in MRC-5 human lung fibroblasts [88, 89]. Cytotoxicity effects in human leukaemia (HL-60) and hepatoma (HepG2) cell lines were related with a decrease in GSH and an increase in ROS [90]. Cell viability and actin and tubulin deformations caused oxidative stress in C17.2 and PC12 cells [91]. Increased oestrogen accumulation in Granulosa cells of the ovary [92]. Influences the viability and motility of human spermatozoa [93].	BALB/c mouse liver tissue apoptosis and inflammation [94, 95]. Caused observable oxidative damage to blood, histopathological alterations, IL-6 upregulation, Nrf2 gene expression, DNA fragmentation, and a substantial drop in antibody titer against avian influenza (AI) and Newcastle disease (ND) in broiler chickens [96]. Neuronal system damage in mice [97]. Citrate Capped- AuNPs caused *Drosophila melanogaster* to exhibit DNA fragmentation, a sharp reduction in fertility and life span, and a significant overexpression of stress proteins [98, 99]. Reduced body weight, spleen index, and RBC in mice [100].
Titanium dioxide NPs	In human amnion epithelial (WISH) cells, there was a decrease in cell viability, morphological changes, an impaired antioxidant system, intracellular ROS generation, and severe DNA damage [101]. Degussa P25 (anatase (70%) and rutile (30%) forms of TiO_2) induces ROS in immortalized mouse microglia brain cells and damages the neurons rapidly [102].	When administered intravenously to pregnant mice, create difficulties during pregnancy. TiO_2 nanoparticles (35 nm) were discovered in the embryonic brain, liver, and placenta. In comparison to untreated controls, mice treated with these nanoparticles had smaller uteri and fetuses [103]. Genotoxicity, inflammation, and oxidative DNA damage in a mouse model [104].
Silica NPs	Pro-inflammatory reactions, DNA damage, autophagy, cell-cycle arrest, and cell death were observed. Endothelial damage is caused by mitochondrial malfunction, changes in mitochondrial dynamics, and biogenesis [105 - 107].	Major damage was shown in the heart, lung, and spleen of CD1 mouse organs after injection with 115 nm Stöber nanoparticles at 450 mg kg1. The damage was linked to mechanical constriction of tiny capillaries rather than a particular interaction between the cells and the silica [108]. When administered intravenously to pregnant mice, create difficulties during pregnancy. Si nanoparticles (70 nm) were discovered in the foetal liver, brain, and placenta. In comparison to untreated controls, mice treated with these nanoparticles had smaller uteri and foetuses [103].

NPs	*In vitro* Toxicity	*In vivo* Toxicity
Carbon based NPs	**SWCNTs** Single- and double-strand DNA damages in V79 cell lines of Chinese hamster fibroblasts [109]. Cell adhesion was reduced and cell growth was suppressed in human embryonic kidney cells (HEK293T) [110]. DNA damage, cell death, and ROS production in normal and malignant human mesothelial cells [111]. **MWCNTs** Induce apoptosis in mouse embryonic stem cells by activating the P53 protein, induce DNA damage [112 - 114]. Penetrated the cell membrane and changed the level of gene expression of several proteins in HEK [115]. In human skin fibroblasts (HSF42), an increase in apoptosis and necrosis disrupts intracellular signalling networks, cell metabolism, and cellular transport [116]. **C60** Raised the quantity of oxidized purines significantly in FE1-Muta mouse lung epithelial cells without affecting DNA strands [117]. A549 cells exhibit a higher frequency of micronuclei [118]. **CQD** Human bronchial epithelial cells (16HBE) exhibited decreased cell viability, owing to oxidative stress [119].	**SWCNTs** Upon inhalation induced genotoxicity in mice (C57BL), instantaneous inflammatory response, fibrosis, oxidative stress, and hyperplasia were observed [120]. Male ICR mice had increased macrophage infiltration and the development of foamy macrophages in the alveolar region [121]. Inflammatory markers such IL-1, IL-6, and TNF-α were found to be present at higher levels in broncho alveolar lavage fluid (BALF), and both male and female SPF Wistar rats showed increased Transgelin 2 gene expression [122]. Increased the amount of neutrophils, lymphocytes, and eosinophils in the lungs of male ICR mice, as well as the increased release of IL-6 and MCP-1 [123]. **MWCNTs** Damages the DNA of mouse leukocytes, bone marrow, and lung cell [124, 125]. Cell viability and alveolar macrophage count in the BALF significantly decreased, while cell count, lymphocytes, neutrophils, lactate dehydrogenase, protein, alkaline phosphatase, and cytokines (tumour necrosis factor-alpha (TNF-α) and interleukin 4 (IL-4)) significantly increased after inhalation. Inflammation, granulomas, and fibrosis in the lungs of male Wistar rats have also been documented [126]. Male guinea pigs exhibited pneumonitis and mild peribronchiolar fibrosis [127]. **C60** Major histocompatibility complex (MHC)-mediated immunity and metalloendopeptidase activity were both increased. In Male Wistar rats, elevated genes were implicated in oxidative damage, inflammation, and apoptosis [128]. Mutant frequencies in the lungs of gpt delta transgenic mice were significantly enhanced (2-3 times) [118]. **CQDs** In zebrafish, zooplankton, and phytoplankton, it caused oxidative stress and water acidification, hindered photosynthesis, and reduced nutrition absorption [129]. In male and female embryos/larvae of rare minnows, yolk agglutination, reduced spontaneous movements, increased heart rate, and enhanced hatching rate were observed [130]. **GQDs** The embryonic development was disrupted. In AB strains of wild-type zebrafish embryo/larva, the hatching rate and heart rate decreased, but mortality increased [131].

CONCLUSION

Nanodrugs can be delivered orally, transdermally, intravenously, or by inhalation. The physicochemical properties of these ingested nanoparticles are influenced by the protein corona, which has an impact on how well they interact with biological systems. Hence developing nanomedicines involves difficulties as their physicochemical properties could change after exposure. Understanding how cells absorb substances is essential for maximizing therapeutic benefits and preventing negative effects. In order to ensure effective treatment, it is possible to identify cell types more prone to consume nanoparticles by understanding internalization routes. The two main routes of entry into the cell are endocytosis and direct fusion with the plasma membrane. Lipids and transport proteins control a number of endocytosis processes, including clathrin-dependent endocytosis, caveolin-dependent endocytosis, clathrin- and caveolin-independent endocytosis, phagocytosis, and macropinocytosis, which allow nanoparticles to enter cells. Nanoparticles may also directly translocate into the cytoplasm, fuse with lipids, or be electroporated *via* cell plasma membranes. Nanoparticle excretion from cells is less studied, but exocytosis is cell-dependent, size-dependent, shape-dependent, and surface chemistry dependent. Exocytosis of NPs is crucial for maintaining homeostasis and receptor operation.

By taking into account aspects including material composition, size, surface chemistry, form, and dose, the field of nanotoxicology investigates the toxicity of nanomaterials used in medicine. Nanoparticles interact with different biomolecules, forming protein coronas and possibly causing toxicity. Reactive oxygen species (ROS) can cause damages to DNA, cell membranes, and protein in addition to oxidative stress and inflammation. Nanoparticles may hinder protein synthesis and differentiation, disrupt cellular processes, and cause neurotoxicity. To assess the *in vivo* and *in vitro* toxicity of various nanoparticles, much research has been conducted.

PRACTICE QUESTIONS

1. What are the major methods of nanoparticles entering the body?
2. Explain the two routes that particles are internalized into a cell.
3. Compare and contrast the five different endocytic pathways of particle internalization into a cell.
4. Explain the route of a nanoparticle, using a flow chart, until excretion after entering the body.
5. List out the main mechanisms of nanoparticle induced cytotoxicity.
6. State the different mechanisms scientists have adopted to reduce the toxicity of nanoparticles in nano medicine.

REFERENCES

[1] Chenthamara, D.; Subramaniam, S.; Ramakrishnan, S.G.; Krishnaswamy, S.; Essa, M.M.; Lin, F.H.; Qoronfleh, M.W. Therapeutic efficacy of nanoparticles and routes of administration. *Biomater. Res.,* **2019**, *23*(1), 20.
[http://dx.doi.org/10.1186/s40824-019-0166-x] [PMID: 31832232]

[2] Donahue, N.D.; Acar, H.; Wilhelm, S. Concepts of nanoparticle cellular uptake, intracellular trafficking, and kinetics in nanomedicine. *Adv. Drug Deliv. Rev.,* **2019**, *143*, 68-96.
[http://dx.doi.org/10.1016/j.addr.2019.04.008] [PMID: 31022434]

[3] Panariti, A.; Miserocchi, G.; Rivolta, I. The effect of nanoparticle uptake on cellular behavior: disrupting or enabling functions? *Nanotechnol. Sci. Appl.,* **2012**, *5*, 87-100.
[PMID: 24198499]

[4] Clift, M.J.D.; Brandenberger, C.; Rothen-Rutishauser, B.; Brown, D.M.; Stone, V. The uptake and intracellular fate of a series of different surface coated quantum dots *in vitro. Toxicology,* **2011**, *286*(1-3), 58-68.
[http://dx.doi.org/10.1016/j.tox.2011.05.006] [PMID: 21619910]

[5] Sabourian, P.; Yazdani, G.; Ashraf, S.S.; Frounchi, M.; Mashayekhan, S.; Kiani, S.; Kakkar, A. Effect of physico-chemical properties of nanoparticles on their intracellular uptake. *Int. J. Mol. Sci.,* **2020**, *21*(21), 8019.
[http://dx.doi.org/10.3390/ijms21218019] [PMID: 33126533]

[6] Sahay, G.; Alakhova, D.Y.; Kabanov, A.V. Endocytosis of nanomedicines. *J. Control. Release,* **2010**, *145*(3), 182-195.
[http://dx.doi.org/10.1016/j.jconrel.2010.01.036] [PMID: 20226220]

[7] Gilleron, J.; Querbes, W.; Zeigerer, A.; Borodovsky, A.; Marsico, G.; Schubert, U.; Manygoats, K.; Seifert, S.; Andree, C.; Stöter, M.; Epstein-Barash, H.; Zhang, L.; Koteliansky, V.; Fitzgerald, K.; Fava, E.; Bickle, M.; Kalaidzidis, Y.; Akinc, A.; Maier, M.; Zerial, M. Image-based analysis of lipid nanoparticle–mediated siRNA delivery, intracellular trafficking and endosomal escape. *Nat. Biotechnol.,* **2013**, *31*(7), 638-646.
[http://dx.doi.org/10.1038/nbt.2612] [PMID: 23792630]

[8] Mout, R.; Ray, M.; Tay, T.; Sasaki, K.; Yesilbag Tonga, G.; Rotello, V.M. General strategy for direct cytosolic protein delivery *via* protein–nanoparticle co-engineering. *ACS Nano,* **2017**, *11*(6), 6416-6421.
[http://dx.doi.org/10.1021/acsnano.7b02884] [PMID: 28614657]

[9] Tang, R.; Kim, C.S.; Solfiell, D.J.; Rana, S.; Mout, R.; Velázquez-Delgado, E.M.; Chompoosor, A.; Jeong, Y.; Yan, B.; Zhu, Z.J.; Kim, C.; Hardy, J.A.; Rotello, V.M. Direct delivery of functional proteins and enzymes to the cytosol using nanoparticle-stabilized nanocapsules. *ACS Nano,* **2013**, *7*(8), 6667-6673.
[http://dx.doi.org/10.1021/nn402753y] [PMID: 23815280]

[10] McMahon, H.T.; Boucrot, E. Molecular mechanism and physiological functions of clathrin-mediated endocytosis. *Nat. Rev. Mol. Cell Biol.,* **2011**, *12*(8), 517-533.
[http://dx.doi.org/10.1038/nrm3151] [PMID: 21779028]

[11] Muñoz, A.; Costa, M. Elucidating the mechanisms of nickel compound uptake: A review of particulate and nano-nickel endocytosis and toxicity. *Toxicol. Appl. Pharmacol.,* **2012**, *260*(1), 1-16.
[http://dx.doi.org/10.1016/j.taap.2011.12.014] [PMID: 22206756]

[12] Kaksonen, M.; Roux, A. Mechanisms of clathrin-mediated endocytosis. *Nat. Rev. Mol. Cell Biol.,* **2018**, *19*(5), 313-326.
[http://dx.doi.org/10.1038/nrm.2017.132] [PMID: 29410531]

[13] Mattila, J.P.; Shnyrova, A.V.; Sundborger, A.C.; Hortelano, E.R.; Fuhrmans, M.; Neumann, S.; Müller, M.; Hinshaw, J.E.; Schmid, S.L.; Frolov, V.A. A hemi-fission intermediate links two mechanistically distinct stages of membrane fission. *Nature,* **2015**, *524*(7563), 109-113.

[http://dx.doi.org/10.1038/nature14509] [PMID: 26123023]

[14] Blanco, E.; Shen, H.; Ferrari, M. Principles of nanoparticle design for overcoming biological barriers to drug delivery. *Nat. Biotechnol.*, **2015**, *33*(9), 941-951.
[http://dx.doi.org/10.1038/nbt.3330] [PMID: 26348965]

[15] Carver, L.A.; Schnitzer, J.E. Caveolae: mining little caves for new cancer targets. *Nat. Rev. Cancer*, **2003**, *3*(8), 571-581.
[http://dx.doi.org/10.1038/nrc1146] [PMID: 12894245]

[16] Anderson, R.G.W. The caveolae membrane system. *Annu. Rev. Biochem.*, **1998**, *67*(1), 199-225.
[http://dx.doi.org/10.1146/annurev.biochem.67.1.199] [PMID: 9759488]

[17] Frank, P.G.; Pavlides, S.; Lisanti, M.P. Caveolae and transcytosis in endothelial cells: role in atherosclerosis. *Cell Tissue Res.*, **2009**, *335*(1), 41-47.
[http://dx.doi.org/10.1007/s00441-008-0659-8] [PMID: 18688651]

[18] Wang, Z.; Tiruppathi, C.; Minshall, R.D.; Malik, A.B. Size and dynamics of caveolae studied using nanoparticles in living endothelial cells. *ACS Nano*, **2009**, *3*(12), 4110-4116.
[http://dx.doi.org/10.1021/nn9012274] [PMID: 19919048]

[19] Lajoie, P.; Nabi, I.R. Regulation of raft-dependent endocytosis. *J. Cell. Mol. Med.*, **2007**, *11*(4), 644-653.
[http://dx.doi.org/10.1111/j.1582-4934.2007.00083.x] [PMID: 17760830]

[20] Sathe, M.; Muthukrishnan, G.; Rae, J.; Disanza, A.; Thattai, M.; Scita, G.; Parton, R.G.; Mayor, S. Small GTPases and BAR domain proteins regulate branched actin polymerisation for clathrin and dynamin-independent endocytosis. *Nat. Commun.*, **2018**, *9*(1), 1835.
[http://dx.doi.org/10.1038/s41467-018-03955-w] [PMID: 29743604]

[21] Martínez-Riaño, A.; Bovolenta, E.R.; Mendoza, P.; Oeste, C.L.; Martín-Bermejo, M.J.; Bovolenta, P.; Turner, M.; Martínez-Martín, N.; Alarcón, B. Antigen phagocytosis by B cells is required for a potent humoral response. *EMBO Rep.*, **2018**, *19*(9), e46016.
[http://dx.doi.org/10.15252/embr.201846016] [PMID: 29987136]

[22] Tavano, R.; Gabrielli, L.; Lubian, E.; Fedeli, C.; Visentin, S.; Polverino De Laureto, P.; Arrigoni, G.; Geffner-Smith, A.; Chen, F.; Simberg, D.; Morgese, G.; Benetti, E.M.; Wu, L.; Moghimi, S.M.; Mancin, F.; Papini, E. C1q-Mediated Complement Activation and C3 Opsonization Trigger Recognition of Stealth Poly(2-methyl-2-oxazoline)-Coated Silica Nanoparticles by Human Phagocytes. *ACS Nano*, **2018**, *12*(6), 5834-5847.
[http://dx.doi.org/10.1021/acsnano.8b01806] [PMID: 29750504]

[23] Chen, F.; Wang, G.; Griffin, J.I.; Brenneman, B.; Banda, N.K.; Holers, V.M.; Backos, D.S.; Wu, L.; Moghimi, S.M.; Simberg, D. Complement proteins bind to nanoparticle protein corona and undergo dynamic exchange *in vivo*. *Nat. Nanotechnol.*, **2017**, *12*(4), 387-393.
[http://dx.doi.org/10.1038/nnano.2016.269] [PMID: 27992410]

[24] Stuart, L.M.; Ezekowitz, R.A.B. Phagocytosis. *Immunity*, **2005**, *22*(5), 539-550.
[http://dx.doi.org/10.1016/j.immuni.2005.05.002] [PMID: 15894272]

[25] Li, Y.; Kröger, M.; Liu, W.K. Endocytosis of PEGylated nanoparticles accompanied by structural and free energy changes of the grafted polyethylene glycol. *Biomaterials*, **2014**, *35*(30), 8467-8478.
[http://dx.doi.org/10.1016/j.biomaterials.2014.06.032] [PMID: 25002266]

[26] Mercer, J.; Helenius, A. Virus entry by macropinocytosis. *Nat. Cell Biol.*, **2009**, *11*(5), 510-520.
[http://dx.doi.org/10.1038/ncb0509-510] [PMID: 19404330]

[27] Conner, S.D.; Schmid, S.L. Regulated portals of entry into the cell. *Nature*, **2003**, *422*(6927), 37-44.
[http://dx.doi.org/10.1038/nature01451] [PMID: 12621426]

[28] Falcone, S.; Cocucci, E.; Podini, P.; Kirchhausen, T.; Clementi, E.; Meldolesi, J. Macropinocytosis: Regulated coordination of endocytic and exocytic membrane traffic events. *J. Cell Sci.*, **2006**, *119*(22), 4758-4769.

[http://dx.doi.org/10.1242/jcs.03238] [PMID: 17077125]

[29]   Cullis, J.; Siolas, D.; Avanzi, A.; Barui, S.; Maitra, A.; Bar-Sagi, D. Macropinocytosis of nab-paclitaxel drives macrophage activation in pancreatic cancer. *Cancer Immunol. Res., 2017, 5*(3), 182-190.
       [http://dx.doi.org/10.1158/2326-6066.CIR-16-0125] [PMID: 28108630]

[30]   Diken, M.; Kreiter, S.; Selmi, A.; Britten, C.M.; Huber, C.; Türeci, Ö.; Sahin, U. Selective uptake of naked vaccine RNA by dendritic cells is driven by macropinocytosis and abrogated upon DC maturation. *Gene Ther., 2011, 18*(7), 702-708.
       [http://dx.doi.org/10.1038/gt.2011.17] [PMID: 21368901]

[31]   Van Lehn, R.C.; Atukorale, P.U.; Carney, R.P.; Yang, Y.S.; Stellacci, F.; Irvine, D.J.; Alexander-Katz, A. Effect of particle diameter and surface composition on the spontaneous fusion of monolayer-protected gold nanoparticles with lipid bilayers. *Nano Lett., 2013, 13*(9), 4060-4067.
       [http://dx.doi.org/10.1021/nl401365n] [PMID: 23915118]

[32]   Hinde, E.; Thammasiraphop, K.; Duong, H.T.T.; Yeow, J.; Karagoz, B.; Boyer, C.; Gooding, J.J.; Gaus, K. Pair correlation microscopy reveals the role of nanoparticle shape in intracellular transport and site of drug release. *Nat. Nanotechnol., 2017, 12*(1), 81-89.
       [http://dx.doi.org/10.1038/nnano.2016.160] [PMID: 27618255]

[33]   Wang, T.; Bai, J.; Jiang, X.; Nienhaus, G.U. Cellular uptake of nanoparticles by membrane penetration: a study combining confocal microscopy with FTIR spectroelectrochemistry. *ACS Nano, 2012, 6*(2), 1251-1259.
       [http://dx.doi.org/10.1021/nn203892h] [PMID: 22250809]

[34]   Jiang, Y.; Huo, S.; Mizuhara, T.; Das, R.; Lee, Y.W.; Hou, S.; Moyano, D.F.; Duncan, B.; Liang, X.J.; Rotello, V.M. The Interplay of Size and Surface Functionality on the Cellular Uptake of Sub-10 nm Gold Nanoparticles. *ACS Nano, 2015, 9*(10), 9986-9993.
       [http://dx.doi.org/10.1021/acsnano.5b03521] [PMID: 26435075]

[35]   Verma, A.; Uzun, O.; Hu, Y.; Hu, Y.; Han, H.S.; Watson, N.; Chen, S.; Irvine, D.J.; Stellacci, F. Surface-structure-regulated cell-membrane penetration by monolayer-protected nanoparticles. *Nat. Mater., 2008, 7*(7), 588-595.
       [http://dx.doi.org/10.1038/nmat2202] [PMID: 18500347]

[36]   He, S.; Fan, W.; Wu, N.; Zhu, J.; Miao, Y.; Miao, X.; Li, F.; Zhang, X.; Gan, Y. Lipid-based liquid crystalline nanoparticles facilitate cytosolic delivery of siRNA *via* Structural transformation. *Nano Lett., 2018, 18*(4), 2411-2419.
       [http://dx.doi.org/10.1021/acs.nanolett.7b05430] [PMID: 29561622]

[37]   Kube, S.; Hersch, N.; Naumovska, E.; Gensch, T.; Hendriks, J.; Franzen, A.; Landvogt, L.; Siebrasse, J.P.; Kubitscheck, U.; Hoffmann, B.; Merkel, R.; Csiszár, A. Fusogenic Liposomes as Nanocarriers for the Delivery of Intracellular Proteins. *Langmuir, 2017, 33*(4), 1051-1059.
       [http://dx.doi.org/10.1021/acs.langmuir.6b04304] [PMID: 28059515]

[38]   Saulis, G.; Saulė, R. Size of the pores created by an electric pulse: Microsecond vs millisecond pulses. *Biochim. Biophys. Acta Biomembr., 2012, 1818*(12), 3032-3039.
       [http://dx.doi.org/10.1016/j.bbamem.2012.06.018] [PMID: 22766475]

[39]   Khalil, I.A.; Kogure, K.; Futaki, S.; Harashima, H. High density of octaarginine stimulates macropinocytosis leading to efficient intracellular trafficking for gene expression. *J. Biol. Chem., 2006, 281*(6), 3544-3551.
       [http://dx.doi.org/10.1074/jbc.M503202200] [PMID: 16326716]

[40]   Selby, L.I.; Cortez-Jugo, C.M.; Such, G.K.; Johnston, A.P.R. Nanoescapology: Progress toward understanding the endosomal escape of polymeric nanoparticles. *Wiley Interdiscip. Rev. Nanomed. Nanobiotechnol., 2017, 9*(5), e1452.
       [http://dx.doi.org/10.1002/wnan.1452] [PMID: 28160452]

[41]   Varkouhi, A.K.; Scholte, M.; Storm, G.; Haisma, H.J. Endosomal escape pathways for delivery of

biologicals. *J. Control. Release,* **2011**, *151*(3), 220-228.
[http://dx.doi.org/10.1016/j.jconrel.2010.11.004] [PMID: 21078351]

[42]   Ahmad, A.; Khan, J.M.; Haque, S. Strategies in the design of endosomolytic agents for facilitating endosomal escape in nanoparticles. *Biochimie,* **2019**, *160*, 61-75.
[http://dx.doi.org/10.1016/j.biochi.2019.02.012] [PMID: 30797879]

[43]   Pack, D.W.; Hoffman, A.S.; Pun, S.; Stayton, P.S. Design and development of polymers for gene delivery. *Nat. Rev. Drug Discov.,* **2005**, *4*(7), 581-593.
[http://dx.doi.org/10.1038/nrd1775] [PMID: 16052241]

[44]   Acar, H.; Samaeekia, R.; Schnorenberg, M.R.; Sasmal, D.K.; Huang, J.; Tirrell, M.V.; LaBelle, J.L. Cathepsin-Mediated Cleavage of Peptides from Peptide Amphiphiles Leads to Enhanced Intracellular Peptide Accumulation. *Bioconjug. Chem.,* **2017**, *28*(9), 2316-2326.
[http://dx.doi.org/10.1021/acs.bioconjchem.7b00364] [PMID: 28771332]

[45]   Jeena, M.T.; Palanikumar, L.; Go, E.M.; Kim, I.; Kang, M.G.; Lee, S.; Park, S.; Choi, H.; Kim, C.; Jin, S.M.; Bae, S.C.; Rhee, H.W.; Lee, E.; Kwak, S.K.; Ryu, J.H. Mitochondria localization induced self-assembly of peptide amphiphiles for cellular dysfunction. *Nat. Commun.,* **2017**, *8*(1), 26.
[http://dx.doi.org/10.1038/s41467-017-00047-z] [PMID: 28638095]

[46]   García, I.; Henriksen-Lacey, M.; Calvo, J.; de Aberasturi, D.J.; Paz, M.M.; Liz-Marzán, L.M. Size-Dependent Transport and Cytotoxicity of Mitomycin-Gold Nanoparticle Conjugates in 2D and 3D Mammalian Cell Models. *Bioconjug. Chem.,* **2019**, *30*(1), 242-252.
[http://dx.doi.org/10.1021/acs.bioconjchem.8b00898] [PMID: 30566340]

[47]   Qu, Q.; Ma, X.; Zhao, Y. Targeted delivery of doxorubicin to mitochondria using mesoporous silica nanoparticle nanocarriers. *Nanoscale,* **2015**, *7*(40), 16677-16686.
[http://dx.doi.org/10.1039/C5NR05139H] [PMID: 26400067]

[48]   Yang, C.; Uertz, J.; Yohan, D.; Chithrani, B.D. Peptide modified gold nanoparticles for improved cellular uptake, nuclear transport, and intracellular retention. *Nanoscale,* **2014**, *6*(20), 12026-12033.
[http://dx.doi.org/10.1039/C4NR02535K] [PMID: 25182693]

[49]   Cubillos-Ruiz, J.R.; Silberman, P.C.; Rutkowski, M.R.; Chopra, S.; Perales-Puchalt, A.; Song, M.; Zhang, S.; Bettigole, S.E.; Gupta, D.; Holcomb, K.; Ellenson, L.H.; Caputo, T.; Lee, A.H.; Conejo-Garcia, J.R.; Glimcher, L.H. ER Stress Sensor XBP1 Controls Anti-tumor Immunity by Disrupting Dendritic Cell Homeostasis. *Cell,* **2015**, *161*(7), 1527-1538.
[http://dx.doi.org/10.1016/j.cell.2015.05.025] [PMID: 26073941]

[50]   Sakhtianchi, R.; Minchin, R.F.; Lee, K.B.; Alkilany, A.M.; Serpooshan, V.; Mahmoudi, M. Exocytosis of nanoparticles from cells: Role in cellular retention and toxicity. *Adv. Colloid Interface Sci.,* **2013**, *201-202*, 18-29.
[http://dx.doi.org/10.1016/j.cis.2013.10.013] [PMID: 24200091]

[51]   Chu, Z.; Huang, Y.; Tao, Q.; Li, Q. Cellular uptake, evolution, and excretion of silica nanoparticles in human cells. *Nanoscale,* **2011**, *3*(8), 3291-3299.
[http://dx.doi.org/10.1039/c1nr10499c] [PMID: 21743927]

[52]   Fröhlich, E. Cellular elimination of nanoparticles. *Environ. Toxicol. Pharmacol.,* **2016**, *46*, 90-94.
[http://dx.doi.org/10.1016/j.etap.2016.07.003] [PMID: 27442891]

[53]   Takahashi, S.; Kubo, K.; Waguri, S.; Yabashi, A.; Shin, H.W.; Katoh, Y.; Nakayama, K. Rab11 regulates exocytosis of recycling vesicles at the plasma membrane. *J. Cell Sci.,* **2012**, *125*(Pt 17), jcs.102913.
[http://dx.doi.org/10.1242/jcs.102913] [PMID: 22685325]

[54]   Yang, W.; Wang, L.; Mettenbrink, E.M.; DeAngelis, P.L.; Wilhelm, S. Nanoparticle Toxicology. *Annu. Rev. Pharmacol. Toxicol.,* **2021**, *61*(1), 269-289.
[http://dx.doi.org/10.1146/annurev-pharmtox-032320-110338] [PMID: 32841092]

[55]   Egbuna, C.; Ifemeje, J.C. Oxidative stress and nutrition. *Tropical Journal of Applied Natural Sciences,*

2017, *2*(1), 110-116.
[http://dx.doi.org/10.25240/TJANS.2017.2.1.19]

[56] Ifemeje, J.C.; Gbolakoro, J.T.; Gbolakoro, J.T.; Arazu, V.N. Comparative study of antioxidant properties and free radical scavenging capacity of Annona muricata and citrus. *Tropical Journal of Applied Natural Sciences,* **2018**, *2*(2), 135-140.
[http://dx.doi.org/10.25240/TJANS.2018.2.2.17]

[57] Egbuna, C.; Kumar, S.; Ifemeje, J.; Kurhekar, J. Pharmacognosy, nanomedicine, and contemporary issues. *Phytochemistry,* **2019**, 131-146.

[58] Kheirallah, D.A.M.; El-Samad, L.M.; Abdel-Moneim, A.M. DNA damage and ovarian ultrastructural lesions induced by nickel oxide nano-particles in Blaps polycresta (Coleoptera: Tenebrionidae). *Sci. Total Environ.,* **2021**, *753*, 141743.
[http://dx.doi.org/10.1016/j.scitotenv.2020.141743] [PMID: 32891989]

[59] Mao, Z.; Xu, B.; Ji, X.; Zhou, K.; Zhang, X.; Chen, M.; Han, X.; Tang, Q.; Wang, X.; Xia, Y. Titanium dioxide nanoparticles alter cellular morphology *via* disturbing the microtubule dynamics. *Nanoscale,* **2015**, *7*(18), 8466-8475.
[http://dx.doi.org/10.1039/C5NR01448D] [PMID: 25891938]

[60] Aziz, T.; Ullah, A.; Fan, H.; Ullah, R.; Haq, F.; Khan, F.U.; Iqbal, M.; Wei, J. Cellulose Nanocrystals Applications in Health, Medicine and Catalysis. *J. Polym. Environ.,* **2021**, *29*(7), 2062-2071.
[http://dx.doi.org/10.1007/s10924-021-02045-1]

[61] Aziz, T.; Ullah, A.; Ali, A.; Shabeer, M.; Shah, M.N.; Haq, F.; Iqbal, M.; Ullah, R.; Khan, F.U. Manufactures of bio-degradable and bio-based polymers for bio-materials in the pharmaceutical field. *J. Appl. Polym. Sci.,* **2022**, *139*(29), e52624.
[http://dx.doi.org/10.1002/app.52624]

[62] Bodewein, L.; Schmelter, F.; Di Fiore, S.; Hollert, H.; Fischer, R.; Fenske, M. Differences in toxicity of anionic and cationic PAMAM and PPI dendrimers in zebrafish embryos and cancer cell lines. *Toxicol. Appl. Pharmacol.,* **2016**, *305*, 83-92.
[http://dx.doi.org/10.1016/j.taap.2016.06.008] [PMID: 27288734]

[63] Yuan, Z.; Li, Y.; Hu, Y.; You, J.; Higashisaka, K.; Nagano, K.; Tsutsumi, Y.; Gao, J. Chitosan nanoparticles and their Tween 80 modified counterparts disrupt the developmental profile of zebrafish embryos. *Int. J. Pharm.,* **2016**, *515*(1-2), 644-656.
[http://dx.doi.org/10.1016/j.ijpharm.2016.10.071] [PMID: 27826026]

[64] Ali, I.; Alsehli, M.; Scotti, L.; Tullius Scotti, M.; Tsai, S.T.; Yu, R.S.; Hsieh, M.F.; Chen, J.C. Progress in Polymeric Nano-Medicines for Theranostic Cancer Treatment. *Polymers (Basel),* **2020**, *12*(3), 598.
[http://dx.doi.org/10.3390/polym12030598] [PMID: 32155695]

[65] Sukhanova, A.; Bozrova, S.; Sokolov, P.; Berestovoy, M.; Karaulov, A.; Nabiev, I. Dependence of nanoparticle toxicity on their physical and chemical properties. *Nanoscale Res. Lett.,* **2018**, *13*(1), 44.
[http://dx.doi.org/10.1186/s11671-018-2457-x] [PMID: 29417375]

[66] De Matteis, V.; Malvindi, M.A.; Galeone, A.; Brunetti, V.; De Luca, E.; Kote, S.; Kshirsagar, P.; Sabella, S.; Bardi, G.; Pompa, P.P. Negligible particle-specific toxicity mechanism of silver nanoparticles: The role of Ag+ ion release in the cytosol. *Nanomedicine,* **2015**, *11*(3), 731-739.
[http://dx.doi.org/10.1016/j.nano.2014.11.002] [PMID: 25546848]

[67] Lee, Y.S.; Kim, D.W.; Lee, Y.H.; Oh, J.H.; Yoon, S.; Choi, M.S.; Lee, S.K.; Kim, J.W.; Lee, K.; Song, C.W. Silver nanoparticles induce apoptosis and G2/M arrest *via* PKCζ-dependent signaling in A549 lung cells. *Arch. Toxicol.,* **2011**, *85*(12), 1529-1540.
[http://dx.doi.org/10.1007/s00204-011-0714-1] [PMID: 21611810]

[68] Wang, X.; Ji, Z.; Chang, C.H.; Zhang, H.; Wang, M.; Liao, Y.P.; Lin, S.; Meng, H.; Li, R.; Sun, B.; Winkle, L.V.; Pinkerton, K.E.; Zink, J.I.; Xia, T.; Nel, A.E. Use of coated silver nanoparticles to understand the relationship of particle dissolution and bioavailability to cell and lung toxicological

potential. *Small,* **2014**, *10*(2), 385-398.
[http://dx.doi.org/10.1002/smll.201301597] [PMID: 24039004]

[69] Gaiser, B.K.; Hirn, S.; Kermanizadeh, A.; Kanase, N.; Fytianos, K.; Wenk, A.; Haberl, N.; Brunelli, A.; Kreyling, W.G.; Stone, V. Effects of silver nanoparticles on the liver and hepatocytes *in vitro.* *Toxicol. Sci.,* **2013**, *131*(2), 537-547.
[http://dx.doi.org/10.1093/toxsci/kfs306] [PMID: 23086748]

[70] Faedmaleki, F.; H Shirazi, F.; Salarian, A-A.; Ahmadi Ashtiani, H.; Rastegar, H. Toxicity effect of silver nanoparticles on mice liver primary cell culture and HepG2 cell line. *Iranian journal of pharmaceutical research. Iran. J. Pharm. Res.,* **2014**, *13*(1), 235-242.
[PMID: 24734076]

[71] Kaiser, J.P.; Roesslein, M.; Diener, L.; Wick, P. Human health risk of ingested nanoparticles that are added as multifunctional agents to paints: an *in vitro* study. *PLoS One,* **2013**, *8*(12), e83215.
[http://dx.doi.org/10.1371/journal.pone.0083215] [PMID: 24358264]

[72] Samberg, M.E.; Oldenburg, S.J.; Monteiro-Riviere, N.A. Evaluation of silver nanoparticle toxicity in skin *in vivo* and keratinocytes *in vitro.* *Environ. Health Perspect.,* **2010**, *118*(3), 407-413.
[http://dx.doi.org/10.1289/ehp.0901398] [PMID: 20064793]

[73] Lin, C.X.; Yang, S.Y.; Gu, J.L.; Meng, J.; Xu, H.Y.; Cao, J.M. The acute toxic effects of silver nanoparticles on myocardial transmembrane potential, I_{Na} and I_{K1} channels and heart rhythm in mice. *Nanotoxicology,* **2017**, *11*(6), 1-11.
[http://dx.doi.org/10.1080/17435390.2017.1367047] [PMID: 28830271]

[74] He, W.; Liu, X.; Kienzle, A.; Müller, W.E.G.; Feng, Q. *In vitro* uptake of silver nanoparticles and their toxicity in human mesenchymal stem cells derived from bone marrow. *J. Nanosci. Nanotechnol.,* **2016**, *16*(1), 219-228.
[http://dx.doi.org/10.1166/jnn.2016.10728] [PMID: 27398448]

[75] Sung, J.H.; Ji, J.H.; Park, J.D.; Yoon, J.U.; Kim, D.S.; Jeon, K.S.; Song, M.Y.; Jeong, J.; Han, B.S.; Han, J.H.; Chung, Y.H.; Chang, H.K.; Lee, J.H.; Cho, M.H.; Kelman, B.J.; Yu, I.J. Subchronic inhalation toxicity of silver nanoparticles. *Toxicol. Sci.,* **2009**, *108*(2), 452-461.
[http://dx.doi.org/10.1093/toxsci/kfn246] [PMID: 19033393]

[76] Seiffert, J.; Buckley, A.; Leo, B.; Martin, N.G.; Zhu, J.; Dai, R.; Hussain, F.; Guo, C.; Warren, J.; Hodgson, A.; Gong, J.; Ryan, M.P.; Zhang, J.J.; Porter, A.; Tetley, T.D.; Gow, A.; Smith, R.; Chung, K.F. Pulmonary effects of inhalation of spark-generated silver nanoparticles in Brown-Norway and Sprague–Dawley rats. *Respir. Res.,* **2016**, *17*(1), 85.
[http://dx.doi.org/10.1186/s12931-016-0407-7] [PMID: 27435725]

[77] Campagnolo, L.; Massimiani, M.; Vecchione, L.; Piccirilli, D.; Toschi, N.; Magrini, A.; Bonanno, E.; Scimeca, M.; Castagnozzi, L.; Buonanno, G.; Stabile, L.; Cubadda, F.; Aureli, F.; Fokkens, P.H.B.; Kreyling, W.G.; Cassee, F.R.; Pietroiusti, A. Silver nanoparticles inhaled during pregnancy reach and affect the placenta and the foetus. *Nanotoxicology,* **2017**, *11*(5), 687-698.
[http://dx.doi.org/10.1080/17435390.2017.1343875] [PMID: 28618895]

[78] Holland, N.; Becak, D.; Shannahan, J. H.; Brown, J.; Carratt, S.; Winkle, L.; Pinkerton, K.; Wang, C.; Munusamy, P.; Baer, D. R. *Cardiac ischemia reperfusion injury following instillation of 20 nm citrate-capped nanosilver.,* **2015**.

[79] Ferdous, Z.; Al-Salam, S.; Greish, Y.E.; Ali, B.H.; Nemmar, A. Pulmonary exposure to silver nanoparticles impairs cardiovascular homeostasis: Effects of coating, dose and time. *Toxicol. Appl. Pharmacol.,* **2019**, *367*, 36-50.
[http://dx.doi.org/10.1016/j.taap.2019.01.006] [PMID: 30639276]

[80] Ebabe Elle, R.; Gaillet, S.; Vidé, J.; Romain, C.; Lauret, C.; Rugani, N.; Cristol, J.P.; Rouanet, J.M. Dietary exposure to silver nanoparticles in Sprague–Dawley rats: Effects on oxidative stress and inflammation. *Food Chem. Toxicol.,* **2013**, *60*, 297-301.
[http://dx.doi.org/10.1016/j.fct.2013.07.071] [PMID: 23933361]

[81] Lafuente, D.; Garcia, T.; Blanco, J.; Sánchez, D.J.; Sirvent, J.J.; Domingo, J.L.; Gómez, M. Effects of oral exposure to silver nanoparticles on the sperm of rats. *Reprod. Toxicol.,* **2016**, *60*, 133-139.
[http://dx.doi.org/10.1016/j.reprotox.2016.02.007] [PMID: 26900051]

[82] Fennell, T.R.; Mortensen, N.P.; Black, S.R.; Snyder, R.W.; Levine, K.E.; Poitras, E.; Harrington, J.M.; Wingard, C.J.; Holland, N.A.; Pathmasiri, W.; Sumner, S.C.J. Disposition of intravenously or orally administered silver nanoparticles in pregnant rats and the effect on the biochemical profile in urine. *J. Appl. Toxicol.,* **2017**, *37*(5), 530-544.
[http://dx.doi.org/10.1002/jat.3387] [PMID: 27696470]

[83] Blanco, J.; Tomás-Hernández, S.; García, T.; Mulero, M.; Gómez, M.; Domingo, J.L.; Sánchez, D.J. Oral exposure to silver nanoparticles increases oxidative stress markers in the liver of male rats and deregulates the insulin signalling pathway and p53 and cleaved caspase 3 protein expression. *Food Chem. Toxicol.,* **2018**, *115*, 398-404.
[http://dx.doi.org/10.1016/j.fct.2018.03.039] [PMID: 29604305]

[84] Garcia, T.X.; Costa, G.M.J.; França, L.R.; Hofmann, M.C. Sub-acute intravenous administration of silver nanoparticles in male mice alters Leydig cell function and testosterone levels. *Reprod. Toxicol.,* **2014**, *45*, 59-70.
[http://dx.doi.org/10.1016/j.reprotox.2014.01.006] [PMID: 24447867]

[85] Nam, G.; Purushothaman, B.; Rangasamy, S.; Song, J.M. Investigating the versatility of multifunctional silver nanoparticles: preparation and inspection of their potential as wound treatment agents. *Int. Nano Lett.,* **2016**, *6*(1), 51-63.
[http://dx.doi.org/10.1007/s40089-015-0168-1]

[86] Wen, H.; Dan, M.; Yang, Y.; Lyu, J.; Shao, A.; Cheng, X.; Chen, L.; Xu, L. Acute toxicity and genotoxicity of silver nanoparticle in rats. *PLoS One,* **2017**, *12*(9), e0185554.
[http://dx.doi.org/10.1371/journal.pone.0185554] [PMID: 28953974]

[87] Ng, C.T.; Li, J.J.E.; Gurung, R.L.; Hande, M.P.; Ong, C.N.; Bay, B.H.; Yung, L.Y.L. Toxicological profile of small airway epithelial cells exposed to gold nanoparticles. *Exp. Biol. Med.,* **2013**, *238*(12), 1355-1361.
[http://dx.doi.org/10.1177/1535370213505964] [PMID: 24157586]

[88] Li, T.; Albee, B.; Alemayehu, M.; Diaz, R.; Ingham, L.; Kamal, S.; Rodriguez, M.; Whaley Bishnoi, S. Comparative toxicity study of Ag, Au, and Ag–Au bimetallic nanoparticles on Daphnia magna. *Anal. Bioanal. Chem.,* **2010**, *398*(2), 689-700.
[http://dx.doi.org/10.1007/s00216-010-3915-1] [PMID: 20577719]

[89] Li, J.J.; Hartono, D.; Ong, C.N.; Bay, B.H.; Yung, L.Y.L. Autophagy and oxidative stress associated with gold nanoparticles. *Biomaterials,* **2010**, *31*(23), 5996-6003.
[http://dx.doi.org/10.1016/j.biomaterials.2010.04.014] [PMID: 20466420]

[90] Mateo, D.; Morales, P.; Ávalos, A.; Haza, A.I. Oxidative stress contributes to gold nanoparticle-induced cytotoxicity in human tumor cells. *Toxicol. Mech. Methods,* **2014**, *24*(3), 161-172.
[http://dx.doi.org/10.3109/15376516.2013.869783] [PMID: 24274460]

[91] Soenen, S.J.; Manshian, B.; Montenegro, J.M.; Amin, F.; Meermann, B.; Thiron, T.; Cornelissen, M.; Vanhaecke, F.; Doak, S.; Parak, W.J.; De Smedt, S.; Braeckmans, K. Cytotoxic effects of gold nanoparticles: a multiparametric study. *ACS Nano,* **2012**, *6*(7), 5767-5783.
[http://dx.doi.org/10.1021/nn301714n] [PMID: 22659047]

[92] Stelzer, R.; Hutz, R.J. Gold nanoparticles enter rat ovarian granulosa cells and subcellular organelles, and alter in-vitro estrogen accumulation. *J. Reprod. Dev.,* **2009**, *55*(6), 685-690.
[http://dx.doi.org/10.1262/jrd.20241] [PMID: 19789424]

[93] Moretti, E.; Terzuoli, G.; Renieri, T.; Iacoponi, F.; Castellini, C.; Giordano, C.; Collodel, G. *In vitro* effect of gold and silver nanoparticles on human spermatozoa. *Andrologia,* **2013**, *45*(6), 392-396.
[http://dx.doi.org/10.1111/and.12028] [PMID: 23116262]

[94]   Cho, W.S.; Cho, M.; Jeong, J.; Choi, M.; Cho, H.Y.; Han, B.S.; Kim, S.H.; Kim, H.O.; Lim, Y.T.; Chung, B.H.; Jeong, J. Acute toxicity and pharmacokinetics of 13 nm-sized PEG-coated gold nanoparticles. *Toxicol. Appl. Pharmacol.,* **2009**, *236*(1), 16-24.
[http://dx.doi.org/10.1016/j.taap.2008.12.023] [PMID: 19162059]

[95]   Cho, E.C.; Xie, J.; Wurm, P.A.; Xia, Y. Understanding the role of surface charges in cellular adsorption versus internalization by selectively removing gold nanoparticles on the cell surface with a I2/KI etchant. *Nano Lett.,* **2009**, *9*(3), 1080-1084.
[http://dx.doi.org/10.1021/nl803487r] [PMID: 19199477]

[96]   Hassanen, E.I.; Morsy, E.A.; Hussien, A.M.; Ibrahim, M.A.; Farroh, K.Y. The effect of different concentrations of gold nanoparticles on growth performance, toxicopathological and immunological parameters of broiler chickens. *Biosci. Rep.,* **2020**, *40*(3), BSR20194296.
[http://dx.doi.org/10.1042/BSR20194296] [PMID: 32124930]

[97]   Chen, Y.S.; Hung, Y.C.; Hong, M.Y.; Onischuk, A.A.; Chiou, J.C.; Sorokina, I.V.; Tolstikova, T.; Steve Huang, G. Control of *in vivo* transport and toxicity of nanoparticles by tea melanin. *J. Nanomater.,* **2012**, *2012*, 1-11.
[http://dx.doi.org/10.1155/2012/746960]

[98]   Pompa, P.P.; Vecchio, G.; Galeone, A.; Brunetti, V.; Sabella, S.; Maiorano, G.; Falqui, A.; Bertoni, G.; Cingolani, R. *In Vivo* toxicity assessment of gold nanoparticles in Drosophila melanogaster. *Nano Res.,* **2011**, *4*(4), 405-413.
[http://dx.doi.org/10.1007/s12274-011-0095-z]

[99]   Vecchio, G.; Galeone, A.; Brunetti, V.; Maiorano, G.; Rizzello, L.; Sabella, S.; Cingolani, R.; Pompa, P.P. Mutagenic effects of gold nanoparticles induce aberrant phenotypes in Drosophila melanogaster. *Nanomedicine,* **2012**, *8*(1), 1-7.
[http://dx.doi.org/10.1016/j.nano.2011.11.001] [PMID: 22094122]

[100]   Zhang, X-D.; Wu, H-Y.; Wu, D.; Wang, Y-Y.; Chang, J-H.; Zhai, Z-B.; Meng, A-M.; Liu, P-X.; Zhang, L-A.; Fan, F-Y. Toxicologic effects of gold nanoparticles *in vivo* by different administration routes. *Int. J. Nanomedicine,* **2010**, *5*, 771-781.
[http://dx.doi.org/10.2147/IJN.S8428] [PMID: 21042423]

[101]   Saquib, Q.; Al-Khedhairy, A.A.; Siddiqui, M.A.; Abou-Tarboush, F.M.; Azam, A.; Musarrat, J. Titanium dioxide nanoparticles induced cytotoxicity, oxidative stress and DNA damage in human amnion epithelial (WISH) cells. *Toxicol. In Vitro,* **2012**, *26*(2), 351-361.
[http://dx.doi.org/10.1016/j.tiv.2011.12.011] [PMID: 22210200]

[102]   Long, T.C.; Tajuba, J.; Sama, P.; Saleh, N.; Swartz, C.; Parker, J.; Hester, S.; Lowry, G.V.; Veronesi, B. Nanosize titanium dioxide stimulates reactive oxygen species in brain microglia and damages neurons *in vitro. Environ. Health Perspect.,* **2007**, *115*(11), 1631-1637.
[http://dx.doi.org/10.1289/ehp.10216] [PMID: 18007996]

[103]   Yamashita, K.; Yoshioka, Y.; Higashisaka, K.; Mimura, K.; Morishita, Y.; Nozaki, M.; Yoshida, T.; Ogura, T.; Nabeshi, H.; Nagano, K.; Abe, Y.; Kamada, H.; Monobe, Y.; Imazawa, T.; Aoshima, H.; Shishido, K.; Kawai, Y.; Mayumi, T.; Tsunoda, S.; Itoh, N.; Yoshikawa, T.; Yanagihara, I.; Saito, S.; Tsutsumi, Y. Silica and titanium dioxide nanoparticles cause pregnancy complications in mice. *Nat. Nanotechnol.,* **2011**, *6*(5), 321-328.
[http://dx.doi.org/10.1038/nnano.2011.41] [PMID: 21460826]

[104]   Trouiller, B.; Reliene, R.; Westbrook, A.; Solaimani, P.; Schiestl, R.H. Titanium dioxide nanoparticles induce DNA damage and genetic instability *in vivo* in mice. *Cancer Res.,* **2009**, *69*(22), 8784-8789.
[http://dx.doi.org/10.1158/0008-5472.CAN-09-2496] [PMID: 19887611]

[105]   Hsiao, I.L.; Fritsch-Decker, S.; Leidner, A.; Al-Rawi, M.; Hug, V.; Diabaté, S.; Grage, S.L.; Meffert, M.; Stoeger, T.; Gerthsen, D.; Ulrich, A.S.; Niemeyer, C.M.; Weiss, C. Biocompatibility of amine-functionalized silica nanoparticles: the role of surface coverage. *Small,* **2019**, *15*(10), 1805400.
[http://dx.doi.org/10.1002/smll.201805400] [PMID: 30721573]

[106] Chen, L.; Liu, J.; Zhang, Y.; Zhang, G.; Kang, Y.; Chen, A.; Feng, X.; Shao, L. The toxicity of silica nanoparticles to the immune system. *Nanomedicine,* **2018,** *13*(15), 1939-1962.
[http://dx.doi.org/10.2217/nnm-2018-0076] [PMID: 30152253]

[107] Guo, C.; Wang, J.; Jing, L.; Ma, R.; Liu, X.; Gao, L.; Cao, L.; Duan, J.; Zhou, X.; Li, Y.; Sun, Z. Mitochondrial dysfunction, perturbations of mitochondrial dynamics and biogenesis involved in endothelial injury induced by silica nanoparticles. *Environ. Pollut.,* **2018,** *236,* 926-936.
[http://dx.doi.org/10.1016/j.envpol.2017.10.060] [PMID: 29074197]

[108] Yu, T.; Hubbard, D.; Ray, A.; Ghandehari, H. *In vivo* biodistribution and pharmacokinetics of silica nanoparticles as a function of geometry, porosity and surface characteristics. *J. Control. Release,* **2012,** *163*(1), 46-54.
[http://dx.doi.org/10.1016/j.jconrel.2012.05.046] [PMID: 22684119]

[109] Kisin, E.R.; Murray, A.R.; Keane, M.J.; Shi, X.C.; Schwegler-Berry, D.; Gorelik, O.; Arepalli, S.; Castranova, V.; Wallace, W.E.; Kagan, V.E.; Shvedova, A.A. Single-walled carbon nanotubes: geno- and cytotoxic effects in lung fibroblast V79 cells. *J. Toxicol. Environ. Health A,* **2007,** *70*(24), 2071-2079.
[http://dx.doi.org/10.1080/15287390701601251] [PMID: 18049996]

[110] Cui, D.; Tian, F.; Ozkan, C.S.; Wang, M.; Gao, H. Effect of single wall carbon nanotubes on human HEK293 cells. *Toxicol. Lett.,* **2005,** *155*(1), 73-85.
[http://dx.doi.org/10.1016/j.toxlet.2004.08.015] [PMID: 15585362]

[111] Pacurari, M.; Yin, X.J.; Zhao, J.; Ding, M.; Leonard, S.S.; Schwegler-Berry, D.; Ducatman, B.S.; Sbarra, D.; Hoover, M.D.; Castranova, V.; Vallyathan, V. Raw Single-Wall Carbon Nanotubes Induce Oxidative Stress and Activate MAPKs, AP-1, NF-κB, and Akt in Normal and Malignant Human Mesothelial Cells. *Environ. Health Perspect.,* **2008,** *116*(9), 1211-1217.
[http://dx.doi.org/10.1289/ehp.10924] [PMID: 18795165]

[112] Muller, J.; Decordier, I.; Hoet, P.H.; Lombaert, N.; Thomassen, L.; Huaux, F.; Lison, D.; Kirsch-Volders, M. Clastogenic and aneugenic effects of multi-wall carbon nanotubes in epithelial cells. *Carcinogenesis,* **2008,** *29*(2), 427-433.
[http://dx.doi.org/10.1093/carcin/bgm243] [PMID: 18174261]

[113] Landsiedel, R.; Kapp, M.D.; Schulz, M.; Wiench, K.; Oesch, F. Genotoxicity investigations on nanomaterials: Methods, preparation and characterization of test material, potential artifacts and limitations—Many questions, some answers. *Mutat. Res. Rev. Mutat. Res.,* **2009,** *681*(2-3), 241-258.
[http://dx.doi.org/10.1016/j.mrrev.2008.10.002] [PMID: 19041420]

[114] Zhu, L.; Chang, D.W.; Dai, L.; Hong, Y. DNA damage induced by multiwalled carbon nanotubes in mouse embryonic stem cells. *Nano Lett.,* **2007,** *7*(12), 3592-3597.
[http://dx.doi.org/10.1021/nl071303v] [PMID: 18044946]

[115] Monteiro-Riviere, N.A.; Nemanich, R.J.; Inman, A.O.; Wang, Y.Y.; Riviere, J.E. Multi-walled carbon nanotube interactions with human epidermal keratinocytes. *Toxicol. Lett.,* **2005,** *155*(3), 377-384.
[http://dx.doi.org/10.1016/j.toxlet.2004.11.004] [PMID: 15649621]

[116] Ding, L.; Stilwell, J.; Zhang, T.; Elboudwarej, O.; Jiang, H.; Selegue, J.P.; Cooke, P.A.; Gray, J.W.; Chen, F.F. Molecular characterization of the cytotoxic mechanism of multiwall carbon nanotubes and nano-onions on human skin fibroblast. *Nano Lett.,* **2005,** *5*(12), 2448-2464.
[http://dx.doi.org/10.1021/nl051748o] [PMID: 16351195]

[117] Jacobsen, N.R.; Pojana, G.; White, P.; Møller, P.; Cohn, C.A.; Smith Korsholm, K.; Vogel, U.; Marcomini, A.; Loft, S.; Wallin, H. Genotoxicity, cytotoxicity, and reactive oxygen species induced by single-walled carbon nanotubes and C $_{60}$ fullerenes in the FE1-Muta™Mouse lung epithelial cells. *Environ. Mol. Mutagen.,* **2008,** *49*(6), 476-487.
[http://dx.doi.org/10.1002/em.20406] [PMID: 18618583]

[118] Totsuka, Y.; Higuchi, T.; Imai, T.; Nishikawa, A.; Nohmi, T.; Kato, T.; Masuda, S.; Kinae, N.; Hiyoshi, K.; Ogo, S.; Kawanishi, M.; Yagi, T.; Ichinose, T.; Fukumori, N.; Watanabe, M.; Sugimura,

T.; Wakabayashi, K. Genotoxicity of nano/microparticles in *in vitro* micronuclei, *in vivo* comet and mutation assay systems. *Part. Fibre Toxicol.,* **2009**, *6*(1), 23.
[http://dx.doi.org/10.1186/1743-8977-6-23] [PMID: 19725983]

[119] Zhang, X.; He, X.; Li, Y.; Zhang, Z.; Ma, Y.; Li, F.; Liu, J. A cytotoxicity study of fluorescent carbon nanodots using human bronchial epithelial cells. *J. Nanosci. Nanotechnol.,* **2013**, *13*(8), 5254-5259.
[http://dx.doi.org/10.1166/jnn.2013.7528] [PMID: 23882751]

[120] Shvedova, A.A.; Kisin, E.; Murray, A.R.; Johnson, V.J.; Gorelik, O.; Arepalli, S.; Hubbs, A.F.; Mercer, R.R.; Keohavong, P.; Sussman, N.; Jin, J.; Yin, J.; Stone, S.; Chen, B.T.; Deye, G.; Maynard, A.; Castranova, V.; Baron, P.A.; Kagan, V.E. Inhalation vs. aspiration of single-walled carbon nanotubes in C57BL/6 mice: inflammation, fibrosis, oxidative stress, and mutagenesis. *Am. J. Physiol. Lung Cell. Mol. Physiol.,* **2008**, *295*(4), L552-L565.
[http://dx.doi.org/10.1152/ajplung.90287.2008] [PMID: 18658273]

[121] Chou, C.C.; Hsiao, H.Y.; Hong, Q.S.; Chen, C.H.; Peng, Y.W.; Chen, H.W.; Yang, P.C. Single-walled carbon nanotubes can induce pulmonary injury in mouse model. *Nano Lett.,* **2008**, *8*(2), 437-445.
[http://dx.doi.org/10.1021/nl0723634] [PMID: 18225938]

[122] Lin, Z.; Ma, L.; X, Z.; Zhang, H.; Lin, B. A comparative study of lung toxicity in rats induced by three types of nanomaterials. *Nanoscale Res. Lett.,* **2013**, *8*(1), 521.
[http://dx.doi.org/10.1186/1556-276X-8-521] [PMID: 24321467]

[123] Park, E.J.; Kim, H.; Kim, Y.; Yi, J.; Choi, K.; Park, K. Carbon fullerenes (C60s) can induce inflammatory responses in the lung of mice. *Toxicol. Appl. Pharmacol.,* **2010**, *244*(2), 226-233.
[http://dx.doi.org/10.1016/j.taap.2009.12.036] [PMID: 20064541]

[124] Patlolla, A.K.; Patra, P.K.; Flountan, M.; Tchounwou, P.B. Cytogenetic evaluation of functionalized single-walled carbon nanotube in mice bone marrow cells. *Environ. Toxicol.,* **2016**, *31*(9), 1091-1102.
[http://dx.doi.org/10.1002/tox.22118] [PMID: 25689286]

[125] Patlolla, A.K.; Hussain, S.M.; Schlager, J.J.; Patlolla, S.; Tchounwou, P.B. Comparative study of the clastogenicity of functionalized and nonfunctionalized multiwalled carbon nanotubes in bone marrow cells of Swiss□Webster mice. *Environ. Toxicol.,* **2010**, *25*(6), 608-621.
[http://dx.doi.org/10.1002/tox.20621] [PMID: 20549644]

[126] Francis, A.P.; Ganapathy, S.; Palla, V.R.; Murthy, P.B.; Ramaprabhu, S.; Devasena, T. One time nose-only inhalation of MWCNTs: Exploring the mechanism of toxicity by intermittent sacrifice in Wistar rats. *Toxicol. Rep.,* **2015**, *2*, 111-120.
[http://dx.doi.org/10.1016/j.toxrep.2015.02.003] [PMID: 28962343]

[127] Grubek-Jaworska, H.; Nejman, P.; Czumińska, K.; Przybyłowski, T.; Huczko, A.; Lange, H.; Bystrzejewski, M.; Baranowski, P.; Chazan, R. Preliminary results on the pathogenic effects of intratracheal exposure to one-dimensional nanocarbons. *Carbon,* **2006**, *44*(6), 1057-1063.
[http://dx.doi.org/10.1016/j.carbon.2005.12.011]

[128] Fujita, K.; Morimoto, Y.; Ogami, A.; Myojyo, T.; Tanaka, I.; Shimada, M.; Wang, W.N.; Endoh, S.; Uchida, K.; Nakazato, T.; Yamamoto, K.; Fukui, H.; Horie, M.; Yoshida, Y.; Iwahashi, H.; Nakanishi, J. Gene expression profiles in rat lung after inhalation exposure to C60 fullerene particles. *Toxicology,* **2009**, *258*(1), 47-55.
[http://dx.doi.org/10.1016/j.tox.2009.01.005] [PMID: 19167457]

[129] Yao, K.; Lv, X.; Zheng, G.; Chen, Z.; Jiang, Y.; Zhu, X.; Wang, Z.; Cai, Z. Effects of Carbon Quantum Dots on Aquatic Environments: Comparison of Toxicity to Organisms at Different Trophic Levels. *Environ. Sci. Technol.,* **2018**, *52*(24), 14445-14451.
[http://dx.doi.org/10.1021/acs.est.8b04235] [PMID: 30486644]

[130] Xiao, Y.Y.; Liu, L.; Chen, Y.; Zeng, Y.L.; Liu, M.Z.; Jin, L. Developmental Toxicity of Carbon Quantum Dots to the Embryos/Larvae of Rare Minnow (*Gobiocypris rarus*). *BioMed Res. Int.,* **2016**, *2016*, 1-11.
[http://dx.doi.org/10.1155/2016/4016402] [PMID: 27872851]

[131] Wang, Z.G.; Zhou, R.; Jiang, D.; Song, J.E.; Xu, Q.; Si, J.; Chen, Y.P.; Zhou, X.; Gan, L.; Li, J.Z.; Zhang, H.; Liu, B. Toxicity of Graphene Quantum Dots in Zebrafish Embryo. *Biomed. Environ. Sci.,* **2015**, *28*(5), 341-351.
[PMID: 26055561]

CHAPTER 6

Regulation, Development, and Commercialization of Nano-Based Drugs

Abstract: Nanopharmaceuticals necessitate rigorous, costly testing to address safety concerns, including cytotoxic effects. The lack of toxicity testing protocols and understanding of the interactions of nanomaterials make it difficult to make accurate assessments of health risks. To meet the purpose of regulating and monitoring nano products in pharmaceuticals, various nations have devised their suitable regulatory processes. Approximately two decades are required for drug development, which includes drug discovery, clinical testing, and production approval. However, only when a novel pharmaceutical product can be mass manufactured in industrially substantial quantities is its development considered to be accomplished. At present, nanodrugs have already been introduced successfully to the market, demonstrating their future potential. This chapter will provide comprehensive details about the drug development process covering regulations, development, and commercialization of nano-based drugs

Keywords: Crystalline NPs, Drug development, Drug commercialization, European medicines agency, FDA, Inorganic NPs, lipid-based NPs, Nano-drug regulation, Polymeric NPs.

1. INTRODUCTION

The advent of nanomedicine has been heralded ever since the U.S. Food and Drug Administration (FDA) granted its initial approval for a nanotherapeutic product back in 1995—Doxil, an anticancer medication utilizing PEGylated nano-liposomes. Contrary to popular belief, however, nanotechnology has not yet fundamentally altered how diseases are diagnosed and treated, despite a handful of clinical breakthroughs that have benefited cancer and cardiology in particular. Nanotechnology is expected to make a big contribution to medicines, *in vivo* imaging, and *in vitro* diagnostics, although the technology has not yet shown its full potential. Many contend that this is caused, at least in part, by the ambiguities surrounding the potential health dangers that nanomaterials could bring [1].

Nanopharmaceuticals undergo more thorough and expensive testing due to safety concerns, particularly those pertaining to the cytotoxic effects caused by nanomaterials [2]. Establishing reliable health risk assessments is difficult due to the absence of approved toxicity testing methodologies and the incomplete knowledge of how nanomaterials interact with biological systems [3]. Because of this ambiguity, nanomedicine may not have performed well in clinical trials, which is one of the main reasons it has taken so long for it to be an authorized therapeutic therapy [4, 5].

Different nations have devised appropriate regulatory procedures to achieve the goal of regulating and monitoring nano products. Countries like the United States (US), the United Kingdom (UK), European Union (EU), China, and Japan play a significant role in establishing and regulating standards and guidelines for the safe and successful commercialization of goods based on nanotechnology [6].

The Food and Drug Administration (FDA) in the US oversees the regulation of nanotechnology-related products, including nanomedicines, employing the legal and regulatory framework already in place as well as standards that are particular to each product. To address the challenge of regulating nanotechnology globally, the FDA established the Nanotechnology Task Force and Nanotechnology Interest Group, which was formed of officials from numerous regulatory centers. Although the FDA has not developed specific rules for nanomedicines, the Task Force anticipates that since they are subject to pre-market review and approval as part of the New Drug Application process, the current laws are sufficient for their safe development. This conclusion is predicated on the claim that current regulatory standards would be able to identify toxicity in nanoproducts [7]. In order to address the safety and efficacy issues of licensing complex medications including nanomaterials, the FDA at long last produced a non-binding draft guidance for industry in December 2017. Nevertheless, this creates a lot of ambiguities regarding potential approval paths [8]. In the US, until recent revisions by Frank R. Lautenberg Chemicals Safety for the 21st Century Act, a broad range of nanomaterials were under the Toxic Substances Control Act (TSCA) [9, 10]. They are subject to special regulations, such as premanufacture notices for nanoparticles and a rule requiring information collecting on both new and existing nanomaterials. Manufacturers are required to submit the precise chemical identification, production volumes, manufacturing processes, usage and exposure details, as well as any accessible health and safety data, in accordance with TSCA section 8(A) [11]. This new law applies to many pharmaceutical-grade excipients, and they must abide by its requirements. The Environmental Protection Agency (EPA) of the United States released a draft advice in January 2017 that lists commonly asked questions and the agency's responses to those queries from suppliers of nanoscaled materials [12].

The Medicines and Healthcare products Regulatory Authority (MHRA) handles the regulation of medications in the UK. There has been no specific guidance provided with regard to nano medicine approval, and they appear to be handled on a case-by-case basis, as with the FDA. For assistance and direction throughout the process, researchers developing nano medicines are urged to communicate with the MHRA Innovation Office. Similar to the US, other institutions, including the UK- and EU-based European Nanomedicine characterisation Laboratory (EU-NCL), supply and continuously improve expertise on preclinical characterisation tests of nano medicine [13].

In accordance with European Union regulation (EC) No. 1907/2006 governing registration, evaluation, authorization, and restriction of chemicals (REACH), and regulation (EC) No. 1272/2008 on classification, labelling and packaging of substances and mixtures all chemicals, including excipients used in the manufacture of pharmaceutical products, are regulated by the European Chemicals Agency (ECHA) [14, 15]. These regulations are applicable to all compounds produced or imported at a rate of more than one ton annually and demand for the issuance of a dossier outlining the toxicological, physicochemical, and eco-toxicological features [11]. The second article of REACH specifically excludes from its scope pharmacological drugs, medicinal products, and invasive medical devices regulated by the European Medicines Agency (EMA) [15]. They are extensively assessed on a case-by-case basis throughout the medication approval procedure. In 2012 [16] and 2017 [17], the ECHA produced a number of nanomaterial-specific guideline sheets describing the regulations for chemical registration and testing, including nanomaterials, as defined by the European Commission (EC) [18]. The European Commission established new standards for the registration of nanomaterials on December 3, 2018. According to the new regulations, both the organization and ECHA must conduct a risk assessment of nanoparticles. From January 1st, 2020 onwards, these ECHa modifications become effective [19]. Numerous reflection papers on the standards for human-use nanomedicines, diagnostic iron oxide nanoparticles, generic liposomal products and surface coatings of nanoscaled parenteral dosage forms have been published by the EMA [11, 20, 21].

In South America, a committee of specialists in the field of nanoparticles was established by the Brazilian Health Surveillance Agency (ANVISA), with an emphasis on medications, medical devices, hygiene products, food and diagnostic tools and supplies. The objective was to create a questionnaire for manufacturers eager to register goods with nanomaterials. Without taking any more action, the effort was abandoned in 2016. All pharmaceuticals that include engineered nanoparticles are now assessed on an individual basis. The National Administration for Food, Drugs and Medical Technology (ANMAT) of Argentina's Nanotechnology Working Group published an article in January 2018 that provided an overview of the tests used to characterize and compare nanomedicines. The draft was available for discussion until February 2018, and ANMAT and pharmaceutical industry workshops and training were concluded [11].

In Asia, the industry is supported in reporting the quality characteristics of nanomedicines by a wide range of GB (Guojia Biaozhun, meaning "national standard") standards, with the involvement from major nations like China and Japan [11]. The Pharmaceuticals and Medical Devices Agency (PMDA) and the Ministry of Health, Labour, and Welfare (MHLW) supervise the regulation of medications in Japan. A reflection paper on polymeric micelles was released by the Japanese MHLW in association with EMA [22] and its own guidelines for the development of liposomes were released in 2016 [23]. The Indian Ministry of Science and Technology published the first draft of a guideline for the assessment of nanopharmaceuticals in March 2019 [24]. It only applies to engineered nanomaterials and is not applicable to goods used in cell-based treatment, tissue engineering, *in vitro* diagnostics, or medical devices. The definition of "nano pharmaceuticals" in the guideline is given as products comprising nanomaterials with a size between 1 and 100 nm. A product is also referred to as nanopharmaceutical if it has altered pharmaceutical properties as a result of the application of certain size-related features and falls within the range of 100 nm to 1000 nm. The marketing authorisation of all nanopharmaceuticals involves a case-by-case analysis, comparable to what it does with conventional medicinal products.

Currently, it might take up to two decades for a medicine to reach the market following its original discovery or development [25]. Drug development involves a number of steps, including drug discovery, clinical testing, and production approval (Fig. **1**). The process of discovering new drugs is a protracted, expensive, and a difficult one that takes years and costs millions of dollars. Identification of the target, lead discovery, lead optimization, and preclinical testing are the steps in this procedure. Clinical testing has a 15% success rate, despite spending a lot of time and money on it. Poor pharmacokinetic features (absorption, distribution, metabolism, excretion, and toxicity [ADMET]) account for around 50% of drug discovery failures [26]. Early signs of a drug's pharmacological activity, safety, and side effects are identified during phase I of clinical testing. Small groups of healthy individuals participate in phase I studies, and it is during these trials that the medicine will be administered to humans for the first time. These trials occasionally examine the ideal medication administration method. Dose escalation, in which participants are exposed to increasing dosages of the medication, establishes a range of safe doses. This permits testing of the drug's pharmacological effects and helps researchers understand how it is metabolized and tolerated at various levels. Once the drug's initial safety has been demonstrated, phase II studies can begin. These studies test the drug's therapeutic effectiveness and safety in patients with the disease or condition being studied. Patients get the various medication dosages that were shown to be safe in the phase I study, allowing for comparison of efficacy and common adverse effects in order to determine the safest dosing schedule. Drug development will go on to phase III if the medication's effectiveness and safety have been established for the illness or condition being studied. Phase III studies sometimes contain a large number of individuals from different countries than those in earlier rounds. A phase III trial's objective is to show the effectiveness and safety of the selected safest dose regimen(s) in a broader population of patients for whom it is designed. A randomised controlled trial will be used to evaluate the new drug's effectiveness and safety to the existing standard treatment(s). Similar to past phases, patients are closely watched for negative effects, and the experiment will be halted if any side effects are severe. The data the phase III study is crucial for determining whether the medicine can be authorized and commercialized. Once the medicine is granted marketing authorization based on the findings of a phase III study, phase IV trials—also known as post marketing studies—start. Pharma firms frequently fund phase IV studies. In order to determine the drug's long-term effectiveness and safety, it is studied in larger patient populations and perhaps in patient subgroups within the population. The medicine might be put up against or paired with other widely used conventional therapies [27].

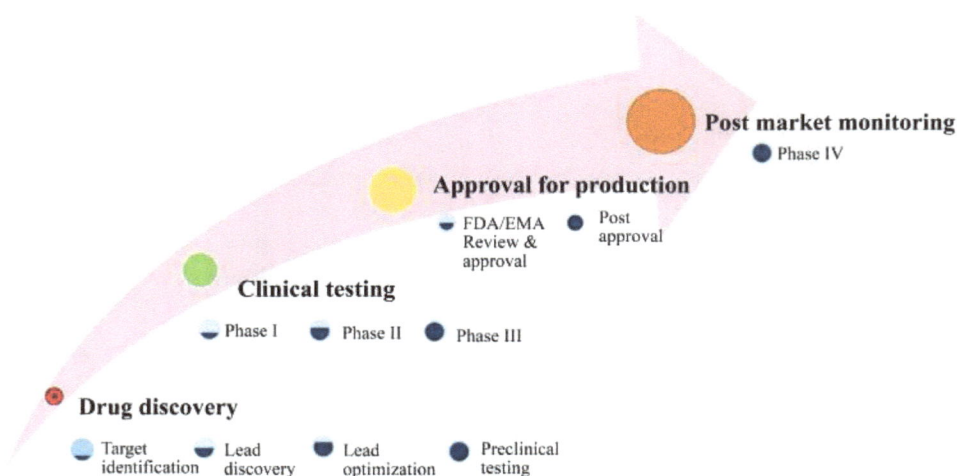

Fig. (1). The processes drug development, marketing and commercialization of pharmaceuticals.

A few factors to take into account during drug development and commercialization include the availability of enough qualified scientists and doctors who are willing to devote a decade or more of their lives to a single project, the need for a novel scientific premise with appropriate intellectual property protection, and the need for an economic business plan that will persuade investors of future financial success. Profit/risk ratios must be sufficiently high and market demands must be accurately assessed. It also has to be clear how the therapeutic compounds are distributed and how long they last [28]. Utilizing skilled market analysis to determine the market's demands and prospects is crucial to lowering the risk of failure. The following sections provide a brief discussion of some of the major obstacles that must be overcome for nanomedicine to go from the lab to the market, including intellectual property, ethics, scalability, repeatability, technological problems, general costs, and environmental effects [29].

It is crucial to submit patents at every stage of the drug research and commercialization process in order to safeguard the firms' and inventors' intellectual property and prevent time and money from being squandered on unnecessary legal proceedings. However, the permitted 20-year period of patent protection (depending on the country) reduces the period of commercial exclusiveness to 12 years or less because it takes so long to obtain regulatory approval for a drug, pass the necessary clinical trials, and finally introduce a new pharmaceutical to the market. Because of this, there are occasions when the company's period of opportunity for profit is too small to warrant investing its resources at risk [30]. The authorities must address this matter, particularly in light of the added difficulties posed by nano pharmaceuticals. The time limit for market exclusivity should be increased considering the ethical concerns, as well as the financial impact that clinical studies have on the overall cost of creating nano pharmaceuticals.

The ability to demonstrate that a product is more effective than alternatives already on the market is one of the key requirements for its successful commercialization. The behaviour of NPs *in vivo*, which is anticipated to differ greatly from their activity *in vitro*, is another major difficulty. The primary problems that require in-depth investigation utilizing various animal (*in vivo*) models are biocompatibility, cellular interactions, diffusion, and tissue transport. It is not simple or inexpensive to carry out these trials to the required degree of efficacy and safety [31]. The majority of human clinical studies in nanomedicine are conducted on individuals with terminal illnesses or those who have tried several therapies without seeing any improvement in their condition [32]. The majority of volunteers in these clinical trials are unlikely to personally gain from their participation, despite the important knowledge that is learned from them.

The key issue here is that the benefit/harm ratio of the health impacts brought on by the nanoformulation remain unclear at this early stage of clinical testing. There will be numerous moral dilemmas in this circumstance. It is undoubtedly necessary to mention the excessive caution used by ethical committees, the inability to offer adequate accurate information about the dangers, advantages, and anticipated outcome of the studies, as well as other humanitarian concerns. These are the key ethical concerns that might impede the conduct of clinical studies as a whole [32 - 34].

Only when a novel pharmaceutical product can be mass manufactured in industrially substantial quantities is its development considered to be accomplished [35]. Since the methods used in the laboratory cannot be replicated on an industrial scale, this stage of product development is extremely important. In order to scale up production while preserving the product's distinctive qualities, technological integration is necessary. Nanosized medicinal products must be scalable while maintaining their nano size and innovative properties.

Nanotechnology-based products are typically difficult to produce using standard manufacturing processes currently in use in this industry. In contrast, in large-scale production, small changes in the manufacturing process can result in significant, detrimental changes in physicochemical properties such as drug composition, size, surface charge, crystallinity, and even therapeutic outcomes. It is simpler to control and optimize a formulation when using small batches. Each and every batch manufactured must be identical in terms of not only physical appearance but also attributes crucial to therapy for a pharmaceutical product to reach the market. Low inter-batch variances are also necessary for nanotech-based products to be accepted in this market since consumers care more that a product "performs" consistently across all batches rather than merely "looking similar." The verified manufacturing technique requires that this repeatability be included into the nano drug system [36].

The success of a novel nanotherapeutic may also be hindered by the high expenses associated with scaling up nanotherapeutics. In addition to the safety of the product containing considerable residual concentrations of the organic solvent, industry also presents additional restrictions such as the limited usage of organic solvent owing to high cost and also due to environmental concerns. Additionally, some preparations may need to be sterilized, thus the production facility has to include an aseptic section that is well-designed [37]. It is crucial that the manufacturing process is planned with consideration for the limitations encountered in the market. Therefore, early in the process in the development of a nanodrug, possible synthesis problems and a cost-benefit analysis should be carefully considered.

The potential environmental effect of nanomedicines during manufacture, usage, and disposal is another aspect to take into account when evaluating their potential impact [38]. Since nanomedicines are anticipated to act similarly to traditional pharmaceuticals, which are commonly acknowledged to eventually be recovered in the environment, there is a possibility that they may have an adverse effect on the environment [39]. The FDA claims that there is a dearth of evidence to assess the safety for humans and the environment, thus they are having difficulty coming up with a standard to assure the safe and effective development of nano-products, whether they be drugs, devices, or biologics. Based on projected environmental consequences, there are inclusion and exclusion criteria used in the evaluation of medicinal items in the USA and the EU. In the EU, the permitted limit for surface water environmental concentrations is 0.01 ppb, and all marketing authorization applications must go through an environmental risk assessment and pre-screening step. As a result, no more environmental risk assessment steps are performed for the product if the anticipated environmental concentration is below this and no other environmental issues are highlighted. If a new medication application is submitted in the USA, the FDA must conduct an environmental assessment unless it is exempted from performing so; however, an exemption cannot be granted if the predicted environmental concentration is greater than 1 ppb [40].

Despite the fact that nanotechnology is still in its early stages of commercialization, the rate of technology enablement is rising significantly, mostly due to the enormous government-mandated funding allocated to nanotechnology [41]. Commercialization is the process of converting novel technologies into lucrative business endeavours. To effectively commercialize a new invention into usable products or services, a variety of experts from the technical, commercial, and economic backgrounds may be involved [42]. The procedure entails a number of steps, beginning with the conception of an idea, its development as technology, and its commercialization; encouraging those ideas to technology development; creating a prototype to verify the viability of the idea; developing a new process or optimizing an existing process; and finally, supplying the market with the proposed deliverables, promoting them, and developing new infrastructures for simplified supply and purchase [43].

Many patients currently use a wide range of nano-based medications that have successfully hit the market. These items, which originate from multiple companies throughout the globe, show the current and (likely) future effectiveness of nanoparticles as medicinal agents. Table **1** lists some of the authorized nano-based medications. (Fig. **2A** and **2B**) illustrates details about the structure and mechanism of action along with the induced effect of some approved nanopharmaceuticals.

Fig. (2A).   Lipid-based approved and marketed nanopharmaceuticals FDA and/or EMA-approved nanomedicines from 1995 to 2022 (last accessed May 2022), catalogued by their nature, encapsulated drug, their mechanism of action, and their induced effects. Adapted from [47] Copyright (2022) Rodríguez, F., *et al.*. Published by MDPI distributed under the terms and conditions of the Creative Commons Attribution (CC BY) license (https://creativecommons.org/licenses/by/4.0/)..

Fig. (2B). Protein- and metallic-based approved and marketed nanopharmaceuticals. FDA and/or EMA-approved nanomedicines from 1995 to 2022 (last accessed May 2022), catalogued by their nature, encapsulated drug, their mechanism of action, and their induced effects. Adapted from [47] Copyright (2022) Rodríguez, F., *et al.*. Published by MDPI distributed under the terms and conditions of the Creative Commons Attribution (CC BY) license (https://creativecommons.org/licenses/by/4.0/).

Table 1. List of some authorized nano-based medications [44-46].

Type	Trade name	Active ingredient	Disease	Approval (Year)
Polymeric NPs	Renagel ® [sevelamer hydrochloride]/Renagel® [sevelamer carbonate]	Cross-linked poly allylamine hydro chloride.	Chronic kidney disease, Hyperphosphatemia	FDA(2000) EMA (2000)
	Eligard®	Leuprolide acetate incorporated in nanoparticles composed of PLGH copolymer.	Advanced hormone-dependent Prostate cancer.	FDA(2004)
	Cimzia®	Certolizumab pegol.	Arthritis, Rheumatoid.	EMA (2009) FDA(2008)
	Adynovate/ Adynovi®	Rurioctocog alfa pegol.	Hemophilia	FDA (2015) EMA (2018)
	Rebinyn/ Refixia®	Polymeric nanoparticles of Coagulation Factor IX (Recombinant), GlycoPEGylated.	Hemophilia B	FDA (2017) EMA (2017)
	Mircera®	Polymeric nanoparticles of Erythropoiesis-stimulating agent (ESA)	Anemia associated with chronic kidney disease in patients from 5 to 17 years old on hemodialysis.	FDA (2018)
	Eysuvis®	Loteprednol etabonate ophthalmic nanosuspension.	Short-term treatment of dry eye disease.	FDA (2020)
Lipid Based NPs	Myocet®	Doxorubicin encapsulated into cligolamellar liposomes.	Metastatic breast cancer.	EMA (2000) FDA (2000)
	Visudyne®	Verteporfin in liposomes.	Age-related macular degeneration.	FDA (2002) EMA (2000)
	Mepact®	Mifamurtide incorporated into a large multilamellar liposomes.	High-grade non-metastatic osteosarcoma.	EMA (2004)
	DepoDur®	Morphine sulfate extended-release liposome injection.	Analgesics	FDA(2004) EMA(2009)
	Onivyde®	Irinotecan in pegylated liposome.	Metastatic adenocarcinoma of the pancreas	FDA (2015) EMA (2016)

Type	Trade name	Active ingredient	Disease	Approval (Year)
-	Vyxeos®	Daunorubicin hydrochloride and cytarabine in liposomes.	Myeloid leukaemia	FDA(2017) EMA(2018)
	Exparel®	Bupivacaine	Acute Pain	EMA (2020) FDA(2011)
	Ikervis®	Ciclosporin	Corneal Diseases	EMA (2015)
	Onpattro Patisiran-LNP®, ALN-TTR02®	Patisiran sodium	Peripheral nerve disease (polyneuropathy) caused by hereditary transthyretin-mediated amyloidosis (hATTR).	FDA(2018) EMA(2018)
	Moderna® COVID-19 Vaccine	CX-024414 (single-stranded, 5'-capped messenger RNA (mRNA) produced using a cell-free *in vitro* transcription from the corresponding DNA templates, encoding the viral spike (S) protein of SARS-CoV-2) spike protein.	COVID-19 virus infection.	EMA (2022) FDA (2020)
	Pfizer®-BioNTech COVID-19 Vaccine	Nucleoside modified mRNA BNT162b2, encoding SARS-CoV-2 spike protein.	COVID-19 virus infection.	FDA (2021,2023) EMA(2020)
	Vyxeos®	Liposomal formulation of cytarabine and daunorubicin.	Acute myeloid leukaemia.	FDA (2017) EMA (2018)
	Zilretta®	Poly-(d,l-lactic acid-c--glycolic acid hydrogel/Triamcinolone acetonide extended-release injectable suspension.	Osteoarthritis pain syndrome.	FDA (2017)
	Shingrix® (zoster vaccine recombinant, adjuvanted)	Liposomal nanoparticles/Recombinant glycoprotein E with an adjuvant system	Herpes Zoster, Prophylaxis	FDA (2017) (2021—for immunocompromised adults) EMA (2018)
	Sublocade®	PLGA nanoparticles of buprenorphine & naloxone	Opioid use disorder (OUD)	FDA (2017) EMA (2006)

(Table 1) cont.....

Type	Trade name	Active ingredient	Disease	Approval (Year)
Inorganic NPs	Feraheme ®	Super Paramagnetic Iron Oxide Nanoparticles (SPION) coated with dextran	Iron deficiency in adult CKD patients	FDA (2009) EMA(withdrawn)
	Ferumoxytol®	Ferumoxytol	Iron deficiency in adult CKD patients	FDA (2021)
	Injectafter/Ferinject®	Iron carboxymaltose colloid	Iron deficient anaemia	FDA (2013)
Crystalline NPs	Ritalin LA®	Methylphenidate hydrochloride. Central nervous system stimuli.	Mental stimuli. Attention Deficit Hyperactivity Disorder (ADHD)	FDA (2002) EMA (2009)
	Tricor®	Fenofibrate	Hypercholesterolemia and hypertriglyceridemia.	FDA (2004) EMA (2018)
	Ryanodex®	Dantrolene sodium	Malignant hyperthermia	FDA (2014) EMA (2016)
	NBTXR3®, Hensify® Nanobiotix	Hafnium oxide crystalline NPs	Soft tissue sarcoma, hepatocellular carcinoma, head and neck squamous cell carcinoma, and advanced solid malignancies with lung or liver metastases.	FDA (2017) EMA (2019)
	Brixadi/ Buvidal	Liquid crystalline System (buprenorphine)	Opioid use disorder	FDA (2021) EMA (2018)
Protein-based NPs	Ontak	Interleukin-2 receptor and diphtheria toxin	Cutaneous T-Cell lymphoma.	FDA (1999)
	Abraxane®/ABI-007	Protein bound paclitaxel	Breast cancer, non-small cell lung cancer, and pancreatic cancer.	FDA (2005, 2012, 2013, 2019) EMA (2008)
	Kadcyla	Trastuzumab Emtansine	Metastatic breast cancer	FDA (2013)

CONCLUSION

Comprehensive, expensive testing is necessary for nanopharmaceuticals to address safety issues, particularly cytotoxic effects. It is challenging to create accurate health risk assessments due to a lack of recognized toxicity testing procedures and a lack of knowledge about the interactions of nanomaterials.

Different countries have established their own appropriate regulatory procedures to achieve the goal of regulating and monitoring nano products.

Drug development takes about two decades and involves various steps, including drug discovery, clinical testing, and production approval. During drug discovery, the process consists of four steps: target identification, lead discovery, lead optimization, and preclinical testing. Phase I, in clinical testing, involves the identification of early signs of a drug's pharmacological activity, safety, and side effects. Phase II studies test the drug's therapeutic effectiveness and safety in patients, while phase III evaluates the drug's effectiveness and safety in a broader population. Phase IV trials, funded by pharma firms, evaluate the drug's long-term effectiveness and safety in larger patient populations and subgroups.

Commercialization is the process of converting cutting-edge technologies into successful business endeavours with the assistance of professionals from the scientific, business, and economic fields. Idea generation, technology development, prototype development, process optimization, market supply, advertising, and infrastructure development are all included. Nano-based medications have successfully entered the market and are widely used by patients worldwide, showcasing their effectiveness as medicinal agents and their potential for future use.

REFERENCES

[1]   Agarwal, V.; Bajpai, M.; Sharma, A. Patented and Approval Scenario of Nanopharmaceuticals with Relevancy to Biomedical Application, Manufacturing Procedure and Safety Aspects. *Recent Pat. Drug Deliv. Formul.,* **2018**, *12*(1), 40-52.
        [http://dx.doi.org/10.2174/1872211312666180105114644] [PMID: 29303083]

[2]   Venkatraman, S. Has nanomedicine lived up to its promise? *Nanotechnology,* **2014**, *25*(37), 372501.
        [http://dx.doi.org/10.1088/0957-4484/25/37/372501] [PMID: 25148691]

[3]   Halappanavar, S.; Vogel, U.; Wallin, H.; Yauk, C.L. Promise and peril in nanomedicine: the challenges and needs for integrated systems biology approaches to define health risk. *Wiley Interdiscip. Rev. Nanomed. Nanobiotechnol.,* **2018**, *10*(1), e1465.
        [http://dx.doi.org/10.1002/wnan.1465] [PMID: 28294555]

[4]   Youn, Y.S.; Bae, Y.H. Perspectives on the past, present, and future of cancer nanomedicine. *Adv. Drug Deliv. Rev.,* **2018**, *130*, 3-11.
        [http://dx.doi.org/10.1016/j.addr.2018.05.008] [PMID: 29778902]

[5]   Weissig, V.; Guzman-Villanueva, D. Nanopharmaceuticals (part 2): products in the pipeline. *Int. J. Nanomedicine,* **2015**, *10*, 1245-1257.
        [http://dx.doi.org/10.2147/IJN.S65526] [PMID: 25709446]

[6]   Ali, F.; Neha, K.; Parveen, S. Current regulatory landscape of nanomaterials and nanomedicines: A global perspective. *J. Drug Deliv. Sci. Technol.,* **2022**, 104118.

[7]   Bawa, R. Regulating nanomedicine can the FDA handle it? *Curr. Drug Deliv.,* **2011**, *8*(3), 227-234.
        [http://dx.doi.org/10.2174/156720111795256156] [PMID: 21291376]

[8]   Emily, M.; Ioanna, N.; Scott, B.; Beat, F. Reflections on FDA Draft Guidance for Products Containing Nanomaterials: Is the Abbreviated New Drug Application (ANDA) a Suitable Pathway for

Nanomedicines? *AAPS J.,* **2018**, *20*(5), 92.
[http://dx.doi.org/10.1208/s12248-018-0255-0] [PMID: 30128758]

[9]   Congress, U.S. Toxic substances control act. *Public Law,* **1976**, *94*(469), 90.

[10]   Congress, U. S.; Congress, U. S. Public Law 114-182-Frank R. Lautenberg Chemical Safety for the 21st Century Act. 2016.

[11]   Marques, M.R.C.; Choo, Q.; Ashtikar, M.; Rocha, T.C.; Bremer-Hoffmann, S.; Wacker, M.G. Nanomedicines Tiny particles and big challenges. *Adv. Drug Deliv. Rev.,* **2019**, *151-152*, 23-43.
[http://dx.doi.org/10.1016/j.addr.2019.06.003] [PMID: 31226397]

[12]   A., (EPA), Chemical substances when manufactured or processed as nanoscale materials: TSCA reporting and recordkeeping requirements. *Fed. Regist.,* **2015**, *80*, 18330.

[13]   Bremer-Hoffmann, S.; Halamoda-Kenzaoui, B.; Borgos, S.E. Identification of regulatory needs for nanomedicines. *J. Interdiscip. Nanomed.,* **2018**, *3*(1), 4-15.
[http://dx.doi.org/10.1002/jin2.34]

[14]   Union, P. Regulation (EC) No 1223/2009 of the european parliament and of the council. *Off. J. Eur. Union L,* **2009**, *342*, 59.

[15]   Se, D.; Schöpf, T. J.; Renner, N. Regulation (EC) No. 1907/2006 of the European Parliament and of the Council of 18 December 2006 concerning the Registration, Evaluation, Authorisation and Restriction of Chemicals (REACH). 2019.

[16]   Tanarro, C. *Guidance on information requirements and chemical safety assessment-Appendix R14-4 Recommendations for nanomaterials.,* 2012.

[17]   ECHA. Guidance on information requirements and chemical safety assessment: Appendix R7-1 for nanomaterials applicable to chapter R7a endpoint specific guidance. Version 2.0. Helsinki, Finland. 2017.

[18]   European Medicines Agency. Reflection paper on the data tequirements for intravenous liposomal products developed with reference to an innovator liposomal product-Final. http://www. ema. europa. eu/docs/en_GB/document_library/Scientific_guideline/2013/03/WC500140351. pdf

[19]   Nanomaterials, E.C.H.A. https://echa.europa.eu/regulations/nanomaterials

[20]   Committee for Medicinal Products for Human. U., *Reflection paper on surface coatings: General issues for consideration regarding parenteral administration of coated nanomedicine products*; European Medicines Agency, Committee for Medicinal Products for Human Use: London, UK, **2013**.

[21]   CHMP. E. M. A. SWP (2013) Draft reflection paper on the data requirements for intravenous iron-based nano-colloidal products developed with reference to an innovator medicinal product: EMA; CHMP/SWP/620008/2012.

[22]   Joint MHLW/EMA reflection paper on the development of block copolymer micelle medicinal products-Draft. http://www.ema.europa.eu/docs/en_GB/document_library/Scientific_guideline/2013/02/WC500138390.pdf

[23]   MHLW. Guideline for the Development of Liposome Drug Products. **2016**.

[24]   BM Gupta, G.; SM Dhawan, D.; Ahmed, K.K.M.; Mamdapur, G.M. Nanomedicine Research in India: A Bibliometric Assessment of Publications Output during 2002-20. *Int. J. Pharm. Investig.,* **2021**, *11*(2), 143-153.
[http://dx.doi.org/10.5530/ijpi.2021.2.27]

[25]   Bawa, R.; Melethil, S.; Simmons, W.J.; Harris, D. Nanopharmaceuticals: patenting issues and FDA regulatory challenges. *SciTech Lawyer,* **2008**, *5*(2), 10-15.

[26]   Zhang, Y.; Luo, M.; Wu, P.; Wu, S.; Lee, T.Y.; Bai, C. Application of Computational Biology and Artificial Intelligence in Drug Design. *Int. J. Mol. Sci.,* **2022**, *23*(21), 13568.
[http://dx.doi.org/10.3390/ijms232113568] [PMID: 36362355]

[27]   Sedgwick, P. Phases of clinical trials. *BMJ,* **2011**, 343.
        [PMID: 24906716]

[28]   Eaton, M.A.W. Improving the translation in Europe of nanomedicines (a.k.a. drug delivery) from academia to industry. *J. Control. Release,* **2012**, *164*(3), 370-371.
        [http://dx.doi.org/10.1016/j.jconrel.2012.06.016] [PMID: 22721816]

[29]   Windheim, J.; Myers, B. A lab-to-market roadmap for early-stage entrepreneurship. *Translational Materials Research,* **2014**, *1*(1), 016001.
        [http://dx.doi.org/10.1088/2053-1613/1/1/016001]

[30]   Bosetti, R.; Vereeck, L. The impact of effective patents on future innovations in nanomedicine. *Pharm. Pat. Anal.,* **2012**, *1*(1), 37-43.
        [http://dx.doi.org/10.4155/ppa.11.4] [PMID: 24236712]

[31]   Farjadian, F.; Ghasemi, A.; Gohari, O.; Roointan, A.; Karimi, M.; Hamblin, M.R. Nanopharmaceuticals and nanomedicines currently on the market: challenges and opportunities. *Nanomedicine (Lond.),* **2019**, *14*(1), 93-126.
        [http://dx.doi.org/10.2217/nnm-2018-0120] [PMID: 30451076]

[32]   Mhaske, A.; Dighe, S.; Ghosalkar, S.; Tanna, V.; Ravikumar, P.; Sawarkar, S.P. Limitations of Current Cancer Theranostics. *Nanotechnology in the Life Sciences,* **2021**, *2*, 305-332.
        [http://dx.doi.org/10.1007/978-3-030-76263-6_12]

[33]   van de Poel, I. How should we do nanoethics? A network approach for discerning ethical issues in nanotechnology. *NanoEthics,* **2008**, *2*(1), 25-38.
        [http://dx.doi.org/10.1007/s11569-008-0026-y]

[34]   Satalkar, P.; Elger, B.S.; Hunziker, P.; Shaw, D. Challenges of clinical translation in nanomedicine: A qualitative study. *Nanomedicine,* **2016**, *12*(4), 893-900.
        [http://dx.doi.org/10.1016/j.nano.2015.12.376] [PMID: 26772431]

[35]   Muller, F.L.; Latimer, J.M. Anticipation of scale up issues in pharmaceutical development. *Comput. Chem. Eng.,* **2009**, *33*(5), 1051-1055.
        [http://dx.doi.org/10.1016/j.compchemeng.2008.09.015]

[36]   Kaur, I.P.; Kakkar, V.; Deol, P.K.; Yadav, M.; Singh, M.; Sharma, I. Issues and concerns in nanotech product development and its commercialization. *J. Control. Release,* **2014**, *193*, 51-62.
        [http://dx.doi.org/10.1016/j.jconrel.2014.06.005] [PMID: 24933600]

[37]   Desai, N. Challenges in development of nanoparticle-based therapeutics. *AAPS J.,* **2012**, *14*(2), 282-295.
        [http://dx.doi.org/10.1208/s12248-012-9339-4] [PMID: 22407288]

[38]   Mahapatra, I.; Clark, J.R.A.; Dobson, P.J.; Owen, R.; Lynch, I.; Lead, J.R. Expert perspectives on potential environmental risks from nanomedicines and adequacy of the current guideline on environmental risk assessment. *Environ. Sci. Nano,* **2018**, *5*(8), 1873-1889.
        [http://dx.doi.org/10.1039/C8EN00053K]

[39]   Baun, A.; Hansen, S. F. *Environmental challenges for nanomedicine.,* **2008**.
        [http://dx.doi.org/10.2217/17435889.3.5.605]

[40]   Foulkes, R.; Man, E.; Thind, J.; Yeung, S.; Joy, A.; Hoskins, C. The regulation of nanomaterials and nanomedicines for clinical application: current and future perspectives. *Biomater. Sci.,* **2020**, *8*(17), 4653-4664.
        [http://dx.doi.org/10.1039/D0BM00558D] [PMID: 32672255]

[41]   Domingues, C.; Santos, A.; Alvarez-Lorenzo, C.; Concheiro, A.; Jarak, I.; Veiga, F.; Barbosa, I.; Dourado, M.; Figueiras, A. Where Is Nano Today and Where Is It Headed? A Review of Nanomedicine and the Dilemma of Nanotoxicology. *ACS Nano,* **2022**, *16*(7), 9994-10041.
        [http://dx.doi.org/10.1021/acsnano.2c00128] [PMID: 35729778]

[42]   Reamer, A. *Technology transfer and commercialization: their role in economic development.*, www. eda. gov/PDF/eda_ttc. pdf**2003**.

[43]   Markman, G.D.; Siegel, D.S.; Wright, M. Research and technology commercialization. *J. Manage. Stud.*, **2008**, *45*(8), 1401-1423.
[http://dx.doi.org/10.1111/j.1467-6486.2008.00803.x]

[44]   Namiot, E.D.; Sokolov, A.V.; Chubarev, V.N.; Tarasov, V.V.; Schiöth, H.B. Nanoparticles in Clinical Trials: Analysis of Clinical Trials, FDA Approvals and Use for COVID-19 Vaccines. *Int. J. Mol. Sci.*, **2023**, *24*(1), 787.
[http://dx.doi.org/10.3390/ijms24010787] [PMID: 36614230]

[45]   Paredes, K.O.; Ruiz-Cabello, J.; Alarcón, D.I.; Filice, M. *The state of the art of investigational and approved nanomedicine products for nucleic acid delivery*; Nucleic Acid Nanotheranostics, **2019**, pp. 421-456.
[http://dx.doi.org/10.1016/B978-0-12-814470-1.00015-0]

[46]   Mohamed, N.A.; Marei, I.; Crovella, S.; Abou-Saleh, H. Recent Developments in Nanomaterials-Based Drug Delivery and Upgrading Treatment of Cardiovascular Diseases. *Int. J. Mol. Sci.*, **2022**, *23*(3), 1404.
[http://dx.doi.org/10.3390/ijms23031404] [PMID: 35163328]

[47]   Rodríguez, F.; Caruana, P.; De la Fuente, N.; Español, P.; Gámez, M.; Balart, J.; Llurba, E.; Rovira, R.; Ruiz, R.; Martín-Lorente, C.; Corchero, J.L.; Céspedes, M.V. Nano-Based Approved Pharmaceuticals for Cancer Treatment: Present and Future Challenges. *Biomolecules*, **2022**, *12*(6), 784.
[http://dx.doi.org/10.3390/biom12060784] [PMID: 35740909]

CHAPTER 7

Future of Nanotechnology-Based Drug Discovery

Abstract: By enhancing drug administration and diagnostics, nanotechnology is transforming the healthcare industry. Novel approaches to drug design are being driven by combining cutting-edge technologies such as nanorobots and artificial intelligence. Healthcare can benefit from the potential of nanotechnology through the development of multifunctional nanotherapeutics, which could close gaps in the current therapeutic field.

Powered by integrated circuits, sensors, and data storage, nanorobots can increase efficiency and lessen systemic effects while follow-up care for cancer patients is made simpler by nanosensors. Additionally, nanotherapeutics have gained their way in developing novel therapeutics to overcome cancer drug resistance by targeting the mechanisms that induce the drug resistance. Another upcoming field in nanomedicine is the utilization of 3D printing techniques in order to create solid dosage forms based on nanomedicine. By enabling flexible design and on-demand manufacture of customized dosages, enhancing bioavailability, and other attributes, 3D printing technology has revolutionized the pharmaceutical industry. The futuristic applications of nanotechnology hybridized with novel techniques will be discussed in this chapter.

Keywords: Artificial intelligence, Drug resistance, Nanorobots, Nanosensors, Nanodrugs, 3-D drug printing, Patient follow-up care, Personalized medicine, Solid dosages.

1. INTRODUCTION

Nanotechnology is changing healthcare practices, and it is expected to have a huge impact in the future and enhance healthcare facilities. It has contributed to both diagnostics and the viability of therapeutic medication administration. The most cutting-edge technologies are being hybridized to take nanotechnology-based drug designing to new heights. For instance, by using artificial intelligence to assist the construction of nanostructures and the use of nanorobots, breakthroughs in nanotechnology have taken a fresh direction. In addition, the creation of multifunctional nano therapeutics has significant potential to close the gaps in the current therapeutic field. This section will discuss how pharmaceutical companies using nanotechnology are moving towards more sophisticated drug design strategies.

Laksiri Weerasinghe, Imalka Munaweera and Senuri Kumarage

2. FUTURE OF NANOTECHNOLOGY IN DISEASE DIAGNOSIS AND THERAPY

Pharmaceutical companies are among the first to benefit from artificial intelligence (AI), which has lately begun to ramp up its application in a variety of societal domains. AI and nanotechnology are two disciplines that are assisting in achieving precision medicine's objective of designing the optimum therapy for each patient. Recent crossover between these two fields has improved patient data collecting and improved nanomaterial design for precision cancer treatment.

The capacity to customize a nanomedicine for every patient is a commonly posed query when addressing precision medicine treatments. Although current technologies allow for the flexible attachment of any desired antibody to nanoparticles as well as versatility in the choice of cargo there are still a number of additional barriers that must be overcome before this strategy can be successfully used [1]. Along with the challenging clinical approval procedure for personalized nanomedicine, concerns must be raised about the drawbacks of present manufacturing methods and the expensive research and development expenses of nanomedicine. By creating a combinatorial therapy strategy for each patient that concurrently targets many pathways, more precise usage of already available medications may be achieved through the use of precision diagnostic platforms and customized drug-tailoring procedures. By doing so, it will be possible to overcome medication resistance and boost treatment effectiveness. The formation, development, and use of these nanomedications will heavily rely on artificial intelligence (AI) and other computational models in the future [2].

By adjusting the drug release rate to the unique pharmacokinetic and pharmacodynamic characteristics of the patient, nanomaterials can enable controlled drug dosage. External stimuli are utilized for this goal in a way similar to the targeted technique. In order to tailor the treatment, dosing management is not always enough, because patients with diverse pharmacogenomic profiles react differently to various medication dosages. In these circumstances, AI can be used to determine the relationship between drug dosage and the effectiveness of the treatment. For instance artificial neural networks that are capable of developing specific radiotherapy regimens for cancer patients in accordance with the treatment's objective, radiation's physical requirements and the patients' physiological and anatomical data have been generated [3].

Numerous issues with formulation development may be resolved by combining AI with nanotechnology [4]. By analyzing the energy released during the interaction between the drug molecules and keeping focus on any circumstances that can cause the formulation to aggregate, a methotrexate nano suspension was created computationally [5]. The analysis of drug-dendrimer interactions and the assessment of drug encapsulation within the dendrimer can be aided by coarse-grained simulation in conjunction with chemical computation. Additionally, tools like LAMMPS and GROMACS 4 may be used to analyze how surface chemistry affects the ingestion of nanoparticles into cells [5]. The creation of silicasomes—a mix of irinotecan-loaded multifunctional mesoporous silica nanoparticles and the tumour-penetrating peptide iRGD— has been aided by AI. Since iRGD enhances silicasome transcytosis, improving treatment outcomes and overall survival, it consequently increased the absorption of silicasomes [6].

Although tailored omics data analysis has advanced, it is still challenging to predict a patient's reaction to treatment solely based on omics. This challenge is particularly evident in the realm of cancer, where it is necessary to take into consideration the heterogeneity of the tumour and metastases as well as the emergence of resistance over time when projecting the tumour's response [7]. The course of treatment can be optimized by evaluating a potential medicine within the patient's body to determine its response. Such *in situ* diagnostics are made possible by nanotechnology. The efficacy of a medicine may be predicted in a patient's tumour by using barcoded liposomes, which each containing a drug and a unique DNA barcode [8, 9]. For instances, murine breast cancer models were injected with unique DNA barcoded liposomes containing four potential medications (gemcitabine, cisplatin, doxorubicin, and caffeine) at dosages less than 0.1% [10]. After 24 hours, a biopsy of the tumour was performed, and the distribution of barcodes between live and dead tumour cells was examined. Higher concentrations of barcodes corresponding to medications with high efficacy were discovered in dead tumour cells compared to low amounts in living cells. Taking a direct count of the barcodes and the percentage of the liposomes delivered to the live and dead cells was the method of analysis in this approach. By taking into account intricate patterns of barcode distribution, integrating AI algorithms into the data analysis process might broaden its application and enable the detection of combinatorial treatment effects [2].

The outcomes of the *in situ* nano-based screening can also be enhanced by using computational approaches for in silico drug screening as the first step [11]. For instance a researcher used a random forest classifier learning-based algorithm to categorize mutational cancer drivers according to their mode of action [12, 13]. The foundation of this method is a mix of decision trees that assess certain attributes once the algorithm has been trained on prior data. An automated fitting of therapeutic agents to each patient's mutational landscape was done after creating a dataset of medications that are currently on the market and are capable of targeting these cancer drivers based on drug-target interactions. This computational technique gives a distinct viewpoint on potential treatment approaches despite its drawbacks, which may include inaccurate mutation categorization, disregard for the combinatorial impact of medications, and intratumour heterogeneity.

Another crucial factor in boosting the success rate of targeted medicines is the incorporation of computer modelling during the nanoparticle design phase. It is now obvious that just attaching a targeting moiety to drug-loaded nanoparticles does not guarantee effective release and delivery to the diseased location. Computational techniques can greatly enhance our understanding of how the characteristics of nanomedicine affect interactions with plasma, the vascular endothelium, and cellular membranes. For instance, a computer model that determined the binding free energy of nanoparticles using a Metropolis Monte Carlo approach predicted the ideal antibody coverage on the surface of nanoparticles for particular vascular endothelium binding [14]. The approach starts with a randomly chosen state of the nanoparticle and ligand system and develops a probability distribution of the system configurations by randomly changing the defined variables. By altering the initial parameter in the computer model and modelling the changes in the system's states, it was possible to determine the impact of the antibody surface coverage of the nanoparticles on the binding energy of the system. The results, which showed optimum targeting at a coverage ratio of more than 100 antibodies per nanoparticle, agreed with the experimental data collected from both cell culture and *in vivo* mouse models. Additionally, it is indispensable to use computer models to forecast how well nanoparticles will be able to navigate obstacles on their journey to the intended organ. The blood-brain barrier-crossing capability of nanoparticles as well as their potential toxicity have been predicted using a variety of model types [15]. The formulations of brain-targeting nanoparticles can be improved using these models. Due to the tremendous complexity of the permeation process, however, building these models is incredibly challenging, necessitating powerful computing power as well as knowledge of the fundamental concepts underlying biological and physical phenomena. Recently, a machine learning method for predicting blood-brain permeability was described and it was based on the chemical makeup, side effects, and indications of the drugs [16]. Other computational techniques took into account the best form and size for drug release and nanoparticle binding [17]. The size and initial burst rates of poly(lactic-co-glycolic acid) (PLGA) nanoparticles, for instance, were predicted using an artificial neural network [18].

Nanorobots are another futuristic achievement in nanomedicine. The major components processed by nanorobots are a power source, integrated circuits, sensors, and a safe data backup and are maintained by computational technologies such as AI [19, 20]. In order to avoid collisions, recognize targets, locate and attach to them, and subsequently expel from the body, they have been programmed. The development of nano- and microrobots allows them to move to the desired location depending on physiological factors like pH, increasing efficacy and minimizing harmful systemic effects [19]. Issues including dosage adjustment, regulated release, and sustained release must be taken into account while building implanted nanorobots for the controlled delivery of medications and genes. Automating the medication release process using AI technologies like neural networks, integrators and fuzzy logic, is necessary [21]. Implants with microchips are used for both programmed release and to locate the implant in the body [22].

To organize and maximize the site-specificity for chemotherapy and other treatments like radiation therapy, photodynamic therapy, and thermotherapy, it is necessary to construct drug carriers based on nanomaterials. Although metal-based nanoparticles offer many advantages, their toxicity is still a major concern. Thus, when creating efficient cancer therapy techniques, it is also necessary to take into account the nano-toxicological features. In addition, the difficulties of drug resistance and the non-druggability of proteins implicated in many types of malignancies may be resolved by nano-carriers with a combination of drug regimens [23]. Thus, further research should be done at the preclinical and clinical levels on combination therapies. In order to satisfy the demands of precise cancer detection and therapy, modified and functionalized nanomaterials also face hurdles with regard to well-established formulation, better localisation, bio-distribution, biocompatibility, and effectiveness. Diagnostics and targeted treatments will be integrated into a single, centralized system for treatment in the coming years of nanomedicine. With the use of this innovative theranostic approach, it may be possible to treat cancer and other chronic diseases in a highly selective, efficient, and reasonably sensitive manner. This might lead to customized chemotherapy and better patient outcomes [24].

3. PATIENT FOLLOW-UP AFTER TREATMENTS

In contrast to the diagnostic and therapy phases, patient follow-up after the completion of the treatment is another crucial topic that is not frequently mentioned. The many cancer types, stages of therapy, and treatment regimens covered by current long-term patient follow-up procedures cause disagreements among medical teams [25]. The sensitivity and accuracy of the tests that are executed, as well as their price, complexity, time commitment, and patient compliance, are key determinants of the effectiveness of long-term follow-up. Many of the sensing technologies created for diagnostic uses may be modified for use in follow-up applications. Nanosensors that are portable and simple to use can facilitate the execution of follow-up procedures for cancer patients.

Flexibility and self-healing nanomaterials should make it possible to create electrical skin nanosensors that can continuously monitor specific biomarkers through sweating, saliva, and non-invasive blood analysis [26]. A flexible sensor array for electrolyte and sweat metabolite detection was created by Gao *et al.*, and Bluetooth-connected to a smartphone app [27]. The sweat profile of the individual was continuously monitored using an on-body nanosensor under various physiological circumstances. Additionally, combining microfluidic technologies with smartphone integration platforms can be invaluable in streamlining patient-operated devices that will enable more frequent follow-up without adding to the workload for medical teams [28].

4. NANOTECHNOLOGY IN OVERCOMING CANCER DRUG RESISTANCE

Although conventional chemotherapy is still a highly effective treatment for malignant cancer, its limitations make the development of alternative treatment modalities imperative [29]. The efficacy of numerous medications that have demonstrated established anticancer qualities in preclinical research is limited in clinical settings due to several factors such as clonal evolution, multi-drug resistance (MDR), transcriptional alterations, tumour heterogeneity, and systemic toxicity [30]. The development of cancer nanotherapeutics aimed to address the intrinsic drawbacks of conventional chemotherapeutics. Over the past few decades, clinical evaluation of meticulously planned nanoparticulate delivery methods has made cancer nanotherapeutics an unmatched opportunity to comprehend and overcome drug resistance [31].

Due to their unique and innate characteristics, cancer stem cells (CSCs) have drawn attention as major contributors to treatment resistance in recent years. These include the ability of CSCs to self-renew, proliferate, and differentiate, as well as their ability to adopt distinct phenotypes in response to changes in their environment caused by anticancer drugs. Other unique characteristics include the expression of specific surface markers, enhanced DNA repairability, hypoxic stability, increased expression of ATP binding cassette (ABC) transporters like P-glycoprotein (P-gp), which efflux chemotherapeutics, and overexpression of antiapoptotic proteins, all of which contribute to drug resistance [31 - 35]. The dormant mode of CSCs enables them to evade the effects of radiation and chemotherapy, which exacerbates drug resistance [36]. Therefore, in order to overcome cancer treatment resistance, it is imperative that better therapeutic regimens for cancer therapy be developed.

Nanomedicine provides novel, durable, and adaptable drug design and delivery options based on genetic profiling of individual patients to enable tailored treatment of cancer MDR, therefore addressing the shortcomings of current therapy and treatment [37, 38]. Through increased efficacy and less harmful effects, the intriguing physicochemical features of nanomaterials improve the therapeutic index of possible chemotherapeutic medicines. In terms of anti-tumour MDR, NPs have demonstrated significant benefits as they offer platforms for drug combination treatment and block the action of specific drug resistance mechanisms, such as cell membrane efflux transporters [39]. It has been suggested that using nanoparticle-based treatment might help treat MDR in a number of cancer types, such as prostate, ovarian, and breast cancer [40 - 42].

The pharmacokinetics and biodistribution of chemotherapeutic medicines in multidrug-resistant cancer cells have been demonstrated to be enhanced by multimodal nanoformulations functionalized with targeting molecules/peptides and ABC efflux pump inhibitors [43]. P-gp inhibitors are released from nanocarriers into cancer cells, where they attach to the drug-binding pocket in the efflux transporters' transmembrane domains (TMDs) and prevent the drug from being effluxed. Creating NPs that include both chemotherapeutics and efflux pump inhibitors will enable the implementation of this tactic. It has been observed that using this strategy will increase the anticancer medications' therapeutic effectiveness [44, 45]. Moreover, in order to counteract apoptotic pathway-mediated medication resistance, anti-apoptotic proteins such B-cell lymphoma 2 (Bcl-2) and nuclear factor kappa B (NF-κB) can be suppressed utilizing anti-apoptotic protein inhibitors and pro-apoptotic chemicals can be activated [46 - 48]. Ceramide can restore wild-type p53 protein expression, a crucial tumour suppressor, by modulating alternative pre-mRNA splicing. Nanoparticles (NPs) can effectively deliver ceramide into cancer cells carrying p53 missense mutations, potentially overcoming drug resistance in cancer by reinstating p53 function [49].

In addition, drug delivery methods based on NPs have the ability to simultaneously block efflux pumps and encourage apoptosis. Drug-resistant liver cancer cell proliferation was inhibited by using an amphiphilic cationic NP complex, which also activated apoptosis and hampered P-gp-induced drug efflux [50]. Furthermore, doxorubicin-resistant breast cancer cells demonstrated notable cytotoxicity upon co-delivery of resveratrol and doxorubicin in NPs, which resulted in apoptosis by down-regulating the expression of NF-κB and Bcl-2 [51].

Multidrug resistance is further exacerbated by hypoxia which is frequent in cancer cells due to atypical blood vessels and the elevated oxygen requirement of rapidly dividing cancer cells. Tumour drug resistance is induced by hypoxia in a variety of ways such as the evading of the slowly dividing cancer cells from cytotoxic chemotherapeutics. Moreover the tumour heterogeneity induced by the gradient of oxygen created by hypoxia also encourages the production of more aggressive phenotypes within the tumour. Furthermore, the upregulation of drug efflux proteins has also been demonstrated to be mediated by hypoxia [52]. One method to prevent a hypoxic environment is to silence the hypoxia-inducible factor 1α (HIF-1α), which is overexpressed in many types of human malignancies. Numerous research works have documented the efficacy of HIF-1α siRNA-containing nanosystems in surmounting MDR in cancer [52, 53].

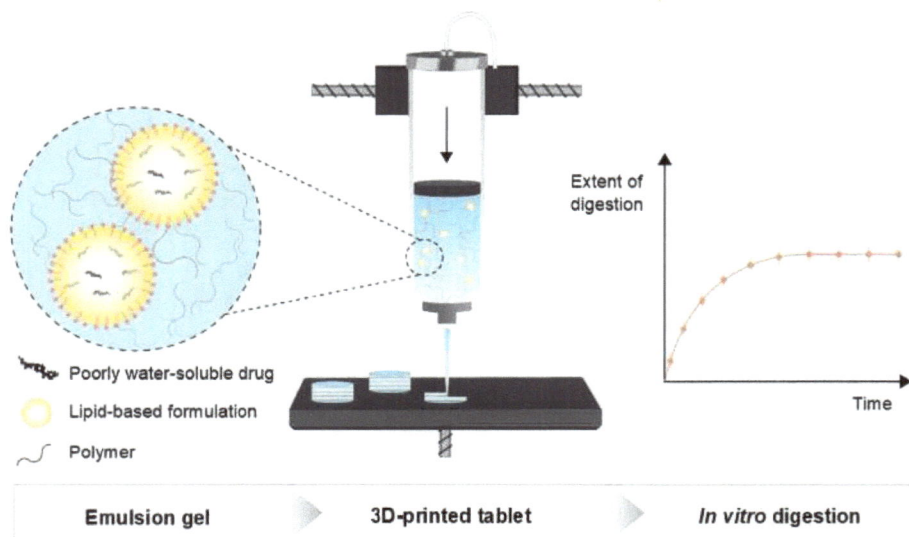

Fig. (1). 3-D printing of lipid-based nanoemulsion using a Semi solid extrusion method. Reproduced with permission from [74] © 2021, Johannesson, J. *et al.* published by Elsevier, distributed under the terms of the Creative Commons Attribution 4.0 International. https://creativecommons.org/licenses/by/4.0.

In the future, multidrug resistance reversal may be improved by nanoparticles that target several pathways of cancer drug resistance. In addition, more and more nanoparticles are being created to target the processes underlying tumour drug resistance that are being identified. Furthermore, new research has begun to explore the function of nanoparticles in immunotherapy, which is a more significant aspect of cancer treatment. Generating NPs loaded with immunomodulatory factors might increase the efficacy of vaccinations used in immunotherapy. Therefore, for the purpose of drug design and delivery, a deeper comprehension of the tumour microenvironment and more research into the interaction between NP-based drug delivery systems and tumour immunity are required [45]. Combining immunology, photodynamics, acoustic dynamics, and other techniques can increase the effectiveness of nano drug delivery systems in MDR malignancies [31, 54, 55]. This might be a major research focus for the future.

5. TRANSLATION OF NANOMEDICINE INTO SOLID DOSAGES

Traditional tablet machines struggle with flexible tablet forms and sizes for tailored drug administration, limiting the potential of future medicine for personalized dosages and regulated release characteristics [56, 57]. With its considerable flexibility in design according to size and on-demand creation of customized dosages for personalized medication distribution, 3D (three-dimensional) printing technology has revolutionized traditional drug manufacturing technique [58, 59]. With the US-FDA's 2015 approval of the Spritam (levetiracetam) by Aprecia Pharmaceuticals, researchers are investigating 3D printing as a possible technology for creating pharmaceutical items [58]. 3D printing technology uses CAD (computer-aided design) to create layer-by-layer 3D objects [60, 61]. With an emphasis on tailored delivery of drugs, the 3D printing process produces pharmaceuticals with a variety of shapes and altered drug release properties [62, 63]. Deposition-based inkjet printing [64, 65], pressure-assisted microsyringe (PAM) technique [66, 67], powder bed deposition [68, 69], laser-based selective laser sintering (SLS) [70], extrusion-based fused deposition modelling (FDM) [71, 72], and stereolithography (SLA) [73] techniques are just a few of the numerous types of 3D printing processes that have been extensively employed in the pharmaceutical industry.

In order to create solid dosage forms based on nanomedicine, the 3D printing technique has been used. Utilizing 3D printing as a type of solid dose for a nanomedicine-based drug, the nanomedicine created through nanotechnology is further made into a solid dosage tablet (Fig **1**). The most widely used technologies for creating solid dosage forms based on nanomedicine are extrusion-based 3D printing processes like FDM and PAM.

Polymeric particles/nanoparticles [75], nanosuspension [76] lipid-based nanoemulsions [74], liposomes [77], and SNEDDS [78, 79], which are drug delivery systems as well as drug candidates have been 3D-printed to pharmaceutical products. For patient administration, the nano formulations were often conveyed as liquid injectables, transdermal delivery devices or filled oral capsules. Through the advancement of 3D printing technology, it has become feasible to distribute poorly soluble drugs locally and systemically in solid dosage forms, notably in the form of oral tablets that are 3D printed [78, 79] and as suppositories [80]. These nano drug formulations have been successfully created using 3D printing technology into a durable solid dosage form without impairing the nanonization properties of the loaded drugs.

When a polymeric nanocapsule carrier system is transformed into a solid dosage form using the conventional tableting method, the strong compression force utilized in the conventional method may impair the system's nano characteristics. Overall characteristics, medication delivery, and overall effectiveness might all be affected due to changes in the nanocarrier size and form when fabricated *via* conventional approaches. However, several initiatives have been undertaken to generate solid dosage forms of polymeric nanocapsules by wet granulation [81], freeze-drying [82] and spray drying [83]. It was reported that polymeric nanocapsules developed using wet granulation resulted in low drug loading of 0.083% w/w capabilities [84]. There is yet no information on producing freeze-dried or spray-dried polymeric nanocapsules into tablets. Thus, using traditional procedures, turning polymeric nanocapsules into solid dosage forms remains a problem for formulation experts. Nevertheless, a polymeric nanocapsule may be effectively transformed into a 3D printed solid dosage form using the hot-melt extrusion (HME) technique [85].

Additionally, the 3D-printed nanopharmaceutical products might be utilized to create customized medications and enhance the bioavailability and properties of pharmaceuticals that are not well soluble in the body. However, this intriguing field has not received enough in-depth research yet. According to the literature study, clinical research must yet be done before these techniques may be successfully applied to humans. In order to successfully translate 3D printed nanomedicine based solid dosage forms into clinical settings, further research is still necessary in this field [86].

CONCLUSION

Nanotechnology is transforming medical procedures and advancing diagnosis and pharmaceutical use. Drug design is being revolutionized by hybridized technologies like nanorobots and artificial intelligence. Pharmaceutical companies are focused on more advanced drug developing methodologies as multifunctional nano therapies have the ability to fill gaps in the present therapeutic area. AI and computational models will play a crucial role in personalized nanomedications, adjusting drug release rates to patient characteristics and determining treatment effectiveness. Understanding the interactions of nanomedicine with plasma, vascular endothelium, and cellular membranes can be improved by computational approaches. Nano robots, powered by integrated circuits, sensors, and data backup, are a futuristic achievement in nano medicine. Based on physiological parameters, they can migrate to appropriate regions, enhancing effectiveness and reducing systemic impacts. AI technologies are required for implanted nanorobots to release medications under regulated conditions, with microchips being used for implant location and programmed release.

After treatment, it is important to follow up with patients. In order to avoid the workload for medical teams by cumbersome long-term follow-up procedures due to the variety of cancer types, treatment stages, and treatment regimens, nano sensors which can simplify follow-up treatments for patience, are being developed.

Nanoparticles targeting cancer drug resistance pathways could improve multidrug resistance reversal by focusing on the processes underlying tumour drug resistance such as overexpression of drug efflux transporters, defective apoptotic pathways, and hypoxic environment. Over the past few decades, the clinical evaluation of meticulously planned nanoparticulate delivery methods has made cancer nanotherapeutics an unmatched opportunity to comprehend and overcome drug resistance. Combining immunology, photodynamics, and acoustic dynamic techniques could increase the effectiveness of nano drug delivery systems in MDR malignancies, making this a major research focus for the future.

In order to create solid dosage forms based on nanomedicine, the 3D printing technique has been used. By enabling flexible design and on-demand fabrication of personalized dosages, 3D printing technology has transformed conventional drug manufacturing. With the aid of this technique, medications that are poorly soluble in the body can have their bioavailability and other qualities improved. However, more research is needed to fully comprehend this appealing field.

REFERENCES

[1] Kedmi, R.; Veiga, N.; Ramishetti, S.; Goldsmith, M.; Rosenblum, D.; Dammes, N.; Hazan-Halevy, I.; Nahary, L.; Leviatan-Ben-Arye, S.; Harlev, M.; Behlke, M.; Benhar, I.; Lieberman, J.; Peer, D. A modular platform for targeted RNAi therapeutics. *Nat. Nanotechnol.,* **2018**, *13*(3), 214-219.
[http://dx.doi.org/10.1038/s41565-017-0043-5] [PMID: 29379205]

[2] Adir, O.; Poley, M.; Chen, G.; Froim, S.; Krinsky, N.; Shklover, J.; Shainsky-Roitman, J.; Lammers, T.; Schroeder, A. Integrating Artificial Intelligence and Nanotechnology for Precision Cancer Medicine. *Adv. Mater.,* **2020**, *32*(13), 1901989.
[http://dx.doi.org/10.1002/adma.201901989] [PMID: 31286573]

[3] Valdes, G.; Simone, C.B., II; Chen, J.; Lin, A.; Yom, S.S.; Pattison, A.J.; Carpenter, C.M.; Solberg, T.D. Clinical decision support of radiotherapy treatment planning: A data-driven machine learning strategy for patient-specific dosimetric decision making. *Radiother. Oncol.,* **2017**, *125*(3), 392-397.
[http://dx.doi.org/10.1016/j.radonc.2017.10.014] [PMID: 29162279]

[4] Sacha, G.M.; Varona, P. Artificial intelligence in nanotechnology. *Nanotechnology,* **2013**, *24*(45), 452002.
[http://dx.doi.org/10.1088/0957-4484/24/45/452002] [PMID: 24121558]

[5] Mehta, C.H.; Narayan, R.; Nayak, U.Y. Computational modeling for formulation design. *Drug Discov. Today,* **2019**, *24*(3), 781-788.
[http://dx.doi.org/10.1016/j.drudis.2018.11.018] [PMID: 30502513]

[6] Ho, D.; Wang, P.; Kee, T. Artificial intelligence in nanomedicine. *Nanoscale Horiz.,* **2019**, *4*(2), 365-377.
[http://dx.doi.org/10.1039/C8NH00233A] [PMID: 32254089]

[7]   Gerlinger, M.; Rowan, A.J.; Horswell, S.; Larkin, J.; Endesfelder, D.; Gronroos, E.; Martinez, P.; Matthews, N.; Stewart, A.; Tarpey, P.; Varela, I.; Phillimore, B.; Begum, S.; McDonald, N.Q.; Butler, A.; Jones, D.; Raine, K.; Latimer, C.; Santos, C.R.; Nohadani, M.; Eklund, A.C.; Spencer-Dene, B.; Clark, G.; Pickering, L.; Stamp, G.; Gore, M.; Szallasi, Z.; Downward, J.; Futreal, P.A.; Swanton, C.; Swanton, C. Intratumor heterogeneity and branched evolution revealed by multiregion sequencing. *N. Engl. J. Med.,* **2012,** *366*(10), 883-892.
[http://dx.doi.org/10.1056/NEJMoa1113205] [PMID: 22397650]

[8]   Yaari, Z.; da Silva, D.; Zinger, A.; Goldman, E.; Kajal, A.; Tshuva, R.; Barak, E.; Dahan, N.; Hershkovitz, D.; Goldfeder, M.; Roitman, J.S.; Schroeder, A. Theranostic barcoded nanoparticles for personalized cancer medicine. *Nat. Commun.,* **2016,** *7*(1), 13325.
[http://dx.doi.org/10.1038/ncomms13325] [PMID: 27830705]

[9]   Dahlman, J.E.; Kauffman, K.J.; Xing, Y.; Shaw, T.E.; Mir, F.F.; Dlott, C.C.; Langer, R.; Anderson, D.G.; Wang, E.T. Barcoded nanoparticles for high throughput *in vivo* discovery of targeted therapeutics. *Proc. Natl. Acad. Sci. USA,* **2017,** *114*(8), 2060-2065.
[http://dx.doi.org/10.1073/pnas.1620874114] [PMID: 28167778]

[10]   Yaari, Z.; da Silva, D.; Zinger, A.; Goldman, E.; Kajal, A.; Tshuva, R.; Barak, E.; Dahan, N.; Hershkovitz, D.; Goldfeder, M.; Roitman, J.S.; Schroeder, A. Theranostic barcoded nanoparticles for personalized cancer medicine. *Nat. Commun.,* **2016,** *7*(1), 13325.
[http://dx.doi.org/10.1038/ncomms13325] [PMID: 27830705]

[11]   Majumder, B.; Baraneedharan, U.; Thiyagarajan, S.; Radhakrishnan, P.; Narasimhan, H.; Dhandapani, M.; Brijwani, N.; Pinto, D.D.; Prasath, A.; Shanthappa, B.U.; Thayakumar, A.; Surendran, R.; Babu, G.K.; Shenoy, A.M.; Kuriakose, M.A.; Bergthold, G.; Horowitz, P.; Loda, M.; Beroukhim, R.; Agarwal, S.; Sengupta, S.; Sundaram, M.; Majumder, P.K. Predicting clinical response to anticancer drugs using an *ex vivo* platform that captures tumour heterogeneity. *Nat. Commun.,* **2015,** *6*(1), 6169.
[http://dx.doi.org/10.1038/ncomms7169] [PMID: 25721094]

[12]   Schroeder, M.P.; Rubio-Perez, C.; Tamborero, D.; Gonzalez-Perez, A.; Lopez-Bigas, N. OncodriveROLE classifies cancer driver genes in loss of function and activating mode of action. *Bioinformatics,* **2014,** *30*(17), i549-i555.
[http://dx.doi.org/10.1093/bioinformatics/btu467] [PMID: 25161246]

[13]   Rubio-Perez, C.; Tamborero, D.; Schroeder, M.P.; Antolín, A.A.; Deu-Pons, J.; Perez-Llamas, C.; Mestres, J.; Gonzalez-Perez, A.; Lopez-Bigas, N. In silico prescription of anticancer drugs to cohorts of 28 tumor types reveals targeting opportunities. *Cancer Cell,* **2015,** *27*(3), 382-396.
[http://dx.doi.org/10.1016/j.ccell.2015.02.007] [PMID: 25759023]

[14]   Liu, J.; Weller, G.E.R.; Zern, B.; Ayyaswamy, P.S.; Eckmann, D.M.; Muzykantov, V.R.; Radhakrishnan, R. Computational model for nanocarrier binding to endothelium validated using *in vivo, in vitro,* and atomic force microscopy experiments. *Proc. Natl. Acad. Sci. USA,* **2010,** *107*(38), 16530-16535.
[http://dx.doi.org/10.1073/pnas.1006611107] [PMID: 20823256]

[15]   Shityakov, S.; Roewer, N.; Broscheit, J.A.; Förster, C. In silico models for nanotoxicity evaluation and prediction at the blood-brain barrier level: A mini-review. *Comput. Toxicol.,* **2017,** *2*, 20-27.
[http://dx.doi.org/10.1016/j.comtox.2017.02.003]

[16]   Gao, Z.; Chen, Y.; Cai, X.; Xu, R. Predict drug permeability to blood–brain-barrier from clinical phenotypes: drug side effects and drug indications. *Bioinformatics,* **2017,** *33*(6), 901-908.
[http://dx.doi.org/10.1093/bioinformatics/btw713] [PMID: 27993785]

[17]   Shah, S.; Liu, Y.; Hu, W.; Gao, J. Modeling particle shape-dependent dynamics in nanomedicine. *J. Nanosci. Nanotechnol.,* **2011,** *11*(2), 919-928.
[http://dx.doi.org/10.1166/jnn.2011.3536] [PMID: 21399713]

[18]   Baghaei, B.; Saeb, M.R.; Jafari, S.H.; Khonakdar, H.A.; Rezaee, B.; Goodarzi, V.; Mohammadi, Y. Modeling and closed-loop control of particle size and initial burst of PLGA biodegradable

nanoparticles for targeted drug delivery. *J. Appl. Polym. Sci.,* **2017**, *134*(33), 45145.
[http://dx.doi.org/10.1002/app.45145]

[19] Luo, M.; Feng, Y.; Wang, T.; Guan, J. Micro-/Nanorobots at Work in Active Drug Delivery. *Adv. Funct. Mater.,* **2018**, *28*(25), 1706100.
[http://dx.doi.org/10.1002/adfm.201706100]

[20] Hassanzadeh, P.; Atyabi, F.; Dinarvand, R. The significance of artificial intelligence in drug delivery system design. *Adv. Drug Deliv. Rev.,* **2019**, *151-152*, 169-190.
[http://dx.doi.org/10.1016/j.addr.2019.05.001] [PMID: 31071378]

[21] Fu, J.; Yan, H. Controlled drug release by a nanorobot. *Nat. Biotechnol.,* **2012**, *30*(5), 407-408.
[http://dx.doi.org/10.1038/nbt.2206] [PMID: 22565965]

[22] Paul, D.; Sanap, G.; Shenoy, S.; Kalyane, D.; Kalia, K.; Tekade, R.K. Artificial intelligence in drug discovery and development. *Drug Discov. Today,* **2021**, *26*(1), 80-93.
[http://dx.doi.org/10.1016/j.drudis.2020.10.010] [PMID: 33099022]

[23] Li, Z.; Tan, S.; Li, S.; Shen, Q.; Wang, K. Cancer drug delivery in the nano era: An overview and perspectives. *Oncol. Rep.,* **2017**, *38*(2), 611-624.
[http://dx.doi.org/10.3892/or.2017.5718] [PMID: 28627697]

[24] Tewabe, A.; Abate, A.; Tamrie, M.; Seyfu, A.; Abdela Siraj, E. Targeted Drug Delivery — From Magic Bullet to Nanomedicine: Principles, Challenges, and Future Perspectives. *J. Multidiscip. Healthc.,* **2021**, *14*, 1711-1724.
[http://dx.doi.org/10.2147/JMDH.S313968] [PMID: 34267523]

[25] Hickey, B. E.; James, M. L.; Lehman, M.; Hider, P. N.; Jeffery, M.; Francis, D. P.; See, A. M. Hypofractionated radiation therapy for early breast cancer. *Cochrane Database of Systematic Reviews,* **2016**, (7)
[http://dx.doi.org/10.1002/14651858.CD003860.pub4]

[26] Jin, H.; Huynh, T.P.; Haick, H. Self-healable sensors based nanoparticles for detecting physiological markers *via* skin and breath: toward disease prevention *via* wearable devices. *Nano Lett.,* **2016**, *16*(7), 4194-4202.
[http://dx.doi.org/10.1021/acs.nanolett.6b01066] [PMID: 27328179]

[27] Gao, W.; Emaminejad, S.; Nyein, H.Y.Y.; Challa, S.; Chen, K.; Peck, A.; Fahad, H.M.; Ota, H.; Shiraki, H.; Kiriya, D.; Lien, D.H.; Brooks, G.A.; Davis, R.W.; Javey, A. Fully integrated wearable sensor arrays for multiplexed *in situ* perspiration analysis. *Nature,* **2016**, *529*(7587), 509-514.
[http://dx.doi.org/10.1038/nature16521] [PMID: 26819044]

[28] Osama, M.; Ateya, A.A.; Sayed, M.S.; Hammad, M.; Pławiak, P.; Abd El-Latif, A.A.; Elsayed, R.A. Internet of Medical Things and Healthcare 4.0: Trends, Requirements, Challenges, and Research Directions. *Sensors (Basel),* **2023**, *23*(17), 7435.
[http://dx.doi.org/10.3390/s23177435] [PMID: 37687891]

[29] Copur, M.S.; Crockett, D.; Gauchan, D.; Ramaekers, R.; Mleczko, K. Molecular Testing Guideline for the Selection of Patients With Lung Cancer for Targeted Therapy. *J. Clin. Oncol.,* **2018**, *36*(19), 2006-2006.
[http://dx.doi.org/10.1200/JCO.2018.78.8240] [PMID: 29763342]

[30] Jamal-Hanjani, M.; Quezada, S.A.; Larkin, J.; Swanton, C. Translational implications of tumor heterogeneity. *Clin. Cancer Res.,* **2015**, *21*(6), 1258-1266.
[http://dx.doi.org/10.1158/1078-0432.CCR-14-1429] [PMID: 25770293]

[31] Bukhari, S.N.A. Emerging nanotherapeutic approaches to overcome drug resistance in cancers with update on clinical trials. *Pharmaceutics,* **2022**, *14*(4), 866.
[http://dx.doi.org/10.3390/pharmaceutics14040866] [PMID: 35456698]

[32] Mao, Y.; Qamar, M.; Qamar, S.A.; Khan, M.I.; Bilal, M.; Iqbal, H.M.N. Insight of nanomedicine strategies for a targeted delivery of nanotherapeutic cues to cope with the resistant types of cancer

stem cells. *J. Drug Deliv. Sci. Technol.,* **2021**, *64*, 102681.
[http://dx.doi.org/10.1016/j.jddst.2021.102681]

[33] Zhou, H.M.; Zhang, J.G.; Zhang, X.; Li, Q. Targeting cancer stem cells for reversing therapy resistance: Mechanism, signaling, and prospective agents. *Signal Transduct. Target. Ther.,* **2021**, *6*(1), 62.
[http://dx.doi.org/10.1038/s41392-020-00430-1] [PMID: 33589595]

[34] Garcia-Mayea, Y.; Mir, C.; Masson, F.; Paciucci, R.; Lleonart, M.E. *In Insights into new mechanisms and models of cancer stem cell multidrug resistance*; Elsevier, **2020**, pp. 166-180.

[35] Wang, J.Q.; Yang, Y.; Cai, C.Y.; Teng, Q.X.; Cui, Q.; Lin, J.; Assaraf, Y.G.; Chen, Z.S. Multidrug resistance proteins (MRPs): Structure, function and the overcoming of cancer multidrug resistance. *Drug Resist. Updat.,* **2021**, *54*, 100743.
[http://dx.doi.org/10.1016/j.drup.2021.100743] [PMID: 33513557]

[36] Liu, Y.; Yang, M.; Luo, J.; Zhou, H. Radiotherapy targeting cancer stem cells "awakens" them to induce tumour relapse and metastasis in oral cancer. *Int. J. Oral Sci.,* **2020**, *12*(1), 19.
[http://dx.doi.org/10.1038/s41368-020-00087-0] [PMID: 32576817]

[37] Mi, Y.; Shao, Z.; Vang, J.; Kaidar-Person, O.; Wang, A.Z. Application of nanotechnology to cancer radiotherapy. *Cancer Nanotechnol.,* **2016**, *7*(1), 11.
[http://dx.doi.org/10.1186/s12645-016-0024-7] [PMID: 28066513]

[38] Liu, J.; Wang, T.; Wang, D.; Dong, A.; Li, Y.; Yu, H. Smart nanoparticles improve therapy for drug-resistant tumors by overcoming pathophysiological barriers. *Acta Pharmacol. Sin.,* **2017**, *38*(1), 1-8.
[http://dx.doi.org/10.1038/aps.2016.84] [PMID: 27569390]

[39] Li, W.; Zhang, H.; Assaraf, Y.G.; Zhao, K.; Xu, X.; Xie, J.; Yang, D.H.; Chen, Z.S. Overcoming ABC transporter-mediated multidrug resistance: Molecular mechanisms and novel therapeutic drug strategies. *Drug Resist. Updat.,* **2016**, *27*, 14-29.
[http://dx.doi.org/10.1016/j.drup.2016.05.001] [PMID: 27449595]

[40] Zhang, J.; Wang, L.; You, X.; Xian, T.; Wu, J.; Pang, J. Nanoparticle therapy for prostate cancer: overview and perspectives. *Curr. Top. Med. Chem.,* **2019**, *19*(1), 57-73.
[http://dx.doi.org/10.2174/1568026619666190125145836] [PMID: 30686255]

[41] Wang, H.; Agarwal, P.; Zhao, G.; Ji, G.; Jewell, C.M.; Fisher, J.P.; Lu, X.; He, X. Overcoming ovarian cancer drug resistance with a cold responsive nanomaterial. *ACS Cent. Sci.,* **2018**, *4*(5), 567-581.
[http://dx.doi.org/10.1021/acscentsci.8b00050] [PMID: 29806003]

[42] Alimoradi, H.; Greish, K.; Barzegar-Fallah, A.; ALshaibani, L.; Pittalà, V. Nitric oxide-releasing nanoparticles improve doxorubicin anticancer activity. *Int. J. Nanomedicine,* **2018**, *13*, 7771-7787.
[http://dx.doi.org/10.2147/IJN.S187089] [PMID: 30538458]

[43] Xu, L.; Liu, J.; Xi, J.; Li, Q.; Chang, B.; Duan, X.; Wang, G.; Wang, S.; Wang, Z.; Wang, L. Synergized multimodal therapy for safe and effective reversal of cancer multidrug resistance based on low-level photothermal and photodynamic effects. *Small,* **2018**, *14*(31), 1800785.
[http://dx.doi.org/10.1002/smll.201800785] [PMID: 29931728]

[44] Jin, K.T.; Lu, Z.B.; Chen, J.Y.; Liu, Y.Y.; Lan, H.R.; Dong, H.Y.; Yang, F.; Zhao, Y.Y.; Chen, X.Y. Recent trends in nanocarrier-based targeted chemotherapy: selective delivery of anticancer drugs for effective lung, colon, cervical, and breast cancer treatment. *J. Nanomater.,* **2020**, *2020*, 1-14.
[http://dx.doi.org/10.1155/2020/9184284]

[45] Yao, Y.; Zhou, Y.; Liu, L.; Xu, Y.; Chen, Q.; Wang, Y.; Wu, S.; Deng, Y.; Zhang, J.; Shao, A. Nanoparticle-based drug delivery in cancer therapy and its role in overcoming drug resistance. *Front. Mol. Biosci.,* **2020**, *7*, 193.
[http://dx.doi.org/10.3389/fmolb.2020.00193] [PMID: 32974385]

[46] Choi, K.Y.; Correa, S.; Min, J.; Li, J.; Roy, S.; Laccetti, K.H.; Dreaden, E.; Kong, S.; Heo, R.; Roh, Y.H.; Lawson, E.C.; Palmer, P.A.; Hammond, P.T. Binary Targeting of siRNA to Hematologic Cancer

Cells *In Vivo* Using Layer-by-Layer Nanoparticles. *Adv. Funct. Mater.,* **2019**, *29*(20), 1900018.
[http://dx.doi.org/10.1002/adfm.201900018] [PMID: 31839764]

[47]   Li, W.; Jiang, Z.; Xiao, X.; Wang, Z.; Wu, Z.; Ma, Q.; Cao, L. Curcumin inhibits superoxide dismutase-induced epithelial-to-mesenchymal transition *via* the PI3K/Akt/NF-κB pathway in pancreatic cancer cells. *Int. J. Oncol.,* **2018**, *52*(5), 1593-1602.
[http://dx.doi.org/10.3892/ijo.2018.4295] [PMID: 29512729]

[48]   Ullah, A.; Ullah, N.; Nawaz, T.; Aziz, T. Molecular mechanisms of Sanguinarine in cancer prevention and treatment. *Anti-Cancer Agents in Medicinal Chemistry (Formerly Current Medicinal Chemistry-Anti-Cancer Agents),* **2023**, *23*(7), 765-778.

[49]   Khiste, S.K.; Liu, Z.; Roy, K.R.; Uddin, M.B.; Hosain, S.B.; Gu, X.; Nazzal, S.; Hill, R.A.; Liu, Y.Y. Ceramide–rubusoside nanomicelles, a potential therapeutic approach to target cancers carrying p53 missense mutations. *Mol. Cancer Ther.,* **2020**, *19*(2), 564-574.
[http://dx.doi.org/10.1158/1535-7163.MCT-19-0366] [PMID: 31645443]

[50]   Cheng, H.; Wu, Z.; Wu, C.; Wang, X.; Liow, S.S.; Li, Z.; Wu, Y.L. Overcoming STC2 mediated drug resistance through drug and gene co -delivery by PHB-PDMAEMA cationic polyester in liver cancer cells. *Mater. Sci. Eng. C,* **2018**, *83*, 210-217.
[http://dx.doi.org/10.1016/j.msec.2017.08.075] [PMID: 29208281]

[51]   Zhao, Y.; Huan, M.; Liu, M.; Cheng, Y.; Sun, Y.; Cui, H.; Liu, D.; Mei, Q.; Zhou, S. Doxorubicin and resveratrol co-delivery nanoparticle to overcome doxorubicin resistance. *Sci. Rep.,* **2016**, *6*(1), 35267.
[http://dx.doi.org/10.1038/srep35267] [PMID: 27731405]

[52]   Jing, X.; Yang, F.; Shao, C.; Wei, K.; Xie, M.; Shen, H.; Shu, Y. Role of hypoxia in cancer therapy by regulating the tumor microenvironment. *Mol. Cancer,* **2019**, *18*(1), 157.
[http://dx.doi.org/10.1186/s12943-019-1089-9] [PMID: 31711497]

[53]   Hajizadeh, F.; Moghadaszadeh Ardebili, S.; Baghi Moornani, M.; Masjedi, A.; Atyabi, F.; Kiani, M.; Namdar, A.; Karpisheh, V.; Izadi, S.; Baradaran, B.; Azizi, G.; Ghalamfarsa, G.; Sabz, G.; Yousefi, M.; Jadidi-Niaragh, F. Silencing of HIF-1α/CD73 axis by siRNA-loaded TAT-chitosan-spion nanoparticles robustly blocks cancer cell progression. *Eur. J. Pharmacol.,* **2020**, *882*, 173235.
[http://dx.doi.org/10.1016/j.ejphar.2020.173235] [PMID: 32574672]

[54]   Sun, X.; Zhao, P.; Lin, J.; Chen, K.; Shen, J. Recent advances in access to overcome cancer drug resistance by nanocarrier drug delivery system. *Cancer Drug Resist.,* **2023**, *6*(2), 390-415.
[http://dx.doi.org/10.20517/cdr.2023.16] [PMID: 37457134]

[55]   Yadav, P.; Ambudkar, S.V.; Rajendra Prasad, N. Emerging nanotechnology-based therapeutics to combat multidrug-resistant cancer. *J. Nanobiotechnology,* **2022**, *20*(1), 423.
[http://dx.doi.org/10.1186/s12951-022-01626-z] [PMID: 36153528]

[56]   Pritchard, D.E.; Moeckel, F.; Villa, M.S.; Housman, L.T.; McCarty, C.A.; McLeod, H.L. Strategies for integrating personalized medicine into healthcare practice. *Per. Med.,* **2017**, *14*(2), 141-152.
[http://dx.doi.org/10.2217/pme-2016-0064] [PMID: 29754553]

[57]   Trenfield, S.J.; Awad, A.; Goyanes, A.; Gaisford, S.; Basit, A.W. 3D printing pharmaceuticals: drug development to frontline care. *Trends Pharmacol. Sci.,* **2018**, *39*(5), 440-451.
[http://dx.doi.org/10.1016/j.tips.2018.02.006] [PMID: 29534837]

[58]   Alqahtani, A. A.; Ahmed, M. M.; Mohammed, A. A.; Ahmad, J. 3D Printed Pharmaceutical Systems for Personalized Treatment in Metabolic Syndrome Pharmaceutics. **2023**.

[59]   Awad, A.; Trenfield, S.J.; Goyanes, A.; Gaisford, S.; Basit, A.W. Reshaping drug development using 3D printing. *Drug Discov. Today,* **2018**, *23*(8), 1547-1555.
[http://dx.doi.org/10.1016/j.drudis.2018.05.025] [PMID: 29803932]

[60]   Durga Prasad Reddy, R.; Sharma, V. Additive manufacturing in drug delivery applications: A review. *Int. J. Pharm.,* **2020**, *589*, 119820.
[http://dx.doi.org/10.1016/j.ijpharm.2020.119820] [PMID: 32891718]

[61] Chen, G.; Xu, Y.; Chi Lip Kwok, P.; Kang, L. Pharmaceutical Applications of 3D Printing. *Addit. Manuf.,* **2020**, *34*, 101209.
[http://dx.doi.org/10.1016/j.addma.2020.101209]

[62] Zhang, J.; Thakkar, R.; Zhang, Y.; Maniruzzaman, M. Structure-function correlation and personalized 3D printed tablets using a quality by design (QbD) approach. *Int. J. Pharm.,* **2020**, *590*, 119945.
[http://dx.doi.org/10.1016/j.ijpharm.2020.119945] [PMID: 33027633]

[63] Ayyoubi, S.; Cerda, J.R.; Fernández-García, R.; Knief, P.; Lalatsa, A.; Healy, A.M.; Serrano, D.R. 3D printed spherical mini-tablets: Geometry versus composition effects in controlling dissolution from personalised solid dosage forms. *Int. J. Pharm.,* **2021**, *597*, 120336.
[http://dx.doi.org/10.1016/j.ijpharm.2021.120336] [PMID: 33545280]

[64] Scoutaris, N.; Ross, S.; Douroumis, D. Current Trends on Medical and Pharmaceutical Applications of Inkjet Printing Technology. *Pharm. Res.,* **2016**, *33*(8), 1799-1816.
[http://dx.doi.org/10.1007/s11095-016-1931-3] [PMID: 27174300]

[65] Buanz, A.B.M.; Saunders, M.H.; Basit, A.W.; Gaisford, S. Preparation of personalized-dose salbutamol sulphate oral films with thermal ink-jet printing. *Pharm. Res.,* **2011**, *28*(10), 2386-2392.
[http://dx.doi.org/10.1007/s11095-011-0450-5] [PMID: 21544688]

[66] Yadav, A.K.; Awasthi, A.; Saxena, K.K.; Agrawal, M.K. In Critical Review on 3D Scaffolds Materials. *Trans Tech Publ,* **2022**, 129-143.

[67] Algahtani, M.S.; Mohammed, A.A.; Ahmad, J.; Saleh, E. Development of a 3D Printed Coating Shell to Control the Drug Release of Encapsulated Immediate-Release Tablets. *Polymers,* **2020**, *12*(6), 1395.
[http://dx.doi.org/10.3390/polym12061395] [PMID: 32580349]

[68] Shi, K.; Tan, D.; Nokhodchi, A.; Maniruzzaman, M. Drop-On-Powder 3D Printing of Tablets with an Anti-Cancer Drug, 5-Fluorouracil. *Pharmaceutics,* **2019**, *11*(4), 150.
[http://dx.doi.org/10.3390/pharmaceutics11040150] [PMID: 30939760]

[69] Sen, K.; Mukherjee, R.; Sansare, S.; Halder, A.; Kashi, H.; Ma, A.W.K.; Chaudhuri, B. Impact of powder-binder interactions on 3D printability of pharmaceutical tablets using drop test methodology. *Eur. J. Pharm. Sci.,* **2021**, *160*, 105755.
[http://dx.doi.org/10.1016/j.ejps.2021.105755] [PMID: 33588046]

[70] Manmadhachary, A.; Siva Rama Krishana, L.; Saxena, K. K. Quantification of the accuracy of additive manufactured (3D printed) medical models. *International Journal on Interactive Design and Manufacturing (IJIDeM),* **2022**.

[71] Macedo, J.; Marques, R.; Vervaet, C.; Pinto, J.F. Production of Bi-Compartmental Tablets by FDM 3D Printing for the Withdrawal of Diazepam. *Pharmaceutics,* **2023**, *15*(2), 538.
[http://dx.doi.org/10.3390/pharmaceutics15020538] [PMID: 36839860]

[72] Francis, V.; Garg, S.; Saxena, K. K.; Jain, P. K.; Lade, J.; Kumar, D. Effect of chemical and heat treatment on 3D printed parts: Nanoparticles embedment approach. *Advances in Materials and Processing Technologies,* **2022**, *8* 4, 2277-2288.

[73] Wang, J.; Goyanes, A.; Gaisford, S.; Basit, A.W. Stereolithographic (SLA) 3D printing of oral modified-release dosage forms. *Int. J. Pharm.,* **2016**, *503*(1-2), 207-212.
[http://dx.doi.org/10.1016/j.ijpharm.2016.03.016] [PMID: 26976500]

[74] Johannesson, J.; Khan, J.; Hubert, M.; Teleki, A.; Bergström, C.A.S. 3D-printing of solid lipid tablets from emulsion gels. *Int. J. Pharm.,* **2021**, *597*, 120304.
[http://dx.doi.org/10.1016/j.ijpharm.2021.120304] [PMID: 33540029]

[75] Xu, W.; Jambhulkar, S.; Zhu, Y.; Ravichandran, D.; Kakarla, M.; Vernon, B.; Lott, D.G.; Cornella, J.L.; Shefi, O.; Miquelard-Garnier, G.; Yang, Y.; Song, K. 3D printing for polymer/particle-based processing: A review. *Compos., Part B Eng.,* **2021**, *223*, 109102.
[http://dx.doi.org/10.1016/j.compositesb.2021.109102]

[76]   Cheow, W.S.; Kiew, T.Y.; Hadinoto, K. Combining inkjet printing and amorphous nanonization to prepare personalized dosage forms of poorly-soluble drugs. *Eur. J. Pharm. Biopharm.,* **2015**, *96*, 314-321.
[http://dx.doi.org/10.1016/j.ejpb.2015.08.012] [PMID: 26325060]

[77]   Sarkar, N.; Bose, S. Liposome-encapsulated curcumin-loaded 3D printed scaffold for bone tissue engineering. *ACS Appl. Mater. Interfaces,* **2019**, *11*(19), 17184-17192.
[http://dx.doi.org/10.1021/acsami.9b01218] [PMID: 30924639]

[78]   S Algahtani, M.; Ahmad, J. 3D printing technique in the development of self-nanoemulsifying drug delivery system: Scope and future prospects. *Ther. Deliv.,* **2022**, *13*(3), 135-139.
[http://dx.doi.org/10.4155/tde-2021-0082] [PMID: 34872343]

[79]   Karalia, D.; Siamidi, A.; Karalis, V.; Vlachou, M. 3D-printed oral dosage forms: Mechanical properties, computational approaches and applications. *Pharmaceutics,* **2021**, *13*(9), 1401.
[http://dx.doi.org/10.3390/pharmaceutics13091401] [PMID: 34575475]

[80]   Persaud, S.; Eid, S.; Swiderski, N.; Serris, I.; Cho, H. Preparations of rectal suppositories containing artesunate. *Pharmaceutics,* **2020**, *12*(3), 222.
[http://dx.doi.org/10.3390/pharmaceutics12030222] [PMID: 32131543]

[81]   Friedrich, R.B.; Fontana, M.C.; Bastos, M.O.; Pohlmann, A.R.; Guterres, S.S.; Beck, R.C.R. Drying polymeric drug-loaded nanocapsules: The wet granulation process as a promising approach. *J. Nanosci. Nanotechnol.,* **2010**, *10*(1), 616-621.
[http://dx.doi.org/10.1166/jnn.2010.1732] [PMID: 20352901]

[82]   Schaffazick, S.R.; Pohlmann, A.R.; Dalla-Costa, T.; Guterres, S.S. Freeze-drying polymeric colloidal suspensions: nanocapsules, nanospheres and nanodispersion. A comparative study. *Eur. J. Pharm. Biopharm.,* **2003**, *56*(3), 501-505.
[http://dx.doi.org/10.1016/S0939-6411(03)00139-5] [PMID: 14602195]

[83]   Beck, R.C.; Ourique, A.F.; Guterres, S.S.; Pohlmann, A.R. Spray-dried polymeric nanoparticles for pharmaceutics: a review of patents. *Recent Pat. Drug Deliv. Formul.,* **2012**, *6*(3), 195-208.
[http://dx.doi.org/10.2174/187221112802652651] [PMID: 22845040]

[84]   Friedrich, R.B.; Bastos, M.O.; Fontana, M.C.; Ourique, A.F.; Beck, R.C.R. Tablets containing drug-loaded polymeric nanocapsules: An innovative platform. *J. Nanosci. Nanotechnol.,* **2010**, *10*(9), 5885-5888.
[http://dx.doi.org/10.1166/jnn.2010.2464] [PMID: 21133121]

[85]   Beck, R.C.R.; Chaves, P.S.; Goyanes, A.; Vukosavljevic, B.; Buanz, A.; Windbergs, M.; Basit, A.W.; Gaisford, S. 3D printed tablets loaded with polymeric nanocapsules: An innovative approach to produce customized drug delivery systems. *Int. J. Pharm.,* **2017**, *528*(1-2), 268-279.
[http://dx.doi.org/10.1016/j.ijpharm.2017.05.074] [PMID: 28583328]

[86]   Ahmad, J.; Garg, A.; Mustafa, G.; Mohammed, A.A.; Ahmad, M.Z. 3D Printing Technology as a Promising Tool to Design Nanomedicine-Based Solid Dosage Forms: Contemporary Research and Future Scope. *Pharmaceutics,* **2023**, *15*(5), 1448.
[http://dx.doi.org/10.3390/pharmaceutics15051448] [PMID: 37242690]

SUBJECT INDEX

www.ingramcontent.com/pod-product-compliance
Lightning Source LLC
Chambersburg PA
CBHW050840220326
41598CB00006B/413